UNDER-SERVED

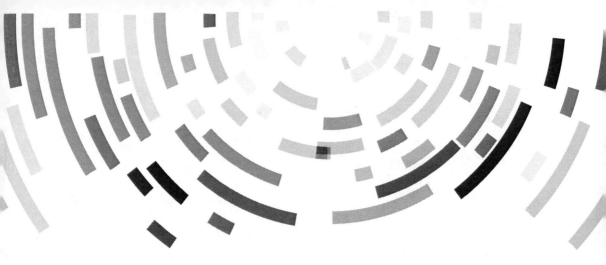

UNDER-SERVED

HEALTH DETERMINANTS OF INDIGENOUS, INNER-CITY, AND MIGRANT POPULATIONS IN CANADA

Edited by **Akshaya Neil Arya** and **Thomas Piggott**

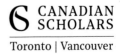

Toronto | Vancouver

Under-Served: Health Determinants of Indigenous, Inner-City, and Migrant Populations in Canada
Edited by Akshaya Neil Arya and Thomas Piggott

First published in 2018 by
Canadian Scholars, an imprint of CSP Books Inc.
425 Adelaide Street West, Suite 200
Toronto, Ontario
M5V 3C1

www.canadianscholars.ca

Copyright © 2018 Akshaya Neil Arya, Thomas Piggott, the contributing authors, and Canadian Scholars.

All rights reserved. No part of this publication may be reproduced, stored in a retrieval system, or transmitted, in any form or by any means, without the prior written permission of Canadian Scholars, under licence or terms from the appropriate reproduction rights organization, or as expressly permitted by law.

Every reasonable effort has been made to identify copyright holders. Canadian Scholars would be pleased to have any errors or omissions brought to its attention.

Library and Archives Canada Cataloguing in Publication

Under-served : health determinants of Indigenous, inner-city, and migrant populations in Canada / edited by Akshaya Neil Arya and Thomas Piggott.

Includes bibliographical references.
Issued in print and electronic formats.
ISBN 978-1-77338-058-2 (softcover).--ISBN 978-1-77338-059-9 (PDF).--
ISBN 978-1-77338-060-5 (EPUB)

1. Native peoples--Health and hygiene--Social aspects--Canada. 2. Immigrants--Health and hygiene--Social aspects--Canada. 3. City dwellers--Health and hygiene--Social aspects--Canada. 4. Marginality, Social Health aspects--Canada. 5. Health--Social aspects--Canada. 6. Social medicine--Canada. 7. Public health--Social aspects--Canada. I. Arya, Akshaya Neil, 1962-, editor II. Piggott, Thomas, 1989-, editor

RA418.3.C3U55 2018   362.10971   C2018-903663-X
                                        C2018-903664-8

Text and cover design by Elisabeth Springate
Typesetting by Brad Horning

Printed and bound in Canada

Canadä

Contents

Foreword   x
David Butler-Jones

Introduction   1
Neil Arya and Thomas Piggott

SECTION I   **INTRODUCING UNDER-SERVED POPULATIONS AND THEIR DETERMINANTS OF HEALTH**   **11**
Section Introduction by Thomas Piggott and Neil Arya

Chapter 1   Deconstructing the Concept of Special Populations for Health Care, Research, and Policy   12
Thomas Piggott and Aaron Orkin

Chapter 2   The Social Determinants of Health of Under-Served Populations in Canada   23
Dennis Raphael

SECTION II   **INDIGENOUS POPULATIONS**   **39**
Section Introduction by Karen Hill

Timeline   Policies and Practices Influencing Indigenous Health   43
Bonnie M. Freeman

Chapter 3   The Impact of Intergenerational Trauma to Health: Policies, Relocation, Reserves, and Residential Schools   45
Bonnie M. Freeman

Chapter 4   Intergenerational Trauma and Indigenous Health in Canada: How Racism Affects the Health of the Indigenous Patient   57
Paul Tomascik, Thomas Dignan, and Barry Lavallée

Chapter 5   Health and Health Service Needs in Urban Indigenous Communities   67
Martin Cooke and Piotr Wilk

Chapter 6   Health for Canadian Indigenous Children   82
Anna Banerji

Chapter 7   Exploring the Development of a Health Care Model Based on Inuit Wellness Concepts as Part of Self-Determination and Improving Wellness in Northern Communities   92
Gwen K. Healey

Chapter 8   Fostering Resilience with Indigenous Youth   105
Bonnie M. Freeman

SECTION III   INNER-CITY AND OTHER SPECIAL POPULATIONS   117
Section Introduction by S. Luckett-Gatopoulos

Timeline   Minimal Supports for the Bottom of the Labour Market   120
Joe Mancini

Chapter 9   Historical Roots—Why in a Time of Unprecedented Wealth and Health Do We Have Homelessness and Ill Health?   121
Joe Mancini

Chapter 10   Poverty, Homelessness, and Ill Health   129
Abe Oudshoorn

Chapter 11   The Forgotten Victims: Impact of Parental Incarceration on the Psychological Health of the Innocent Children Left Behind   141
Jessica Reid

Chapter 12   Approaching the Health and Marginalization of People Who Use Opioids   153
Sharon Koivu and Thomas Piggott

Chapter 13 Pathways to Health Equity for LGBTQ Populations   166
Nathan Lachowsky, Jacqueline Gahagan, and Kelly Anderson

Chapter 14 "Prescribing Income": A Multi-level Approach to Treating Social Determinants for Health Providers   177
Ritika Goel and Gary Bloch

Chapter 15 Models of Primary Care Delivery for Under-Served Populations in Inner-City Settings   185
Dale Guenter, Abe Oudshoorn, and Joe Mancini

SECTION IV REFUGEE AND MIGRANT POPULATIONS   197
Section Introduction by Shpresa Aliu-Berisha

Timeline A Brief History of Migration and Marginalization   200
Neil Arya

Chapter 16 Social Determinants of Refugee Health   204
Michaela Hynie

Chapter 17 Health Issues in Refugee Populations   226
Meb Rashid, Vanessa Redditt, Andrea Hunter, and Kevin Pottie

Chapter 18 Mental Health Impact of Canadian Immigration Detention   246
Hanna Gros

Chapter 19 Migrant Farm Worker Health Care: Unique Strategies for a Unique Population   253
Janet McLaughlin and Michelle Tew

SECTION V RESEARCH FOR UNDER-SERVED POPULATIONS   265
Section Introduction by Thomas Piggott and Neil Arya

Chapter 20 Indigenous Health Research: Lessons from Life in the Arctic   267
Gwen K. Healey

Chapter 21 Overcoming Challenges of Conducting Longitudinal Research in Stigmatized Urban Neighbourhoods   277
Biljana Vasilevska, Angela Di Nello, Erin Bryce, and James R. Dunn

Chapter 22 Practical and Ethical Considerations for Health Research with Refugees   288
Patricia Gabriel

Chapter 23 Engaging Communities to Identify Needs and Develop Solutions: Participatory Research Incorporates Community Voice in All Aspects of Health Research Decision-Making   306
Jon Salsberg, Soultana Macridis, Treena Delormier, Richard Hovey, Neil Andersson, Alex M. McComber, and Ann C. Macaulay

SECTION VI MAKING CHANGE—EDUCATION, ADVOCACY, AND SYSTEM CHANGE   321
Section Introduction by Neil Arya and Thomas Piggott

Chapter 24 Educating Health Professionals to Care for Vulnerable and Marginalized Populations   323
Lesley Cooper, Neil Arya, Mona Negoita, and Ngan Pham

Chapter 25 Thinking Upstream: A Vision for a Healthy Society   341
Ryan Meili and Thomas Piggott

Chapter 26 Reforming Health Systems to Promote Equity and Improve the Health of Under-Served Populations   352
Anne Andermann

Chapter 27 From the Clinics to the Streets: The Fight against Refugee Health Cuts in Canada   364
Philip Berger, Meb Rashid, Alexander Caudarella, Andrea Evans, and Christopher Holcroft

Chapter 28 The Ws of Successful Advocacy for the Under-Served: Lessons from Days of Action for Refugee Health   371
Neil Arya

Conclusion 379
Thomas Piggott and Neil Arya

Glossary   383
Contributor Biographies   390

Foreword

David Butler-Jones

A society is healthy only to the extent that it is healthy as a whole. Those who went before us in shaping the society we have today recognized that basic social structures, how we organize public services, and equitable access to common public goods were essential for social and economic well-being. Clean water, safe nutritious foods, adequate housing, public education, parks and public spaces, public health, and primary health care, among others, were essentials of modern community life. Gaps remain, however, and now the disparities seem to be increasing again, as we take for granted how hard won was the success we achieved and the efforts required to maintain it.

The 1960s, during my adolescence, was a time of renewed social change. Acceptance of traditional authority was challenged, and there was an increased sense of the need for social institutions and programs to level the playing field and improve equity, reduce racism and discrimination, and so forth. As a teen working with the United Church of Canada committees in the latter part of the decade, I came to understand how what we have come to call the "social determinants" impact the health and well-being of communities. It was not only a matter of social justice, as issues of poverty, the rights of women and children, and how we do international development fairly impact the health, well-being, and economy of all. Focusing on what communities actually need, not what we think they need, and working in partnership to assist, not direct, how they move toward a future they want was more successful and meaningful as the communities had greater control. The individuals, who made up those communities, could then contribute overall to successful economies and improved health and social conditions.

In the 1970s, as a medical resident, I was working with a young woman in hospital who had attempted suicide. Over the space of several weeks she journeyed to a point of no longer wanting to end her life. She had told me her story of abuse when she was child, having a limited education, with few friends and no family support, now trying to raise two little girls on welfare, in a neighbourhood that she felt was unsafe. While the counselling and support were helpful in the short term, how could we possibly improve her chances, and those of her children, without tackling the determinants and root causes? As S. Luckett-Gatopoulos described poignantly in the introduction to Section III, "Until you have slept on a park bench, it is hard to understand the series of non-choices that brings people there."

Academic and clinician Sir William Osler noted a century ago, "To prevent disease, to relieve suffering and to heal the sick, this is our work." I do not think his ordering was by accident. And while his comments were addressed to the practice of medicine, they also have a broader application. Public health has always had a primary mandate to address the challenges of those who are marginalized and the under-served.

If our focus is only on those who can afford care, or have the capacity to come to us, or already have power, we are failing our responsibility as health or social service professionals. This perspective is not only the realm of public health practitioners but of all of us, to both understand and to contribute where we can.

Typically reported infant mortality and life expectancy related data, while important, can mask significant disparities. While specific country-to-country or region-to-region comparisons do not provide straightforward answers, they can be telling, in generating the question of and possible solutions to "if there, then why not here?" As we work to better understand and address the challenges of the under-served and marginalized, we need to question our own assumptions of what is doable and how we organize our efforts. For example, it is widely recognized that Sweden has one of the lowest infant mortality rates (IMR) in the 2.5 per 1,000 range in 2011; they also have a relatively small gap between the rate for infants born into the lowest versus highest income quintile, a ratio of 1.41 (Hjern 2012). By comparison, in Canada at that time the overall IMR was 4.5 and the ratio of the gap between highest and lowest was 1.49. This, however, masked an even greater variability in IMR between provinces (Canadian Institute for Health Information 2016).

One might dismiss such differences as Canada is a much larger country, with remote areas lacking access to care. This may be true for many; however, in Canadian urban areas, with access to some of the best teaching hospitals in the world, such discrepancies persist in these settings for Indigenous peoples: "Infant mortality rates were not significantly different across areas for First Nations (10.7, 9.9, 7.9, and 9.7 per 1,000 in rural areas with no, weak, moderate/strong urban influence, and urban areas, respectively), but rates were significantly lower in less isolated areas for non-First Nations (7.4, 6.0, 5.6, and 4.6 per 1,000, respectively)" (Zohng-Chen et al. 2010). And in Vancouver, life expectancy at birth in different neighbourhoods varies from 79 to 85 years (City of Vancouver 2015).

It is essential as practitioners and policy and program managers that we know where, specifically, the challenges are and why, in order to focus resources and services more appropriately. In Chapter 5, Cooke and Wilk demonstrate how such challenges continue for urban Indigenous individuals and communities. In subsequent chapters, other authors address different populations in particular settings that illustrate both parallels and differences in the challenges faced by and appropriate responses to support the under-served and marginalized.

When I speak of public health I describe it in a way adapted from the *Dictionary of Epidemiology*: "Public Health is the organized efforts of society to improve health and well-being and reduce inequalities in health"; or, as I use more commonly, just "reduce inequalities," as health will naturally be one of the positive consequences.

Public health in this understanding takes us back to its roots as the first public good in health for which governments are responsible. Sir Benjamin Disraeli, prime minister of Britain in the early days of public health, spoke to it as "the foundation upon which rests the happiness of the people and welfare of the state." In this context public health is not just a set of programs and services but a way of thinking about health challenges and the need for understanding and ways of working to address the broad social determinants, including "One Health" (the interface of animal, human, environment, and economy). It crosses disciplines and perspectives, requiring efforts at the policy, program, and practice levels. What we recognized when I was Chair of the National Roundtable on Climate and Health in 2000 has been magnified in the years since through evidence and experience. The changing climate, and the rising CO_2 and air pollution, is not only a risk to the sustainability of our future economy as more and more resources go to mitigating the impacts but it also has a disproportionate impact on the poor and marginalized, whether through air pollution, heat stress, flooding, drought, rising sea levels, economic risks, and so on.

Health and economy are a virtuous cycle in that improved economics improve health and better health improves economies. Inequity in access to education, employment, and housing limit the overall success of a society, leading to greater rates of poor health and social disruption, among many other markers of societal dysfunction. The legacy of colonialism and racism, or other forms of discrimination and control, further limits not only individual potential but that potential for those individuals to contribute to the well-being of others. As much as income is important, poverty is a constellation of resources and capacities necessary to succeed. In the end it is not a zero-sum game, in that equal opportunity does benefit all. While I have argued over the years, particularly as my reason for working in public health and preventive medicine, that this is a matter of social justice, the evidence is very clear that there are also rational economic reasons for addressing health determinants.

I have been fortunate in my career to have worked in many parts of the country, from small outpost communities and more northern towns to large cities and regions, at different levels of governance, in both research and practice. All of those experiences have reinforced not only the importance of these issues but practical ways that we can make a difference.

When I was the first Chief Medical Officer in Saskatchewan, we brought together evidence of not only what we know but also what individuals, organizations, and governments can do to address them. These became reference binders for the use of regional health authorities and others in how they plan programs and activities to take into account the determinants. We also brought together NGOs, academics, and federal and provincial funders of health promotion to do joint planning on what would be the most effective and coordinated approaches.

Then as Chief Public Health Officer for Canada and Deputy Minister for the Public Health Agency, I produced annual reports on the state of public health in Canada, mandated in the Public Health Agency of Canada Act to be independent reports to parliament (Butler-Jones 2008, 2009, 2010, 2011, 2012, 2013). These reports had a social determinants focus, illustrating not only the reality faced by those on the margins but ways in which evidence and promising practices work to improve equity. Each year had a different determinants focus, including different stages of life, influences such as sex and gender or infectious diseases, how determinants influence health in different populations, and the particular challenges and approaches for Indigenous and other communities.

I am struck by how the editors and authors of *Under-Served* have brought together a range of perspectives on the issues, including important understandings of the impacts of intergenerational trauma, the impact of migration and being undocumented, and other challenges, along with practical approaches and solutions for communities practitioners and policy-makers. The book both challenges us and offers solutions. Understanding the fostering of resilience, how different communities such as the Inuit conceive of health and healing, how we can better educate professionals to care for vulnerable and marginal populations, pathways to health equity for LGBTQ populations, models of primary care in inner cities, and the impacts of migration are among the many examples you will explore through these chapters.

While all of the determinants are important, there are two things that make a fundamental difference to individual trajectories. The first is whether we have others we love and care about and who love and care about us. Isolation substantially increases our mortality risk at any age, regardless of gender: "individuals with adequate social relationships have a 50% greater likelihood of survival compared to those with poor or insufficient social relationships" (Holt-Lunstad, Smith, and Layton 2010). The second is whether we have choice and some sense that our choices matter to our future. Chandler and Lalonde's (1998) research on community control and culture on reducing the risk of adolescent suicide is but one example. They found that among Indigenous communities in British Columbia that had been engaged in land claims, in those that had a strong focus on culture and influence over the delivery of services such as education, health, and policing, adolescent suicide was rare. Whereas in those communities that lacked a sense of control, adolescent suicide rates were many times that of the province as a whole. Auger's (2016) synthesis of research on cultural continuity presents a fuller picture of the importance of connection to culture.

It is therefore striking that so many past and current policies have done the opposite, whether in how we structure welfare, the residential school system, support for recent migrants and refugees, or how governments have not respected treaties, or self-determination, by Indigenous communities.

MOVING BEYOND UNDERSTANDING TO DEVELOPING PUBLIC POLICY

One of the things I observe is that we're much better at understanding the importance of determinants than practical ways to address them. Most determinants seem large and beyond our individual or organizational mandate or capacity. What can I do about others experiencing poverty, for example? For this reason, I have found it helpful to have a framework for ways in which respond. I like to break action on determinants down into six areas represented by the acronym *PACEM*.

- **P**artner: Who else can we work with, to do it better together? Joining with others rather than duplicating or creating anew. The editors, as one form of partnership, have brought together a broad group of individuals interested in improving the health of under-served populations from across the health sector and beyond to other allied sectors.

- **Advocate:** What needs to be done at a policy, program, or legislative level? Can we bring both evidence and workable solutions, rather than just point out problems for others?
- **Cheerlead:** Encouraging others and not being a barrier to progress or undermining others' good efforts because they aren't ours.
- **Enable:** What we do directly to change or influence the determinants. How we work effectively with others. Adopting reconciliation approaches. Ensuring services are accessible to those who need them most.
- **Mitigate:** Reducing the risks of adverse outcomes. For example, harm reduction, clinical care, or immunization to prevent diseases like hepatitis A, which we know is a result of overcrowding and sanitation issues. Working to minimize or mitigate the harms, while not ignoring that the real solutions are determinant based.

A key to successfully tackling complex issues and challenges is forming partnerships and coalitions with other individuals, groups, and organizations that share a similar concern and goals. To be successful we must consider what we do to be a team sport, requiring a range of skills and perspectives. If we are to be effective in addressing the determinants, we cannot just hope others will do it. There are many factors mitigating against that hope, as any history of our errors and relative inaction will attest.

Each chapter in this book further illustrates both challenges and practical opportunities for each of us as we move forward in the work of addressing the determinants of health in under-served and marginalized populations.

MAKING IT WORK

Having chaired a range of coalitions and intersectoral and intergovernmental processes, and in working with other organizations, I have found four fundamental approaches helpful in making partnerships work, to get at various issues and determinants:

Rule of Three

Often organizations, groups, or committees get bogged down trying to find agreement. I find it helpful to categorize issues as follows:

- Those that we essentially agree on, we do.
- Those issues or solutions that we may differ to some extent, but not enough to oppose, we do.

- And those that we likely will never agree on, we don't ignore, but we don't let them become more than 5 to 10 percent of our time and focus. We need not agree on everything to work effectively on what we do.

Respect

We cannot influence who or what we do not respect. We don't need to like them or want to go to dinner with them, but if we don't respect their position, or understand where they are coming from, we are unlikely to get anywhere.

Make It Practical

It is not enough to outline the problem; rather, have practical solutions or approaches that could be acted on.

Have Something to Offer

It can be quite compelling to, rather than have a request for something more to do with limited resources, have an offer of what we could do and explore what they could then contribute.

The editors have pulled together a range of issues, perspectives, and approaches to address social determinants in marginalized groups. There is much in this to learn, to experience, and to do.

While there is never certainty, I have always appreciated the perspective of Stephen Leacock, Canadian economist, academic, and satirist: "Success is 10% inspiration and 90% perspiration." It is, after all, what we do, not just what we say. And success is a team sport.

David Butler-Jones, MD MHSc LL.D(hc)
FCFPC FRCPC FACPM
Former Chief Public Health Officer of Canada

REFERENCES

Auger, Monique D. 2016. "Cultural Continuity as a Determinant of Indigenous Peoples' Health: A Metasynthesis of Qualitative Research in Canada and the United States." *International Indigenous Policy Journal* 7 (4): article 3.

Butler-Jones, David. 2008. *The Chief Public Health Officer's Report on the State of Public Health in Canada, 2008: Addressing Health Inequalities.* Ottawa: Public Health Agency of Canada.

Butler-Jones, David. 2009. *The Chief Public Health Officer's Report on the State of Public Health in Canada, 2009: Growing Up Well—Priorities for a Healthy Future.* Ottawa: Public Health Agency of Canada.

Butler-Jones, David. 2010. *The Chief Public Health Officer's Report on the State of Public Health in Canada, 2010: Growing Older—Adding Life to Years.* Ottawa: Public Health Agency of Canada.

Butler-Jones, David. 2011. *The Chief Public Health Officer's Report on the State of Public Health in Canada, 2011: Youth and Young Adults—Life in Transition.* Ottawa: Public Health Agency of Canada.

Butler-Jones, David. 2012. *The Chief Public Health Officer's Report on the State of Public Health in Canada, 2012: Influencing Health—The Importance of Sex and Gender.* Ottawa: Public Health Agency of Canada.

Butler-Jones, David. 2013. *The Chief Public Health Officer's Report on the State of Public Health in Canada, 2013: Infectious Disease—The Never-Ending Threat* Ottawa: Public Health Agency of Canada.

Canadian Institute for Health Information. 2016. *Trends in Income Related Health Inequalities in Canada* (2011 data). Last updated July. https://secure.cihi.ca/free_products/trends_in_income_related_inequalities_in_canada_2015_en.pdf.

Chandler, Michael J., and Christopher Lalonde. 1998. "Cultural Continuity as a Hedge against Suicide in Canada's First Nations." *Transcultural Psychiatry* 35 (2): 191–219. https://doi.org/10.1177/136346159803500202.

City of Vancouver. 2015. "Social Indicators and Trends 2014." Last updated April 14. https://vancouver.ca/files/cov/factsheet1-a-good-start.PDF.

Hjern, Anders. 2012. "Health in Sweden: The National Public Health Report 2012. Chapter 2." *Scandinavian Journal of Public Health* 40 (Suppl 9): 23–41. https://doi.org/10.1177/1403494812459458.

Holt-Lunstad, Julianne, Timothy B. Smith, and J. Bradley Layton. 2010. "Social Relationships and Mortality Risk: A Meta-analytic Review." *PLoS Medicine* 7 (7):e1000316. https://doi.org/10.1371/journal.pmed.1000316.

Zhong-Cheng Luo, Russell Wilkins, Maureen Heaman, Patricia Martens, Janet Smylie, Lyna Hart, Fabienne Simonet, et al. 2010. "Birth Outcomes and Infant Mortality by the Degree of Rural Isolation Among First Nations and Non-First Nations in Manitoba, Canada." *Journal of Rural Health* 26 (2): 175–181. https://dx.doi.org/10.1111%2Fj.1748-0361.2010.00279.x.

Introduction

Neil Arya and Thomas Piggott

As Canada marked its 150th birthday last year, it was a time to reflect on how much healthier we had become as a nation during this time frame. Since Confederation, the life expectancy of Canadians increased, on average, from 43 to 82 years (Belshaw 2015; World Bank n.d.). It is not just the duration of life that has increased; the quality of life in Canada has increased as well. According to the US News and World report, Canada is the second-best country in the world to live (U.S. News n.d.). We have much to thank for these advances: the advent of vaccinations, sanitation and public health regulations, and organized universal publicly funded health care. These developments have brought great improvements to both the quality and duration of life in Canada. Yet portions of the Canadian population have not shared in this giant leap forward in health—many remain *under-served*.

The life expectancy of Inuit men is 15 years shorter than the Canadian average (Statistics Canada 2017). Homeless populations have a life expectancy 11 years shorter than the Canadian average (Hwang et al. 2009). Refugees, while often fleeing dire conditions in their home country, arrive to Canada facing a new set of challenges. These stark health inequities are evidence that populations are under-served within our social and health care system. But beyond inequitable health care, these differences are driven by inadequate or prejudicial systems, structures, policies, and practices faced by under-served populations on a daily basis in Canada.

THE ORIGINS

This book has been a long and winding project, allowing us great fortune, as editors, to interact with brilliant minds and passionate advocates working on issues relating to the determinants of health for under-served populations across Canada. It represents the collaborative work of a tremendous number of people from coast to coast to coast. The initial inspiration for this volume for us, as editors, was our involvement, as organizers, in the PEGASUS (Peace, Global Health and Sustainability) conference (see http://www.pegasusconference.ca/), which began in 2014. PEGASUS has become a conference that gathers together academics, practitioners, students, advocates, and policy-makers interested in health issues, globally and locally.

Many of the chapters in this book stem from presentations or connections made at PEGASUS. In this book, we have sought to recreate a spirit of story sharing, collaborative learning, critical questioning, and inspiring insights that is present at the conference. While we editors are both health care providers—and that may reflect the approach the book takes—we have sought out a diverse range of experts to broaden the perspectives presented.

THE EDITORS

Akshaya Neil Arya

Neil Arya is a family doctor in Kitchener, Ontario. After five years of delivering mental health services to people at risk for homelessness in St. John's Kitchen, he founded the CFFM Refugee Health Clinic, which has continued to support Government-Assisted Refugees since 2008, in collaboration with Reception House Waterloo Region. He has lectured and supervised medical and public health students at the University of Waterloo, McMaster University, and Western University, with a focus on under-served populations. As director of the Global Health Office at Western University, he established several community and institutional collaborations. He has also delved into research and advocacy, speaking and writing on topics relating to under-served populations.

Thomas Piggott

Thomas Piggott is a family doctor and is finishing his training in public health and preventive medicine at McMaster University. He completed his Masters in Public Health Economics at the London School of Hygiene and Tropical Medicine and has special interest in health evidence, equity, and economics in primary care and public health. He is the founder of Global Health Sim, a Canadian non-profit focused on innovative education through simulation.

THE LANGUAGE

Throughout the book, you will note the use of varied terms to discuss populations whose health outcomes are diverse and needs vary. As discussed in Piggott and Orkin Chapter 1, it is critical to deconstruct the terminology we use to understand its origins, uses, and implications. Too frequently, terms such as *marginalized* or *vulnerable* are employed without deeper reflection. Throughout the book, we have encouraged authors to reflect critically on the nomenclature they feel most appropriate to use, relating to the content of their writing. Disagreement over terminology was rare, but in some cases the development of the book itself stimulated valuable debate and, often, terminology we could each "live with." As editors, we attempted to be critical in our own use of language.

When it comes to representing the situation of the populations of focus in the book, we explicitly chose the term *under-served*. As defined in the glossary and elaborated on in Chapter 1, *under-served* places the explanatory burden for the differences in health not within a group (e.g., vulnerable) but on Canadian society.

THE POPULATIONS

This book focuses on three key under-served populations in Canada: Indigenous peoples, inner-city populations, and migrant populations. The focus on these populations is far from a comprehensive list of under-served populations in Canada. While other populations including LGBTQ people, children of incarcerated parents, and people who use drugs are discussed, many populations with analogous issues are absent but may be addressed in the online supplement. However, various issues identified might have similar effects on such populations. Furthermore, the division of these populations is in many ways artificial. As discussed by Lachowsky, Gahagan, and Anderson in Chapter 13, intersecting experiences of marginalization may be present at the individual level. Finally, the term *inner city*, used to reflect US city centres in decline in the 80s and 90s, may not be accurate in today's Canada, where poverty is much mor spread out, with great concentrations in inner and outer suburbs.

THE PERSON

As we search to understand challenges to populations, it is quite easy to lose sight of the individuals that compose them. To humanize discussions around issues, we have sought to include personal stories of people whose health has been impacted by being under-served, and those of their health care providers. These stories, which may be heart-wrenching and even empowering, serve to ground the discussion. All of these stories have been shared with expressed consent of the individual to whom they belong. Some individuals wished to make their stories public; others are anonymized aggregations to protect individual identities. As the prolific First Nations author Dr. Thomas King said in his 2003 Massey Lecture, "The truth about stories is that's all we are" (King 2003). Stories are the substance that puts context to complexity and that must guide your journey through this book.

THE CARE

Remaining at the heart of the work of health *care* providers, particularly those who work with under-served populations, is "caring" for the patient. Throughout training to become health care providers, we incessantly "zoom in" to the cellular level. We learn of the microbiological or biochemical "etiology" and pathophysiology of diseases. This biomedical perspective is indeed how most of society experiences health care, and it is where governments often focus their investments.

Even when trying to maintain a focus on caring, as health care providers, we may be transfixed by the treatment of disease, forgetting the role of caring. Our patients' diseases may be confusing, unusual, or academically challenging, but this is where practitioners may feel somewhat in control, where we have models to work with, where cause and effect are apparent. As our health care has evolved, pills seemingly exist for nearly every condition—there are now prescriptions for even those conditions that have been recently insurmountable, such as HIV and some cancers.

Were this actually true, many of our patients would still experience barriers to obtaining such care. Despite Canada's formidable development of a single-payer, publicly funded, universal health care system, great inequities remain in terms of access to health care services. Patients living farther from urban centres, on reserves, or in rural and remote parts of

> ## Marginalization: A Personal Story (Akshaya Neil Arya)
>
> Growing up in small-town Ontario, as the only non-white student in my class for much of my childhood, I (A. N. A.) had a very personal sense of marginalization. I was excluded from the "mainstream." I was a child of refugees who were displaced from what became Pakistan to India in 1947. Then, at one month of age, I, too, was displaced with them from India. During my early years growing up across rural Canada—moving from British Columbia to Saskatchewan to Southwestern Ontario, finally settling in Grey-Bruce Counties by age seven—I often felt alone and isolated; classmates picked on me, and I was called a "Paki."
>
> A brief note about my name: It was partly because of wanting to reduce separateness that my parents added the middle name Neil to Akshaya Arya when I was two, something that happens frequently in immigrant families. It has not only been easier to pronounce for most Canadians but helps me fit in; it became my name to the outside world and is used here. However, Akshaya remains a central part of my identity and within the family and Indian community; it is the name of a famous Indian journalist and freedom fighter, and now is that of an Indian actor, with the meaning (in Sanskrit) of *invincible*, and I choose to keep it on the book cover as I have done with my other three edited collections.
>
> It was not until much later that I began to recognize that my childhood was, in fact, one of relative privilege. In 1972, our family began to assist new ethnic Asian refugees who had been kicked out of Idi Amin's Uganda, arriving in town with literally nothing except the clothes on their backs. From a socioeconomic standpoint, those children who picked on me were perhaps actually more marginalized than I; our community of Wiarton had one of the lowest per capita incomes and levels of education in the province. One classmate of mine, who considered himself the most travelled among our class, had been to Toronto only once in his lifetime. Most of my classmates were not blessed with educated parents. Employed as a teacher, my father gave us exposure to different languages, cultures, and religions, as well as the opportunity to travel overseas.
>
> Even further marginalized were the First Nations people living in a reserve just outside of Wiarton, then called Cape Croker. Later, as a medical student, I had the opportunity to visit this same reserve of the Chippewas of the Nawash Unceded First Nation, part of the Saugeen Ojibway Nation, on medical elective. Their way of life was constantly disparaged by people in town, and they were held responsible for many of the social and security issues that plagued their own community and that of Wiarton. Such experiences have led me to view marginalization as a fluid and relative concept that may exist for each of us, but to vastly different degrees.

Canada experience longer wait lists for services, and sometimes even an inability to access any care. Individuals living with no fixed address, lacking necessary identification, or with a pending decision on whether their claim as refugee is "justified" are frequently turned away from health services—they are treated as unequal. The words of Martin Luther King Jr.

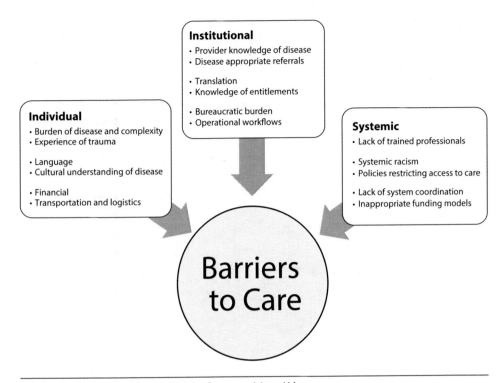

Figure 0.1: Barriers to Refugee Health

Source: Arya, McMurray, and Rashid (2012).

address this divide well: "Of all the forms of inequality, injustice in health care is the most shocking and inhumane" (quoted in Moore 2013).

In our health care *service*, it is all too clear that there are some Canadians we leave *under-served*. Busy health care providers often feel overwhelmed and impeded by such inexplicable structural barriers to service, which impact health outcomes. Barriers to access were classified for refugees, for instance, as individual, institutional, and systemic (see figure 0.1).

Though we may have first-hand experience of these inequities in health care, we are often blind to the upstream issues preceding the diseases to which we bear witness (see Meili and Piggott, Chapter 25, for a discussion of "Thinking Upstream"). These are the root or intermediate causes—the systemic inadequacies that prevent those in need from receiving care. These causes, frequently seen through the lens of the social determinants of health, as presented by Raphael in Chapter 2, are the factors and social conditions that must truly be considered responsible for the diseases that health care providers witness.

When we as health care providers are able to directly address acute issues (see bottom row of figure 0.2), our fixes may be considered "Band-Aid" solutions rather than efforts to deal with the more distal factors, which could prove preventive of recurrences for the individual or others, as well as sustainable.

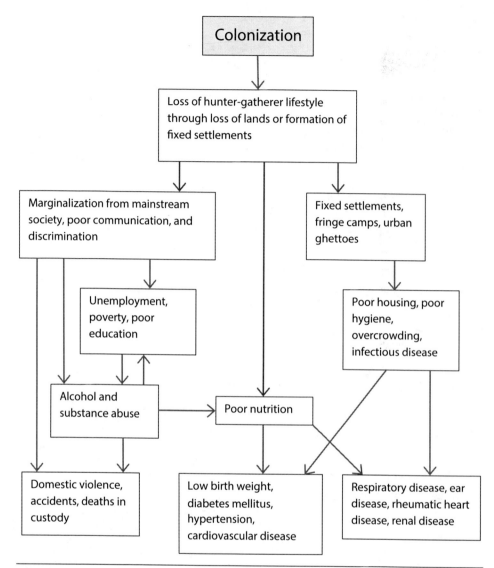

Figure 0.2: Colonization and Health

Source: Mathews (1998).

THE DETERMINANTS

Zooming out from the cellular level—the biomedical focus that is our daily currency as health care providers—the more distal factors, including the social determinants of health, become apparent. These factors, the inevitable pre-conditions to the diseases we see time and time again, are often seen as relegated as "somebody else's" work. All too often, the patterns of disease seen in under-served populations repeat themselves over and over again. Under-served populations incessantly suffer the brunt of these conditions rooted in

> ### My Coming to Understand the Social Determinants (Thomas Piggott)
>
> I (T. P.) came to sense the social determinants of health at an early age, although in less sophisticated terms. In high school, I completed a project to raise awareness about healthy eating, exercise, and childhood obesity that would set me on a pathway to pursuing health care. For the project, I began to tour my school and other schools in my community, talking not only to students but also to administrators about the importance of a healthy lifestyle. I warned of the "epidemic" of childhood obesity.
>
> It was a gratifying project, and I became energized by community mobilization. I was hearing positive feedback. I distinctly remember one overweight ninth-grade student with a beaming smile approaching me after one of my presentations to say, "that was so awesome—I'm going to start running!" However, I soon came to see the issues underlying healthy behaviours as more complex. Several days later, I saw the same kid in the school hallway. Upon seeing me, his face turned sombre as he relayed to me that when he asked his mom if he could buy running shoes to start running, she just laughed him off and said that they "just couldn't afford them."
>
> I realized educating students and administrators could only take the issue so far. From my position of privilege, exercise was easy. My parents taught me to value it from an early age: they enrolled me in sports, and on weekends we would go hiking and camping. For others, I came to realize, it was more complex. I became frustrated by this "great divide" I was witnessing. The kids from families with money were the ones in sports, and the ones who were eating a healthy diet, and the ones of an appropriate weight. Kids from families without the same financial means did not have these same opportunities.

the social determinants of health. Awareness of this suffering and its inevitability can be exhausting for health care providers; it may even fuel caregiver burnout.

Rather than zooming out, we may choose to "zone out." As we hope to make clear in this book, that need not be the case. Zooming out opens us to a whole new world of experiences, which can make us more effective as health care providers.

Understanding the determinants of health and zooming out often requires attention to political decisions that have consequences for the health of under-served populations. Rudolf Virchow wrote that "medicine is a social science and politics is nothing else but medicine on a large scale" (quoted in Friedlander 2018). Health care providers may use this as an impetus for their political action on the determinants of health, without attention to the less quoted corollary penned by Virchow: "Medicine as a social science, as the science of human beings, has the obligation to point out problems and to attempt their theoretical solution; the politician, the practical anthropologist, must find the means for their actual solution" (quoted in Friedlander 2018).

Much of the action taken to improve the social determinants of health of underserved populations must occur elsewhere in society—in education, in economic and social policy-making, in housing development, and so forth. Perceived success of action on the determinants of health may vary across the political spectrum, but no orientation is simply right or wrong; reality is more complicated.

On the political "right," governments sometimes have implemented divisive policies, often devoid of scientific evidence. With the "Common Sense Revolution" in Ontario, Social Services Minister David Tsubouchi sought to aid welfare recipients whose benefits he had cut across the board by 22 percent; he advised them to haggle with shopkeepers and consider a shopping list including pasta without sauce, bread without butter, and a 69-cent on-sale dented tuna can (Harrington 1995).

In Alberta, an inebriated Ralph Klein asked his driver to take him to the Herb Jamieson Centre, a homeless shelter, on December 12, 2001, where he swore at and berated people, tossing coins at them and telling them to get jobs (Purdy 2011). Federal ministers more recently have insinuated that refugees are bogus, privileged freeloaders, out to steal social benefits paid for by hard-working Canadian taxpayers, fuelling a long-standing myth, much like Ronald Reagan's legendary "welfare queen" (Canadian Council for Refugees 2013). Criticizing Ontario for covering claimants, federal Minister Chris Alexander opined that "simply arriving on our shores and claiming hardships isn't good enough. This isn't a self-selection bonanza, or a social program buffet"; his spokesperson, Alexis Pavlich, later elaborated: "Failed asylum claimants and asylum claimants from safe countries no longer receive gold-plated health care benefits that are better than what Canadian taxpayers, including seniors, receive" (quoted in Mas 2014). Indigenous people steretotyped as "dirty, drunk Aboriginals" have been left to die by the police or in hospital waiting areas (*CBC News Online* 2005; Puxley 2013).

On the other hand, those on the political "right" are often more generous with individual charitable donations and have more significant involvement in church groups and service clubs, all of which help to serve such populations, rather than expecting governments to provide solutions. They may have a visceral distaste for giving some people more rights and privilege than others. Despite his, at times, contrary actions, Ralph Klein was one of the more empathic premiers we have had, often referencing his own personal struggles as giving him an understanding of the "common man."

Those on the political "left" are more likely to favour social policy supporting government intervention and investment to counter historical wrongs and give opportunity to those who are vulnerable. However, they may unconsciously stigmatize people as victims, without agency or voice. It should not be forgotten that it was the liberals of the day, and religious organizations, who, in the name of progress, promoted assimilationist policies towards Indigenous communities, including residential schools.

Marginalized people generally do not seek charity but want an equal playing field. They want a hand up, not a handout. People who find themselves marginalized are often proportionately far more generous to others less fortunate than those who have much more.

In addition to the stigma that may impact under-served populations, people who are under-served are frequently left without voice. Szasz, Laing, and Foucault challenged psychiatry to examine its own instruments of oppression, recognizing the political and social roots of mental illness and the systematic marginalization of the discourse of those it wished to ignore. Pathologizing populations in inner cities may act as an extrajudicial mechanism for getting rid of undesirables, instead of seeking reasons for their distress. At the very least, our approach to mental health neglects families and communities who could be involved in promoting resiliency of the individual.

Periodically, headlines relating to the under-served prick the conscience of the Canadian populace, much as the refugee child Alan Kurdi pricked international attention, but most of the stories of institutional prejudice and racism are left untold. While overt stigmatization and prejudice may be receding for marginalized populations in Canada, institutional prejudice and racism, by way of policies, practices, and assumptions embedded in our health care institutions, remain a barrier for many to accessing equitable care. Governments of both the right and left can give and take away voice.

YOU, THE READER

This book furnishes the reader with a variety of perspectives, from front-line health care providers, who provide care to under-served populations, to advocates, researchers, policy-makers, and educators. It presents the issues and tangible actions that can be integrated into your own health care practices or other lines of work. We would like you to remember this is more than a book about trauma and disadvantage, though these are often important to understanding the roots of the problems faced by under-served populations. We hope you will recall the stories of individuals in order to appreciate their resilience in overcoming societal injustices and obstacles, those of health professionals who have gone beyond the status quo, and the policies that truly make an impact on those who are under-served.

Throughout the book, we seek to continually answer the question: What difference will it make? Hearing from front-line health care providers, advocates, and academics working with under-served populations, we hope to convince you that it can indeed make a difference whether you are working in or plan to work in health care provision or public health policy.

If, as editors, we are doing our job, you may at times feel discomforted as you journey through this book. Creating a safe space should not mean avoiding challenging beliefs. The time to challenge is now. The issues are complex, but that cannot negate action. If health equity is to be achieved, we can no longer sit back and zone out while populations go *under-served*. We encourage you to join us and continue the conversation at the book's accompanying website: http://www.underserved.ca.

REFERENCES

Arya, Neil, Josephine McMurray, and Meb Rashid. 2012. "Enter at Your Own Risk: Government Changes to Comprehensive Care for Newly Arrived Canadian Refugees." *CMAJ* 184 (17): 1875–6. https://doi.org/10.1503/cmaj.120938.

Belshaw, John Douglas. 2015. *Canadian History: Pre-Confederation*. BC Open Textbooks. https://opentextbc.ca/preconfederation/.

Canadian Council for Refugees. 2013. "Refugees and Income Assistance—Rebutting the Chain Email ('Pensioners' Myth')." Updated July. http://ccrweb.ca/en/refugees-and-income-assistance-rebutting-chain-email-pensioners-myth.

CBC News Online. 2005. "Neil Stonechild: Timeline." November 3. http://www.cbc.ca/news2/background/stonechild/timeline.html.

Friedlander, E. 2018. "Rudolf Virchow on Pathology Education." *Pathology Guy*, April 15. http://www.pathguy.com/virchow.htm.

Harrington, Denise. 1995. "1995: 'Tsubouchi Diet' Causes Uproar in Ontario." *The National*, October 20. http://www.cbc.ca/archives/entry/1995-tsubouchi-diet-causes-uproar-in-ontario.

Hwang, Stephen, Russell Wilkins, Michael Tjepkema, Patricia J. O'Campo, and James R. Dunn. 2009. "Mortality among Residents of Shelters, Rooming Houses and Hotels in Canada: An 11-Year Follow-Up Study." *BMJ* 339: b4036. https://doi.org/10.1136/bmj.b4036.

King, Thomas. 2003. "The Truth about Stories." The 2003 CBC Massey Lectures, November 7. http://www.cbc.ca/radio/ideas/the-2003-cbc-massey-lectures-the-truth-about-stories-a-native-narrative-1.2946870.

Mas, Susana. 2014. "Chris Alexander Scolds Ontario over Health Care to Refugees." *CBC News*, January 22. http://www.cbc.ca/news/politics/chris-alexander-scolds-ontario-over-health-care-to-refugees-1.2507008.

Mathews, John. 1998. "The Menzies School of Health Research Offers a New Paradigm of Cooperative Research." *Medical Journal of Australia* 169 (11): 625–9. https://www.mja.com.au/journal/1998/169/11/medical-research-perspectives.

Moore, Amanda. 2013. "Tracking Down Martin Luther King, Jr.'s Words on Health Care." *Huffington Post*, January 18. http://www.huffingtonpost.com/amanda-moore/martin-luther-king-health-care_b_2506393.html.

Purdy, Chris. 2011. "Homeless Man Undeterred by Ralph Klein's Slurred Rant." *Globe and Mail*, August 1. Updated September 6, 2012. http://www.theglobeandmail.com/news/national/homeless-man-undeterred-by-ralph-kleins-slurred-rant/article588988/.

Puxley, Chinta. 2013. "Brian Sinclair, Winnipeg Aboriginal Who Died after 34-Hour Hour Hospital Wait, Assumed 'Sleeping It Off.'" *Huffington Post Canada*, August 29. Updated October 29, 2013. http://www.huffingtonpost.ca/2013/08/29/brian-sinclair-winnipeg_n_3837008.html.

Statistics Canada. 2017. "Projected Life Expectancy at Birth by Sex, by Aboriginal Identity." http://www.statcan.gc.ca/pub/89-645-x/2010001/c-g/c-g013-eng.htm.

U.S. News. n.d. "U.S. News Best Countries Ranking." Accessed December 2, 2017. https://www.usnews.com/news/best-countries/rankings-index.

World Bank. n.d. "Life Expectancy at Birth, Total (Years)." Accessed January 17, 2018. https://data.worldbank.org/indicator/SP.DYN.LE00.IN.

SECTION I

INTRODUCING UNDER-SERVED POPULATIONS AND THEIR DETERMINANTS OF HEALTH

SECTION INTRODUCTION BY THOMAS PIGGOTT AND NEIL ARYA

This first section of *Under-Served* introduces fundamental concepts to ground the discussions that will follow through the rest of the book. We hope that the critical lens we present on terminology and the determinants of health will help in framing your understanding of the health of under-served populations in Canada.

In Chapter 1, Piggott and Orkin introduce the concept of terminology related to the populations addressed in this book. As they discuss, the implications of words we apply in conversation and writing regarding under-served population are complex, and too often, terminology is employed without due consideration to its meaning and implications. Terminology, if not given careful attention, may stigmatize. Terminology evolves, and critically assessing terminology may also allow groups take ownership of the discourse; words that have previously been generally accepted may fall out of favour as affected populations react. As is discussed in the sections that follow, *Indigenous* and *LGBTQ* are terms that are accepted today but were foreign to previous generations. As you read this chapter, reflect on the terminology that you use: Do you know the roots and connotations?

In Chapter 2, the leading voice on the social determinants of health in Canada, Dennis Raphael, will provide you with a grounding and framework for understanding and assessing the social determinants of health (SDH) specifically applied to under-served populations. The chapter delves into the evidence regarding the influence of SDH on health outcomes for under-served populations. Whether you are new to the concept of SDH or have encountered it many times before, the framework presented for the resources that make under-served populations healthy or drive disease is key to conceptualizing the chapters that follow.

CHAPTER 1

Deconstructing the Concept of Special Populations for Health Care, Research, and Policy

Thomas Piggott and Aaron Orkin

LEARNING OBJECTIVES

After reading this chapter, you should be able to:

1. Outline terminology identifying special populations, including *marginalized*, *vulnerable*, and *under-served*.
2. Explore the rationales and motivations for identifying certain populations as "special."
3. Discuss the concepts of health inequalities and inequities as they relate to special populations.
4. Explore the implications of terminology for special populations, especially for health care provision.

BACKGROUND

Caring for some people effectively requires more resources than caring for others. This is true in clinical practice, with some patients requiring more time that others even with the same conditions. It is also true in public health and social services, where some need more time, more effort, more money, even in the context of social assistance or other governmental programming meant to correct inequities. The need for additional resources and approaches to care effectively, and the fact that some under-served populations demand even fewer resources, as they may not access care as readily, are central premises of this book.

Some patients have multiple co-morbidities, requiring drugs, tests, frequent clinical monitoring, and interventions, while others live healthily without intervention. Those in need of increased attention have often experienced great adversity, trauma, or barriers through their lifetimes that prevent them from attaining health; these factors impacting health are often termed the social determinants of health (SDH), as described by Raphael in Chapter 2 of this volume and advanced in the seminal work of Sir Michael Marmot (2005; Marmot and the Commission on Social Determinants of Health 2008). This book employs varied terminology to name special populations with worsened health outcomes, including *marginalized*, *vulnerable*, and *under-served*. In this chapter, we explore the terminology identifying special populations and the purpose and utility of such efforts to identify these groups. While others, including authors in this book, might accept it as self-evident that identifying the marginalization, vulnerability, or unique service needs of special populations is a useful or even necessary approach to improving health, this chapter explores legitimate critical perspectives on these assumptions and offers some reflective analyses.

TERMINOLOGY OF SPECIAL POPULATIONS

The appropriate and politically correct terminology for "special" populations is ever-changing. *Marginalized*, *vulnerable*, and *under-served* are among the variety of terms employed throughout this book to capture the special status and circumstances of these special populations. We will begin by presenting definitions of these terms. In this text, the term *under-served* was used after careful reflection and as an intention to illustrate an unmet service need for the populations of focus. However, in this chapter, we use the term *special* populations because we believe it to carry the least connotations, which can serve as distractions as we deconstruct the terminology.

The most common term in the health sciences literature is *vulnerable*. With its Latin origins meaning "to wound," vulnerable, at its most basic, refers to a susceptibility to harm (Schroeder and Gefenas 2009). Hurst (2008, 191) goes on to elaborate that within the context of health, vulnerability refers to an "increased likelihood of incurring additional or greater wrong." Others have further elaborated on this understanding to include individuals who are "susceptible to being harmed, wronged, mistreated, discriminated against or taken advantage of in the context of health care and research" (Ganguli-Mitra and Biller-Andorno 2011, 239) or who have "an inability to protect themselves, either physically or emotionally" (Schroeder and Gefenas 2009, 114). Much of the literature related to vulnerability originates from the research sphere, where vulnerability is a necessary lens in research ethics, and in the process of obtaining informed consent. Others extend the relevance of vulnerability to health care in discussing the power differential between the physician, with the knowledge, power, and capacities to provide treatment, and the vulnerable patient, who is in need of these services (Zaner 2000).

Resilience, on the other hand, can be thought of as the inverse of vulnerability, and "denotes a combination of abilities and characteristics that interact dynamically to allow an individual to bounce back, cope successfully, and function above the norm in spite of significant stress or adversity" (Tusaie and Dyer 2004, 3). Friedli (2009) applies the concept of resiliency to the individual, social, community, geography, and policy levels. A resilient population could be defined as a vulnerable population's opposite.

Marginalized may capture similar individuals to those identified as vulnerable, yet the term carries distinct connotations (*Oxford Living Dictionaries* n.d.). Lynam and Cowley (2007, 146) describe marginalization as "a sense of being overlooked, categorized or misrepresented. It curtails opportunities for capacity-building, and constrains ways in which relationships are established." Many individuals who might be considered vulnerable may also be considered marginalized, yet marginalization emphasizes a societal isolation of the individual as "other," pushed to the periphery or margins (Lynam and Cowley 2007). Where vulnerability might be captured as a statistical risk for an adverse outcome, marginalization refers more directly to a social and inappropriate under-representation or under-recognition.

Kipnis (2001) describes a context-sensitive approach to vulnerability with six categories: cognitive and communicative vulnerability, institutional vulnerability, differential vulnerability, medical vulnerability, economic vulnerability, and social vulnerability. This also suggests that "the vulnerability is not necessarily intrinsic to the individual, but rather sometimes a mismatch between a characteristic of the individual and the context in which she/he finds her/himself" (Ganguli-Mitra and Biller-Andorno 2011, 241).

Under-served implies a lack of adequate provision of service to an individual or group. In the context of health care, it refers to "an increased likelihood that individuals who belong to a certain population (and people can belong to more than one) may experience difficulties in obtaining needed care, receive less care or a lower standard of care, experience different treatment by health care providers, receive treatment that does not adequately meet their needs, or they will be less satisfied with health care services than the general population" (Bowen 2001, 7). Whereas *vulnerable* or *marginalized* identify the problem within the individual, *under-served* points to a system failure that leaves a group of individuals with an unmet need. *Under-served* also creates an avenue for rectifying this unmet need, by way of bridging the gap between needs and services by creating more appropriate or adequate services.

SPECIAL POPULATIONS REPORTED IN THE LITERATURE

Special populations with inequitable health outcomes can be identified on the basis of a wide variety of biological, social, and political characteristics. With reference to vulnerability, Ganguli-Mitra and Biller-Andorno (2011, 240) state that "historically the definition of the term revolved around autonomy (or lack of it) but the use of the term today has become increasingly inclusive of other characteristics, leading to diverse categories and different ethical approaches." Some of these diverse characteristics include experiences in terms of the determinants of health, variations in diseases experienced, and differences in health service access and needs (as shown in figure 1.1). The characteristics of populations requiring special attention overlap—a phenomenon termed *intersectionality*—and many other characteristics do not apply solely to a unique population (for a discussion of intersectionality, see Lachowsky, Gahagan, and Anderson, Chapter 13 in this volume). Furthermore, some characteristics, such as education or housing, are fluid, changing through an individual's life, while others, such as race or the early childhood experiences of an adult, are fixed.

A non-comprehensive list of special populations identified in the literature as "special" includes the following: children, individuals with low education levels, individuals with non-normative gender identities, individuals with inadequate or precarious housing, immigrants, Indigenous populations, those living in low-income countries, visible minorities, people with mental and physical disabilities, pregnant women, prisoners, racialized individuals, refugees, people suffering from serious illness, people who identify as LGBTQ, asexual individuals, those who are socially isolated, people with low socioeconomic status, the unemployed, and, more broadly, women (Ganguli-Mitra and Biller-Andorno 2011; Hurst 2008; Nickel 2006). Such a list prompts a reasonable query: If all of these populations are "special" (marginalized, under-served, or vulnerable), then what section of the population remains, or may be deemed to be "not special"? If everyone is somehow special, what is the term's discriminatory or analytical value?

HEALTH CARE, RESEARCH, AND POLICY

Thus far, we have introduced terminology related to special populations. There is also a rich discourse regarding special populations, the nature of which depends on the field in question. In clinical care, we often neglect to even identify a patient as a part of a particular "population." He or she is a single person or patient presenting for care, not representative of specific groups. It is only in certain activities, such as screening for diseases, attending to risk factors, or accessing restricted services, that a patient's assignment to a population becomes clinically relevant and highly visible.

Special populations also become more central in research processes. Much of the literature on special populations, and on vulnerability in particular, originates from the research field. It is here that rigorous processes of reflecting upon and assessing vulnerability are ingrained in research design, approval, and recruitment processes. In certain studies, researchers may seek to enrol participants because they represent a certain population in question. Particular special populations may prove to be more difficult to enrol or follow up with in research studies.

Research is focused on the creation of knowledge and its advancement for society, yet conducting medical research generally involves recruiting patients on an individual basis. In some instances, a study participant may personally benefit—by having access to a new and effective drug to treat a disease that afflicts them, for example. However, in many instances, the gains are not realized by the individual—only society as a whole will reap the rewards. For this reason, research ethics, especially the issues of informed consent, vulnerability, and coercion, require due consideration (for a discussion of these issues in the context of refugee health research, see Gabriel, Chapter 22 in this volume). Careful consideration of research ethics can, however, have mixed effects. While it is imperative to protect vulnerable populations from malignant or inconsiderate research, such protection may also further marginalize these groups by dissuading researchers from working with them and making much needed "answers" more difficult to come by for these populations.

In contrast to the individual-level focus on vulnerability of participants in research, in the health policy and governance realm, attention may be focused on certain populations. For example, the Ontario government, with its Ontario Public Health Standards, mandates public health organizations to give attention to "priority populations," defined as those groups with a higher disease burden and with members who experience inequities in their health (Tyler and Hassen 2015). Governments must take collective action on health inequities to improve the health of the priority populations they govern.

HEALTH INEQUITIES

We will now further examine the concept of differences in health outcomes—the fundamental basis upon which a population is considered vulnerable, marginalized, or under-served. Some call such variations in health "trends" or "differences." In the United States, the discourse largely revolves around "disparities" (Braveman 2006). *Disparity* tells us more about an individual or group's failure to achieve or receive, whereas *vulnerability* tells us more about features of the community or society that might leave an individual or group with less likelihood to achieve or receive. In the public health literature, there is discussion of "inequalities" and "inequities." The distinction between *unequal* and *inequitable* requires brief disambiguation.

The special populations in Canada discussed in this book are all afflicted with unequal, as well as, arguably, inequitable, health outcomes compared to the general population. Whereas *in-* signifies without, *equal* is defined as same, and *equitable* refers to justice or fairness. *Equity* is grounded in the social principles of distributive justice (Braveman and Gruskin 2003). The argument can be made that discussing health inequalities allows for inclusion of unavoidable differences in outcomes due to biological or genetic differences. For instance, prostate cancer rates differ from men to women because women (without prostates) cannot get prostate cancer. As such, consensus amongst health researchers emphasizes the need to discuss health inequities: the *avoidable* and especially unjust differences in health outcomes (WHO n.d.). Some biological or genetic variables previously presumed fixed and unavoidable are in fact greatly influenced by other social or environmental factors. We conventionally assume that for differences to be inequities and to be unfair, there must be an element of avoidability. Preda and Voigt (2015) question this assumption and propose that unavoidable differences may too be unfair. While they may not be preventable, we might be able to intervene to rectify the differences post hoc (i.e., secondary or tertiary prevention). Instead of focusing on avoidability, Preda and Voigt therefore suggest focus be placed on the amenability of society to correct morally unacceptable differences.

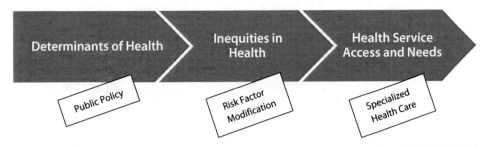

Figure 1.1: Differences in the Health of Special Populations and Interventions

Health inequities may be a symptom of a broader societal inequity simply coming to light as adverse health outcomes. As Sen (2002, 661) has stated,

> health equity cannot but be a central feature of the justice of social arrangements in general.... Health equity cannot be concerned only with health, seen in isolation. Rather it must come to grips with the larger issue of fairness and justice in social arrangements, including economic allocations, paying appropriate attention to the role of health in human life and freedom.

In this context, scholars and practitioners concerned with health inequities and aware of the inextricable nature of health outcomes and matters of justice and fairness must consider whether health or healthiness is best treated as a goal unto itself or as a metric of social or cultural values. Is the goal of advancing health equity to achieve optimal population health or optimal population fairness?

In epidemiology and health care, it seems self-evident that identifying differences and inequities is valuable because it presents a potential intervention point. It is perhaps an opportunity to redress historical wrongs, modify a risk factor for an individual's health, or correct a social determinant of health for future generations. Some of the actions that can be taken on various factors influencing the health of special populations are demonstrated in figure 1.1. The determinants of health are socioeconomic and political and therefore require attention at a political or public policy level.

Increasingly, health is being recognized as a human right, and with this comes an impetus for political provision of opportunities to attain health (Braveman 2010). But in defining health as a human right, the question of what standard of health humans are entitled to attain arises and can act in opposition to equity. As Braveman (2010, 39) writes,

> the right to the highest attainable standard of health could be used by some, in individual-level litigation, to justify unlimited expenditures on expensive medical technology for a few articulate, empowered individuals, to the detriment of investments in more

equitable interventions with greater effectiveness in improving population health and reducing disparities.

Inequities in health occur after the social determinants have already caused differences in health. As Preda and Voigt (2015) have suggested, failing political action, the SDH inequities can be addressed as secondary prevention actions by health care providers—that is, through risk factor modification or by creating and accessing appropriate services. This can include more conventional interventions such as treating hypertension caused by fast food, a sodium-rich diet, or poverty; or it can include broader patient advocacy measures, such as assistance with supported housing or income assistance, as described by Goel and Bloch (Chapter 14 in this volume). Finally, when the two previous actions have failed, specialized health care can address an individual's unique needs once disease strikes.

PITFALLS OF THE IDENTIFICATION OF SPECIAL POPULATIONS

Terminology varies for populations requiring specific attention in health care and public health. Often this terminology is used interchangeably when discussing populations requiring specific attention, yet the implications of each of these terms varies considerably, as has been shown.

In the research field of epidemiology, this varied use of terminology has escalated quickly; yet despite the moral implications of this conversation, it has largely been siloed within the scientific community. Venkatapuram and Marmot (2009) argue that, in philosophy, insufficient exchange has happened with those focused on morality to have deepened the understanding of the causes and responses to inequalities. With this siloed escalation of the focus on special populations, the variety of populations presented as special has expanded widely.

Some have argued that when considering certain classifications of populations requiring specific attention, the scope has expanded so broadly that nearly everyone is included (Hurst 2008; Ganguli-Mitra and Biller-Andorno 2011). As a result, Levine and colleagues (2004, 46) state that the concept of vulnerability on the whole has become "too nebulous to be meaningful."

The implications of this expansion have led to the unfortunate consequence that "the special protection reserved for genuinely vulnerable populations is being lost" (Schroeder and Gefenas 2009, 113). Does the identification of special populations actually lead to improved health outcomes and reduced health inequities? And if so, by what criteria must we identify populations that warrant special attention to avoid the overexpansion, and loss, of special protection or attention?

Identifying special populations is not without harms. Labelling can lead to stigma, as well as loss of independence or autonomy. This is particularly the case with reference to the term *vulnerable*, which implies an individual-level insecurity, while *marginalized* and *under-served* have more systemic implications. Ultimately, we must constantly ask, does the labelling of special populations lead to health benefits and reductions in the underlying vulnerabilities and marginalization? On the whole, is this concept more helpful or harmful? Reducing or mitigating these harms often relies on community-based and participatory approaches, as well as ensuring that the voices, perspectives, and leadership of special populations are heard and prioritized in addressing community needs.

Some scholars have proposed that we abandon terminology such as *vulnerable* altogether, notably when conceptual frameworks and clear definitions for their use are lacking (Wrigley 2015). However, strong arguments remain to retain this lens in a focused and appropriate way, perhaps as a "precautionary principle" that advocates a default of precaution where interventions have the potential to do harm to special populations, and where the evidence is incomplete (Grinnell 2004). With a clearer definition of criteria for characteristics such as *vulnerable*, the utility can be improved. In an effort to provide these criteria, Tavaglione et al. (2015) propose that *vulnerability* consists of denial of legitimate claims to physical integrity, autonomy, freedom, social provision, impartial quality of government, social bases of self-respect, or communal belonging. With this clearer understanding, the vulnerability lens can more effectively be used as a "moral safeguard" (DeMarco 2004, 44) or a "multifaceted concept that can inspire the search for the right moral response" (Ganguli-Mitra and Biller-Andorno 2011, 249) when dealing with special populations.

CONCLUSIONS AND APPLICATIONS TO HEALTH CARE PRACTICE

This chapter has reviewed numerous theoretical frameworks, terminologies, and high-level concepts. Is there in fact a continuum of need for individuals, and does this more appropriately address the manner by which to plan health care and public health activities? When does an individual or group become vulnerable, marginalized, or under-served?

The idea that focusing increased resources on special populations is essential to the task of addressing health inequities is well accepted; however, the manner by which populations are deemed to be special, and the breadth to which special attention should be applied to population groups, remains a matter of unsolved debate. At the level of patient care, we must take each patient's circumstances and history independently. When advocating for increased attention or resources for a patient, health care providers should do so in a culturally safe and non-stigmatizing way. At a research level, the drawbacks and benefits of labelling special populations should be deliberated through the research design, review, and implementation process. At a policy level, governments should be encouraged to support activities that balance programs broadly targeting the SDH with those focusing in on the unique needs of selected populations in consultation with those selected populations.

Terminology for special populations is too often used unconsciously or uncarefully. Although the underlying concepts are perhaps essential and create desperately needed opportunities for intervention, they also bring disadvantages and harms. A more thoughtful attention to these concerns offers a chance to recognize those disadvantages and tackle health inequities with more effective interventions and more appropriate language and discourses.

CRITICAL THINKING QUESTIONS

1. Discuss the terms presented for special populations in this chapter, including *marginalized*, *vulnerable*, and *under-served*.
2. What are the implications of these terms from a health care provider perspective?
3. What are the implications of these terms from a patient perspective?
4. What are the implications of these terms from a policy perspective?
5. How will you reconcile the use of terminology related to special populations in your work?

REFERENCES

Bowen, Sarah. 2001. "Access to Health Services for Underserved Populations in Canada." In *"Certain Circumstances": Issues in Equity and Responsiveness to Health Care in Canada*, 1–60. Ottawa: Health Canada. https://www.canada.ca/content/dam/hc-sc/migration/hc-sc/hcs-sss/alt_formats/hpb-dgps/pdf/pubs/2001-certain-equit-acces/2001-certain-equit-acces-eng.pdf.

Braveman, Paula. 2006. "Health Disparities and Health Equity: Concepts and Measurement." *Annual Review of Public Health* 27: 167–94. https://doi.org/10.1146/annurev.publhealth.27.021405.102103.

Braveman, Paula. 2010. "Social Conditions, Health Equity, and Human Rights." *Health and Human Rights* 12 (2): 31–48.

Braveman, P., and S. Gruskin. 2003. "Defining Equity in Health." *Journal of Epidemiology and Community Health* 57 (4): 254–8. https://doi.org/10.1136/jech.57.4.254.

DeMarco, J. P. 2004. "Vulnerability: A Needed Moral Safeguard." *American Journal of Bioethics* 4 (3): 82–84.

Friedli, Lynne. 2009. *Mental Health, Resilience and Inequalities*. Copenhagen: World Health Organization Europe. http://apps.who.int.libaccess.lib.mcmaster.ca/iris/bitstream/handle/10665/107925/E92227.pdf.

Ganguli-Mitra, Agomoni, and Nikola Biller-Andorno. 2011. "Vulnerability in Health Care and Research Ethics." In *The SAGE Handbook of Health Care Ethics*, edited by Ruth Chadwick, Henk ten Have, and Eric Meslin, 239–50. Thousand Oaks, CA: Sage.

Grinnell, F. 2004. "Subject Vulnerability: The Precautionary Principle in Human Research." *American Journal of Bioethics* 4 (3): 52–53.

Hurst, Samia A. 2008. "Vulnerability in Research and Health Care; Describing the Elephant in the Room?" *Bioethics* 22: 191–202. https://doi.org/10.1111/j.1467-8519.2008.00631.x.

Kipnis, K. 2001. *Vulnerability in Research Subjects: A Bioethical Taxonomy.* Bethesda, MD: National Bioethics Advisory Commission.

Levine, Carol, Ruth Faden, Christine Grady, Dale Hammerschmidt, Lisa Eckenwiler, and Jeremy Sugarman. 2004. "The Limitations of 'Vulnerability' as a Protection for Human Research Participants." *American Journal of Bioethics: AJOB* 4 (3): 44–49. https://doi.org/10.1080/15265160490497083.

Lynam, M. Judith, and Sarah Cowley. 2007. "Understanding Marginalization as a Social Determinant of Health." *Critical Public Health* (2): 137–49. https://doi.org/10.1080/09581590601045907.

Marmot, Michael. 2005. "Social Determinants of Health Inequalities." *Lancet* 365 (9464): 1099–104.

Marmot, Michael, and the Commission on Social Determinants of Health. 2008. *Closing the Gap in a Generation: Health Equity through Action on the Social Determinants of Health.* Geneva: World Health Organization. http://apps.who.int/iris/bitstream/10665/43943/1/9789241563703_eng.pdf.

Nickel, Philip J. 2006. "Vulnerable Populations in Research: The Case of the Seriously Ill." *Theoretical Medicine and Bioethics* 27 (3): 245–64. https://doi.org/10.1007/s11017-006-9000-2.

Oxford Living Dictionaries. n.d. s.v. "Marginalize." Accessed April 18, 2018. http://www.oxforddictionaries.com/definition/english/marginalize.

Preda, Adina, and Kristin Voigt. 2015. "The Social Determinants of Health: Why Should We Care?" *American Journal of Bioethics* 15 (3): 25–36. https://doi.org/10.1080/15265161.2014.998374.

Schroeder, Doris, and Eugenijus Gefenas. 2009. "Vulnerability: Too Vague and Too Broad?" *Cambridge Quarterly of Health Care Ethics* 18 (2): 113–21. https://doi.org/10.1017/S0963180109090203.

Sen, Amartya. 2002. "Why Health Equity?" *Health Economics.* 11: 659–66. https://doi.org/10.1002/hec.762.

Tavaglione, Nicolas, Angela K. Martin, Nathalie Mezger, Sophie Durieux-Paillard, Anne François, Yves Jackson, and Samia A. Hurst. 2015. "Fleshing out Vulnerability." *Bioethics* 29 (2): 98–107. https://doi.org/10.1111/bioe.12065.

Tusaie, Kathleen, and Janyce Dyer. 2004. "Resilience: A Historical Review of the Contruct." *Holistic Nursing Practice* 18 (1): 3–10.

Tyler, Ingrid, and Nadha Hassen. 2015. *Priority Populations Project Technical Report.* Toronto: Public Health Ontario. https://www.publichealthontario.ca/en/eRepository/Priority_Populations_Technical_Report.pdf.

Venkatapuram, Sridhar, and Michael Marmot. 2009. "Epidemiology and Social Justice in Light of Social Determinants of Health Research." *Bioethics* 23 (2): 79–89. https://doi.org/10.1111/j.1467-8519.2008.00714.x.

World Health Organization (WHO). n.d. "Social Determinants of Health: Key Concepts." Accessed May 6, 2015. http://www.who.int/social_determinants/thecommission/finalreport/key_concepts/en/.

Wrigley, Anthony. 2015. "An Eliminativist Approach to Vulnerability." *Bioethics* 29 (7): 478–87. https://doi.org/10.1111/bioe.12144.

Zaner, Richard. 2000. "Power and Hope in the Clinical Encounter: A Meditation on Vulnerability." *Medicine, Health Care and Philosophy: A European Journal* 3 (3): 265–75.

CHAPTER 2

The Social Determinants of Health of Under-Served Populations in Canada

Dennis Raphael

LEARNING OBJECTIVES

After reading this chapter, you should be able to:

1. Appreciate how living and working conditions—not biomedical factors or health-related behaviours—are the primary contributors to health and illness.
2. Identify the key themes that have emerged from the social determinants of health literature.
3. Be knowledgeable about the pathways by which living and working conditions come to shape health.
4. Recognize how Canada's changing public policy environment has worsened the situation of Canadians in general and those found in certain social locations in particular.

Social determinants of health (SDH) are the economic and social factors or, in popular parlance, the living and working conditions that shape our health. These conditions are the primary determinants of whether we stay healthy or become ill (a narrow definition of health) and the extent to which we possess the social and personal resources necessary to achieve personal aspirations, satisfy needs, and cope with the environment (a broader definition of health). SDH are about the quantity and quality of a variety of resources a society chooses to make available to its members. These resources include, but are not limited to, conditions of childhood, income, education, employment security and working conditions, food and housing security, and availability of health and social services.

Social locations such as Indigenous descent, social class, dis/ability, gender, race, and immigrant and refugee status are also SDH, as they specify which individuals have access to these resources. In Canada, many groups experience SDH that threaten their health;

specifically, they experience the material and social deprivation that leads to adverse health outcomes. That so many groups are subject to these effects is due to the public policies that create inequitable distributions of the SDH among the Canadian population.

More and more evidence is accumulating of how the inequitable distribution of SDH results in avoidable and unjust differences in health outcomes—that is, health inequities—among Canadians (Raphael 2016). Nevertheless, these facts continue to be generally unknown to the Canadian public, who is instead warned by governmental authorities, disease associations, and the media about health risks posed by biomedical and behavioural factors such as high cholesterol levels, excessive body weight, lack of physical activity, dietary choices that lack in fruits and vegetables, and tobacco and excessive alcohol use, among others. The impact of these factors upon health pale in comparison to the direct effects of the SDH.

In this chapter, I present the case that since the sources of health are how a society organizes and distributes resources, economic and social policies that promote health are required. I show how numerous groups in Canada have come to be especially susceptible to the material and social deprivation that cause health problems and how public policy creates these situations. I detail numerous grassroots efforts that aim to shift Canadians' ways of thinking about the SDH to pressure governing authorities to implement public policies that promote rather than threaten health.

LIVING AND WORKING CONDITIONS: THE PRIMARY DETERMINANTS OF HEALTH

Not only has it been known since the mid-nineteenth century that living and working conditions are the primary determinants of health; it has also been known that powerful economic and political forces shape these conditions (Raphael 2016). In Canada, numerous studies have demonstrated that the material and social circumstances to which people are exposed are far more important to their health than "lifestyle choices" such as using tobacco or alcohol, choosing to eat fruits and vegetables, or partaking in physical activity (Raphael 2016).

These findings have not gone unnoticed by civil servants working for the Public Health Agency of Canada. Since the mid-1970s, Canadian governmental and public health agencies have produced numerous, though unpublicized, policy documents containing these findings (Butler-Jones 2008; Canadian Population Health Initiative 2008; Health Council of Canada 2010). Despite these efforts, there has been little application of these concepts in the making of Canadian public policy in general and to the situations of those most susceptible to their effects in particular (Bryant et al. 2011).

WHAT ARE SDH?

In 1996, Tarlov identified how inequalities in the quality of "social determinants" of housing, education, social acceptance, employment, and income were translated into disease-related processes. Since then, various approaches to SDH, with many similarities, have appeared. They are presented in table 2.1. These factors are strong predictors of

Table 2.1. Various Conceptualizations of the Social Determinants of Health

World Health Organization (1986)	Dahlgren and Whitehead (1992)	Health Canada (1998)	Wilkinson and Marmot (2003)	Centers for Disease Control and Prevention (2005)	Raphael, Bryant, and Curry-Stevens (2004)
peace	agriculture and food production	income and social status	social gradient	socioeconomic status	Indigenous ancestry
shelter	education	social support networks	stress	transportation	disability
education	work environment	education	early life	housing	early life
food	unemployment	employment and working conditions	social exclusion	access to services	education
stable ecosystem	water and sanitation	physical and social environments	work	discrimination by social grouping	employment and working conditions
income	health care services	healthy child development	unemployment	social or environmental stressors	food security
sustainable resources	housing	health services	social support		gender
social justice		gender	addiction		health care services
equity		culture	food		housing
			transport		income and its distribution
					race
					social safety net
					social exclusion
					unemployment and employment security

health outcomes, such as infant mortality and life expectancy, and the incidence of just about every physical, mental, or social affliction, as well as injuries (Mikkonen and Raphael 2010). Exposures to the SDH as a function of social class, gender, and race lead to differences in health outcomes for these groups. Importantly, these differences in exposures lead to especially adverse health outcomes for Indigenous Canadians, the homeless, and immigrants and refugees.

Raphael's list of 14 SDH is especially relevant to Canadians (Mikkonen and Raphael 2010). These determinants are consistent with most existing formulations, are understandable to the public, and focus on areas of either active governmental policy activity (e.g., health care services, education) or policy inactivity that have provoked criticism (e.g., food and housing security, income inequality, the social safety net). *Social Determinants of Health: Canadian Perspectives* provides an analysis of the current state of these determinants at the national level (Raphael 2016).

THEMES IN THE SDH LITERATURE

Elsewhere, I have identified five SDH-related themes relevant to the issue of the health of the vulnerable in Canada (Raphael 2016). Below, I very briefly summarize these; then I describe the specific SDH situations of three groups especially susceptible to adverse health outcomes due to exposure to the adverse SDH in Canada: Indigenous people, the homeless, and immigrants and refugees in Canada.

Theme 1: Empirical Evidence of the Importance of the SDH

Only a small percentage (10 to 15 percent) of the profound improvement in life expectancy among Canadians since 1900 is due to improved health care (McKinlay and McKinlay 1987). Improvements in behaviour (e.g., reductions in tobacco use and changes in diet) are often hypothesized as responsible for improved longevity, but improvements in health are primarily due to improving the material conditions of early childhood, education, food availability, health and social services, housing, employment security, working conditions, and other SDH (Evans 2002). Indeed, Statistics Canada estimates that 40,000 Canadians each year die prematurely because they do not enjoy the health of the wealthiest 20 percent of Canadians (Tjepkema, Wilkins, and Long 2013).

Theme 2: Mechanisms and Pathways by which SDH Influence Health

The *Black Report* and the *Health Divide* report considered two primary mechanisms for understanding the differences in virtually every health outcome across social classes, ethnic groups, genders, and races in Western nations (Townsend, Davidson, and Whitehead 1992). The cultural/behavioural explanation sees individuals' behavioural choices (e.g., tobacco and alcohol use, diet, physical activity) as responsible for these groups developing and dying from various diseases. The materialist/structuralist explanation sees the material conditions under which people live and work—for example, access to the amenities of life, working conditions, quality of available food and housing—as shaping these group health outcomes. Evidence and expert opinion sides with the materialist/structuralist explanation (Bartley 2016; Graham 2007; Raphael 2016; World Health Organization 2008).

One widely cited model outlines how the organization of society shapes SDH and health itself and lends itself to a materialist/structuralist explanation (Brunner and Marmot 2006; see figure 2.1).

In this model, social structure is a catchall for the organization of society and how it distributes access to resources. Three pathways link social structure with health status. The first is a direct link between social structure, material factors, and health status. Material factors include not only positive exposures to health-enhancing environments or situations and exposures to negative health environments, but also threatening events or situations. In the second pathway, social structure shapes social and work environments to create

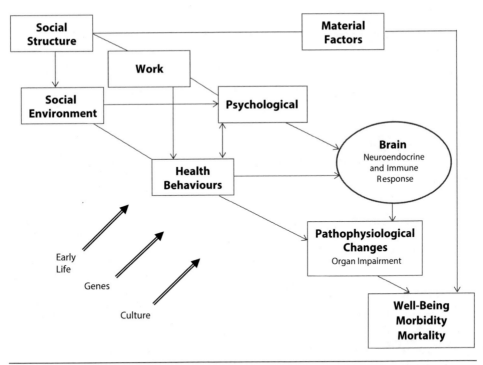

Figure 2.1: Social Determinants of Health

The model links social structure to health and disease via material, psychosocial, and behavioural pathways. Genetics, early life, and cultural factors are further important influences upon population health.

Source: Brunner and Marmot (2006, 9).

psychological and behavioural responses that, operating through brain mechanisms, determine health status. The third pathway sees these same environments creating behavioural coping responses that directly impair bodily organs, thereby determining health. Early life, genes, and culture contribute to these processes at all levels of the model.

Theme 3: The Importance of a Life-Course Perspective

The SDH under which individuals live their lives have a cumulative effect upon their health. This has been repeatedly demonstrated in longitudinal studies that follow individuals across their lives (Blane 1999) and is most clearly demonstrated in the cases of heart disease and stroke and adult-onset diabetes (Raphael et al. 2003; Raphael and Farrell 2002).

Adopting a life-course perspective directs attention to how the range of SDH operates at every level of development—early childhood, childhood, adolescence, and adulthood—to influence health immediately, as well as to provide the basis for health or illness during later stages of the life course. Of course, these circumstances are shaped and influenced by public policy (Raphael 2011, 2013).

Theme 4: The Role of Public Policy and Policy Environments

Health-threatening SDH come about because of public policy decisions (Pal 2006). Early life, for example, is shaped by availability of sufficient material resources to assure adequate educational opportunities, food, and housing, among other factors. Much of this has to do with parents' employment security, wages, and the quality of their working conditions (Raphael 2014). These factors are shaped by public policy decisions and do not usually come under individual control. A policy-oriented approach places such findings within a broader policy context.

Theme 5: Politics, Political Ideology, and the SDH

Why certain nations take up this information and apply it in the formulation of public policy while others, such as Canada, do not can be explained through differing forms of the welfare state. Three distinct types of welfare states exist: social democratic (e.g., Sweden, Norway, Denmark, and Finland), liberal (the United States, the United Kingdom, Canada, and Ireland), and conservative (France, Germany, Netherlands, and Belgium, among others) (Esping-Andersen 1990, 1999).

Social democratic nations provide a wide range of universal and generous benefits and are proactive in developing policies that support workers, families, and gender equity. Liberal nations spend considerably less on supports and services. They offer modest universal transfers and modest social insurance plans. Benefits are provided primarily through means-tested assistance and thus are provided only to the least well-off. Health indicators such as life expectancy, premature years of life lost prior to age 70, teenage pregnancy rates,

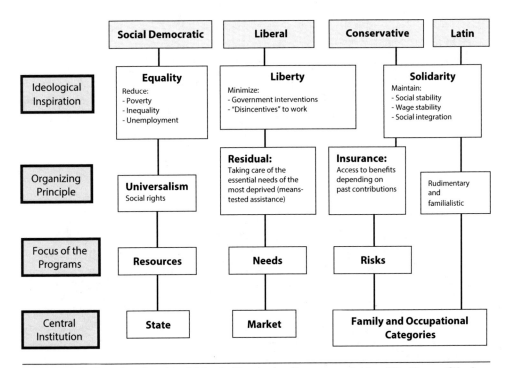

Figure 2.2: Ideological Variations in Forms of the Welfare State

Source: Saint-Arnaud and Bernard (2003, 503, fig. 2).

and infant mortality and low birth-weight rates are better for social democratic nations than for liberal nations (Innocenti Research Centre, 2007, 2013; Navarro 2004).

Two Canadian sociologists succinctly sum up how these differences in political economy can come to be related to the SDH (Saint-Arnaud and Bernard 2003; see figure 2.2).

Within liberal welfare states, minimal government intervention occurs in the marketplace. It is claimed that such interventions provide disincentives to work, breeding "welfare dependence." As a result, meagre benefits are provided to those on social assistance in Canada, and there is weak legislative support for the labour movement, undeveloped policies for assisting those with disabilities, and a general reluctance to provide universal services and programs. Programs that exist are residual, meaning they meet only the most basic needs of the most deprived. Liberal welfare states have the greatest degree of wealth and income inequality, the weakest safety nets, and the poorest population health.

THE SITUATION OF PARTICULAR GROUPS SUSCEPTIBLE TO ADVERSE HEALTH OUTCOMES IN CANADA

There are clear SDH-related effects associated with specific social locations in Canada whereby these groups are more likely to experience both health-threatening SDH and adverse health outcomes. In addition to experiencing material and social deprivation related to SDH, these groups also experience a greater lack of access to health care and other services, which tends to add insult to injury (McGibbon 2016). In this section, I focus on three groups that have been the subject of much attention in research, health, and social services practice: Canadians of Indigenous descent (Smylie and Firestone 2016), the homeless (Bryant 2016), and immigrants and refugees (Hyman and Meinhard 2016).

Indigenous Peoples

Indigenous peoples in Canada are more likely to live in poverty, and this is related to a greater incidence of unemployment, unavailability of full-time employment, and lower income for both full-time and part-time employment (Smylie and Firestone 2016). The 2011 National Household Survey found the average annual income for Indigenous men and women over the age of 15 to be $33,570 and $26,341, respectively. This corresponded to 68 percent of annual income for non-Indigenous men and 79 percent for non-Indigenous women.

Smylie and Firestone (2016) also describe how the unemployment rate for Indigenous peoples in 2009 was 14 percent as compared to 8 percent for non-Indigenous Canadians. For First Nations peoples living on-reserve, the rate of unemployment was 23 percent, compared to a rate of 12.3 percent for First Nations peoples living off-reserve. Unemployment rates were 20 percent for Inuit and 9 percent for Métis. Similar adverse SDH for Indigenous peoples are seen for food security and housing, which manifest in very high rates of illness, injuries, and premature mortality (Smylie and Firestone 2016).

The situation of Indigenous people is a result of Canada's long history of colonialism, the effects of which continue to this day (Smylie and Firestone 2016). Four specific examples of this process include a) the Indian Act, b) disregard for Métis land claims, c) the relocation of Inuit communities, and d) residential schools. Each of these are reflective of deep-seated racism in Canadian society that has led to Indigenous people suffering the material and social deprivation associated with exposures to health-threatening SDH.

Homeless People

Bryant (2016) has reported on how numerous studies find greater incidence of mental illness, HIV infection, physical violence, chronic respiratory diseases, arthritis or rheumatism, hypertension, asthma, epilepsy, and diabetes among the homeless population than those with housing. In terms of life expectancy, Bryant reports that a UK study showed that male street sleepers in London had an average life expectancy of 42 years, and residents of hostels for the homeless had a life expectancy of 63 years—both profoundly shorter than the average life expectancy of housed men.

Homelessness shortens life expectancy by 20 years in the US. In Toronto between 1979 and 1990, 71 percent of homeless people who died were younger than 70 years old as compared to 38 percent in the general population (Bryant 2016). Among nine thousand men using Toronto shelters in 1995, young homeless men in Toronto were eight times more likely to die than men of the same age in the general population. Bryant (2016) reports that "another Canada study found that mortality rates were 515 per 100,000 person-years for homeless women aged 18–44 years and 438 per 100,000 person-years for homeless women aged 45–64 years in Toronto" (367).

Homelessness is a direct effect of Canada's unwillingness to provide many Canadians with the economic resources necessary to attain housing, as well as an unwillingness to create public policy that would provide affordable housing for those whose income may be low. The result is the homelessness crisis associated with the adverse health outcomes described above.

Immigrants and Refugees

Statistics Canada has documented differences in income and employment status of recent and earlier immigrants to Canada (Picot 2004). The rise in low-income status affected immigrants in all education and age groups, including the university-educated. Economic returns to recent immigrants for their work experience and education were diminished compared to those of earlier immigrants. Since 75 percent of these recent immigrants were members of racialized groups, the hypothesis that racism and discrimination is responsible for these diminishing returns must be considered.

Hyman and Meinhard (2016) report that while Canadian immigrants generally experience lower rates of chronic diseases (e.g., cancer, diabetes, heart disease), there is evidence of heterogeneity and changes for the worse over time. Recent immigrants and refugees from South Asia, Latin America, the Caribbean, and Sub-Saharan Africa to Ontario have a two to three times greater risk of developing type 2 diabetes than immigrants and refugees from Western Europe or North America. Hyman and Meinhard (2016) discuss the specific health situation of refugees:

> There is strong evidence from Canadian and international studies that compared to other groups, refugees generally have poorer health due to their experience of displacement and the difficult resettlement process. Refugees may have experienced traumatic events such as war, family separation, physical and psychological torture, refugee camp internment, acute deprivation, periods of prolonged desertion and poor access to health care prior to arrival. (110)

Hyman and Meinhard (2016) also describe the concern that recent immigration policies denying health insurance and creating barriers to welfare and housing are increasing the susceptibility of refugees to health problems.

ANALYSIS

Canada has so many people susceptible to material, economic, and social deprivation because governments do little to manage the economic system and how it distributes economic and social resources. As a result, income and wealth inequality is high, and authorities spend rather little on universal benefits and supports or programs for the groups susceptible to deprivation. Canada's spending on health care is relatively high compared to other OECD (Organisation for Economic Co-operation and Development) nations, but its spending on other programs directed towards families, children, seniors, and working adults is among the lowest of OECD nations (Bryant et al. 2011). This is due to the power and influence of the corporate and business sector that has been very successful in weakening the Canadian welfare state (Langille 2016). It has accomplished this by calling for reduced taxes for the well-off, reduced government spending, and the removal of regulations and legislation that help moderate the sharp edges of unbridled economic capitalism.

Providing health and social services to these susceptible groups is vital (McGibbon 2016); but limiting activities to such provision does little to modify the situations that create their deprivation in the first place (Raphael 2011). As such, it has been argued that the health care and social service sectors must mobilize efforts to influence public policy. Pathways for doing so are provided in the following sections.

EFFORTS TO SHIFT THE DISCOURSE ON SDH

Baum (2007) has argued that achieving health equity requires the application of a nutcracker model by which action is exerted from both above and below. Raphael (2015) has argued that current governmental inaction (from above) on these issues is a result of many factors, the most important being corporate dominance of governmental public policy agendas. This is abetted by the public's lack of awareness of how this corporate agenda—the stressing of minimal governmental intervention in the economy leading to low wages, lack of employment security, and a weak labour sector—is affecting their health. As a result, what is especially required is action from below in the form of mobilizing Canadians through the development of political and social movements.

The purpose of these efforts would be to literally to force governmental ministries of health and other ministries with related mandates—for example, labour, education, finance, and so on—to take these issues seriously. Ultimately, the election of left-leaning governments and influence (e.g., the NDP being elected in Alberta and British Colombia, Ryan Meili being elected as leader of the Saskatchewan NDP, and the earlier elevating of the NDP to the official opposition in Ottawa) is another way to accomplish these goals. Implementing proportional representation in the electoral process would also strengthen the influence of progressive political parties on public policy-making (Raphael and Curry-Stevens 2016).

As noted, it has usually been left to grassroots movements to attempt to shift the public policy agenda. On the public health front, a local public health unit in Ontario created a video animation, "Let's Start a Conversation about Health ... and Not Talk about Health Care at All" (Sudbury and District Health Unit 2011). It has been adapted for use by no fewer than 21 other public health units in Ontario (out of the total 36), numerous others across Canada, and jurisdictions in the United States and Australia (Raphael and Sayani 2017). Raising public awareness can only help move this agenda forward.

Mikkonen and Raphael's (2010) public primer entitled *Social Determinants of Health: The Canadian Facts* has been downloaded over 700,000 times since April 2010; 85 percent of these downloads have been by Canadians. A new Canadian organization, Upstream (2013), aims to create a movement to create a healthy society through dissemination to the public of evidence-based, people-centred ideas. The purpose of these activities is to create a groundswell of public interest that will force policy-makers to take the SDH seriously.

Nevertheless, while the SDH concept has attained greater visibility, there is little evidence that it has contributed to Canadian public policy advances. Part of the problem in Canada is the continuing institutional emphasis on healthy lifestyle messaging at the expense of a social determinants perspective (Kirkland and Raphael 2017).

CONCLUSION

The SDH approach is not new. Its roots are in the critical examination of the causes of illness and disease that date from the mid-nineteenth century. The modern resurgence of interest in how living and working conditions shape health began in the 1970s. British researchers who have investigated the sources of health inequalities identified living and working conditions as the source of these inequalities. Canadians have developed concepts that direct attention to various SDH. However, Canada lags well behind other jurisdictions in *applying* this knowledge to developing economic and social policies in support of health.

Canada is a liberal welfare state where government action takes a backseat to the operation of the economic system, the result of growing influence of the corporate and business sector. Nevertheless, a number of grassroots efforts that have promise for moving a SDH agenda forward are under way. It is unclear as to the extent that these ideas can be translated into public policy action without the election of governments at all levels that are motivated to truly address the SDH of Canadian in general and those particularly susceptible to adverse health outcomes in particular.

CRITICAL THINKING QUESTIONS

1. Reflect upon the degree of familiarity you had with the idea of living and working conditions as primary determinants of health prior to reading the chapter. When you thought of health and its determinants, what did you think of?

2. How have living and working conditions and the public policies that shape them been considered as health issues in your previous studies?
3. What experiences have you personally encountered or observed of people experiencing the social determinants of health? Did these experiences have obvious health or health-related effects?
4. Look at a few days of health-related stories in the *Globe and Mail* or your local newspaper. How often is there an SDH angle on a health story?

RECOMMENDED READINGS

Bartley, Mel. 2016. *Health Inequality: An Introduction to Concepts, Theories, and Methods.* 2nd ed. Cambridge: Polity.

> Large differences in life expectancy exist between the most privileged and the most disadvantaged social groups in industrial societies. This book assists in understanding the four most widely accepted theories of what lies behind inequalities in health: behavioural, psychosocial, material, and life-course approaches.

Canadian Medical Association (CMA). 2013. *What Makes Us Sick?* Ottawa: CMA.

> Throughout the winter and spring of 2013, the CMA conducted wide-ranging consultations to gather input on Canadians' views on the social determinants of health. This report summarizes these findings and puts forth numerous recommendations on how the social determinants can be addressed in the service of improving Canadians' health.

Graham, Hilary. 2004. "Social Determinants of Health and Their Unequal Distribution: Clarifying Policy Understandings." *Milbank Quarterly* 82: 101–24.

> This article outlines some of the emerging issues in the social determinants of health field and details how their consideration influences the framing of problems and their potential solutions.

Health Council of Canada. 2010. *Stepping It Up: Moving the Focus from Health Care in Canada to a Healthier Canada.* Toronto: Health Council of Canada.

> This report examines how health inequalities and the conditions that spawn them (the social determinants of health) play a significant role in health system costs. It concludes that ongoing spending on acute care and programs that encourage a healthy lifestyle are not enough to improve the overall health of Canadians, particularly those who live in or close to poverty. It outlines a series of recommendations by which the social determinants of health can be addressed by governing authorities.

Raphael, Dennis. 2010. *Poverty in Canada: Implications for Health and Quality of Life.* 2nd ed. Toronto: Canadian Scholars' Press.

> This book focuses on how the social determinants of health cluster to create the most disadvantageous life circumstance: poverty. It includes information on the lived experience

of poverty, how public policy shapes its incidence, and how poverty shapes health and the quality of life.

Raphael, Dennis, Toba Bryant, and Marcia H. Rioux. 2010. *Staying Alive: Critical Perspectives on Health, Illness, and Health Care*. 2nd ed. Toronto: Canadian Scholars' Press.

This book provides a range of approaches for understanding health issues. In addition to traditional health sciences and sociological approaches, this text provides human rights and political economy perspectives on health. It focuses on these issues in Canada but provides an international context for these analyses.

RELATED WEBSITES

National Collaborating Centre on the Determinants of Health (NCCDH): http://www.nccdh.ca/

The NCCDH focuses on the social and economic factors that influence the health of Canadians. It translates and shares evidence with public health organizations and practitioners to influence interrelated determinants and advance health equity. Through various products and services, it works to advance knowledge, foster knowledge use, and accelerate network development.

Social Determinants of Health: The Canadian Facts: http://www.thecanadianfacts.org

This website contains a printed document on the social determinants of health situation in Canada that has been downloaded over 700,000 times. It also links to various resources that include reports, media, and other websites that focus on the social determinants of health situation in Canada.

Sudbury and District Health Unit: Health Equity Resources: https://www.sdhu.com/health-topics-programs/health-equity/health-equity-resources

This innovative local public health unit has created a host of materials that introduce the social determinants of health and what public health agencies can do about them. Its video "Let's Start a Conversation about Health … and Not Talk about Health Care at All" overviews the social determinants concept and has been adapted for use by over 20 of the 36 local public health units in Ontario. It has also been adapted across Canada and in many other nations.

Summary of the Senate Subcommittee on Population Health—Final Report: http://www.phn-rsp.ca/pubs/ssphfr-rfscssp/index-eng.php

The Canadian Senate Subcommittee undertook the task to examine and report on the "impact of the multiple factors and conditions that contribute to the health of Canada's population, known collectively as the social determinants of health." This website contains this report and others. It is an important document of what could be—yet isn't being—done to address the social determinants of health in Canada.

World Health Organization Commission on Social Determinants of Health (CSDH): http://www.who.int/social_determinants/thecommission/en/

> The CSDH supports countries and global health partners to address the social factors leading to ill health and inequities. It draws the attention of society to the social determinants of health that are known to be among the worst causes of poor health and inequalities among and within countries.

REFERENCES

Bartley, Mel. 2016. *Understanding Health Inequalities: An Introduction to Concepts, Theories and Methods*. 2nd ed. Oxford: Polity.

Baum, Fran. 2007. "Cracking the Nut of Health Equity: Top Down and Bottom Up Pressure for Action on the Social Determinants of Health." *Promotion and Education* 14 (2): 90–95.

Blane, David. 1999. "The Life Course, the Social Gradient and Health." In *Social Determinants of Health*, edited by Michael G. Marmot and Richard G. Wilkinson, 54–77. Oxford: Oxford University Press.

Brunner, Eric, and Michael Marmot. 2006. "Social Organization, Stress, and Health." In *Social Determinants of Health*, edited by Michael Marmot and Richard G. Wilkinson, 6–30. Oxford: Oxford University Press.

Bryant, Toba. 2016. "Housing and Health." In *Social Determinants of Health: Canadian Perspectives*, 3rd ed., edited by Dennis Raphael, 361–86. Toronto: Canadian Scholars' Press.

Bryant, Toba, Dennis Raphael, Ted Schrecker, and Ronald Labonte. 2011. "Canada: A Land of Missed Opportunity for Addressing the Social Determinants of Health." *Health Policy* 101 (1): 44–58.

Butler-Jones, David. 2008. *Report on the State of Public Health in Canada 2008: Addressing Health Inequalities*. Ottawa: Public Health Agency of Canada.

Canadian Population Health Initiative. 2008. *Reducing Gaps in Health: A Focus on Socio-economic Status in Urban Canada*. Ottawa: Canadian Population Health Initiative.

Esping-Andersen, Gosta. 1990. *The Three Worlds of Welfare Capitalism*. Princeton, NJ: Princeton University Press.

Esping-Andersen, Gosta. 1999. *Social Foundations of Post-industrial Economies*. New York: Oxford University Press.

Evans, Robert D. 2002. *Interpreting and Addressing Inequalities in Health: From Black to Acheson to Blair to …?* London: Office of Health Economics.

Graham, Hilary. 2007. *Unequal Lives: Health and Socioeconomic Inequalities*. New York: Open University Press.

Health Council of Canada. 2010. *Stepping It Up: Moving the Focus from Health Care in Canada to a Healthier Canada*. Toronto: Health Council of Canada.

Hyman, Ilene, and Agnes Meinhard. 2016. "Public Policy, Immigrant Experiences, and Health Outcomes in Canada." In *Immigration, Public Policy, and Health: Newcomer Experiences in Developed Nations*, edited by Dennis Raphael, 97–132. Toronto: Canadian Scholars' Press.

Innocenti Research Centre. 2007. *An Overview of Child Well-Being in Rich Countries*. Florence: Innocenti Research Centre.

Innocenti Research Centre. 2013. *Child Well-Being in Rich Countries: A Comparative Overview*. Florence: Innocenti Research Centre.

Kirkland, Rachel, and Dennis Raphael. 2017. "Perpetuating the Utopia of Health Behaviourism: A Case Study of the Canadian Men's Health Foundation's *Don't Change Much* Initiative." *Social Theory and Health* 16 (1): 1–19. https://doi.org/10.1057/s41285-017-0040-7.

Langille, David. 2016. "Follow the Money: How Business and Politics Shape our Health." In *Social Determinants of Health: Canadian Perspectives*, 3rd ed., edited by Dennis Raphael, 470–90. Toronto: Canadian Scholars' Press.

McGibbon, Elizabeth. 2016. "Oppression and Access to Health Care: Deepening the Conversation" In *Social Determinants of Health: Canadian Perspectives*, 3rd ed., edited by Dennis Raphael, 491–520. Toronto: Canadian Scholars' Press.

McKinlay, John, and Sonja M. McKinlay. 1987. "Medical Measures and the Decline of Mortality." In *Dominant Issues in Medical Sociology*, edited By Howard D. Schwartz, 10–28. New York: Random House.

Mikkonen, Juha, and Dennis Raphael. 2010. *Social Determinants of Health: The Canadian Facts*. Toronto: School of Health Policy and Management, York University. http://thecanadianfacts.org.

Navarro, Vicente, ed. 2004. *The Political and Social Contexts of Health*. Amityville, NY: Baywood.

Pal, Leslie. 2006. *Beyond Policy Analysis: Public Issue Management in Turbulent Times*. Toronto: Nelson.

Picot, Garnett. 2004. *The Deteriorating Economic Welfare of Immigrants and Possible Causes*. Ottawa: Statistics Canada.

Raphael, Dennis. 2011. "Poverty in Childhood and Adverse Health Outcomes in Adulthood." *Maturitas* 69: 22–26.

Raphael, Dennis. 2013. "Adolescence as a Gateway to Adult Health Outcomes." *Maturitas* 75 (2): 137–41.

Raphael, Dennis. 2014. "Social Determinants of Children's Health in Canada: Analysis and Implications." *International Journal of Child, Youth and Family Studies* 5 (2): 220–39.

Raphael, Dennis. 2015. "Beyond Policy Analysis: The Raw Politics behind Opposition to Healthy Public Policy." *Health Promotion International* 30 (2): 380–96.

Raphael, Dennis, ed. 2016. *Social Determinants of Health: Canadian Perspectives*. 3rd ed. Toronto: Canadian Scholars' Press.

Raphael, Dennis, Susan Anstice, Kim Raine, Kerry Mcgannon, Syed Rizvi, and Vanessa Yu. 2003. "The Social Determinants of the Incidence and Management of Type 2 Diabetes Mellitus: Are We Prepared to Rethink Our Questions and Redirect Our Research Activities?" *Leadership in Health Services* 16: 10–20.

Raphael, Dennis, and Ann Curry-Stevens. 2016. "Surmounting the Barriers: Making Action on the Social Determinants of Health a Public Policy Priority." In *Social Determinants of Health: Canadian Perspectives*, 3rd ed., edited by Dennis Raphael, 561–83. Toronto: Canadian Scholars' Press.

Raphael, Dennis, and Evelyn S. Farrell. 2002. "Beyond Medicine and Lifestyle: Addressing the Societal Determinants of Cardiovascular Disease in North America." *Leadership in Health Services* 15: 1–5.

Raphael, Dennis, and Ambreen Sayani. 2017. "Assuming Policy Responsibility for Health Equity: Local Public Health Action in Ontario, Canada." *Health Promotion International* (October): dax073. https://doi.org/10.1093/heapro/dax073.

Saint-Arnaud, Sebastien, and Paul Bernard. 2003. "Convergence or Resilience? A Hierarchical Cluster Analysis of the Welfare Regimes in Advanced Countries." *Current Sociology* 51 (5): 499–527.

Smylie, Janet, and Michelle Firestone. 2016. "The Health of Indigenous Peoples." In *Social Determinants of Health: Canadian Perspectives*, 3rd ed., edited by Dennis Raphael, 434–69. Toronto: Canadian Scholars' Press.

Sudbury and District Health Unit. 2011. "Let's Start A Conversation about Health … and Not Talk about Health Care at All." Sudbury, ON: Sudbury and District Health Unit. https://www.phsd.ca/health-topics-programs/health-equity/health-equity-resources.

Tarlov, Alvin. 1996. "Social Determinants of Health: The Sociobiological Translation." In *Health and Social Organization: Towards a Health Policy for the 21st Century*, edited by David Blane, Eric Brunner, and Richard Wilkinson, 71–93. London: Routledge.

Tjepkema, Michael, Russell Wilkins, and Andrea Long. 2013. "Cause-Specific Mortality by Income Adequacy in Canada: A 16-Year Follow-Up Study." *Health Reports* 24 (7): 14–22.

Townsend, Peter, Nick Davidson, and Margaret Whitehead, eds. 1992. *Inequalities in Health: The Black Report and The Health Divide*. New York: Penguin.

Upstream. 2013. "Upstream is a Movement to Create a Healthy Society through Evidence-Based, People-Centred Ideas." http://www.thinkupstream.net/sign_up_splash?splash=1.

World Health Organization. 2008. *Closing the Gap in a Generation: Health Equity through Action on the Social Determinants of Health*. Geneva: World Health Organization.

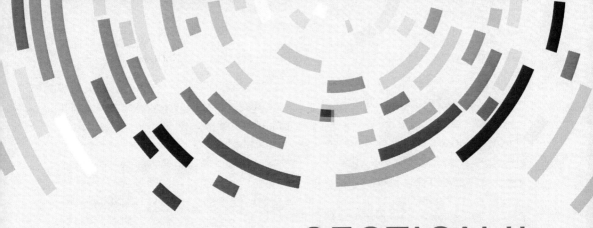

SECTION II

INDIGENOUS POPULATIONS

SECTION INTRODUCTION BY KAREN HILL

I finally came home at 31 years of age. Home was the Six Nations of the Grand River Territory in Southern Ontario. Six Nations is a Rotinonshonni (Iroquois) community. The Six Nations is a confederacy of initially five nations comprising Mohawk, Oneida, Onondaga, Cayuga, and Seneca, later joined by the Tuscarora. I had grown up between Southern Ontario, Western New York, and South Florida, only coming to this reserve for family visits. The birth of my second son led to increasing awareness of missing pieces in my life and a need to know who I was as an Indigenous person. I woke up one morning, put my five-month-old son in his car seat, and drove home.

    As I drove onto the reserve, I noticed how much it had advanced: roads were paved, new homes were built, and in the village of Ohsweken (O-sway-ga), there was an employment centre. I applied for a teaching position with the Six Nations Polytechnic and, surprisingly to me, got the job. During this time, I had the opportunity to work with and learn from several traditional knowledge keepers. They spoke in ways that were new to me, yet somehow familiar. They saw the world so vividly and spoke eloquently about "us" as part of creation itself. The Moon is our Grandmother, Earth our Mother, and the Sun our Eldest Brother. I struggled to truly hear and understand the heart of their words and the Truth they were trying to share. They spoke in ways that were new to me, yet somehow familiar. The more I listened, the more I recognized their teachings as those that I had learned as a child at my Grandfather's feet. Beliefs and values that he shared only in the absence of my Grandmother, whose "Residential School" upbringing taught her that the traditional knowledge was of no use and that some of it was evil and therefore forbidden. This overshadowing of our traditional teachings and my own identity as a Mohawk woman was the result of a process called *colonization* that I had yet to learn. The residential school system my Grandmother attended was a key component in the colonization process and one that hit close to home for me.

One day, when Harvey Longboat, an Onondaga Chief, came to speak, I asked God to help me to hear with my spirit. I put down my pen and opened up my heart to the words he shared. I finally "heard" the meaning of Harvey's words deep in my soul. Through *Kaianereko:wen* (The Great Law—the basis of the founding constitution of the League of the Iroquois, a confederacy of five nations, Mohawk, Oneida, Onondaga, Cayuga, and Seneca, and later joined by the Tuscarora) teachings and his personal wisdom, the message was simple: "Stop waiting for permission to be *Onkwehonwe* [original people]. We are free to be who we are created to be." On that day, I received the healing I had come home to find. I began to see my Grandmother, raised in the Indian residential schools, as more than an angry woman who suffered from mental illness. This woman, who had been the eldest daughter of a hereditary Tuscarora Chief, was forced to deny who she was as a human being, from the age of 6 to 16; yet she came out of residential school still fluent in both Tuscarora and Mohawk languages. I began to see her as a strong survivor. I could finally forgive her and love her and, in doing so, afford the same respect to myself. The decolonization process of reclaiming my true identity as an Indigenous woman had begun.

As my knowing of our "traditional" ways grew, I saw that our people were in need of the same healing I had received. I looked into the health care in my community and what I saw was that there was no real system of health care. Yes, there were programs and services, but none were dedicated to building relationships with the community, so sorely needed. One day at work, as I cleaned out old file boxes left behind by a prior employee, I came across an application form for medical school. At that moment, my unspoken dream of becoming a doctor surfaced and I took this as a sign. I applied to medical school and was admitted, at the age of 37, to McMaster University School of Medicine in Hamilton, Ontario.

While in my medical training, I learned about diseases, their diagnoses, and treatment, but nothing about healing. The only mention of Indigenous peoples of Canada was when a lecturer declared that "being Aboriginal is a risk factor for contracting tuberculosis." Advocacy was being taught as speaking on behalf of "marginalized" populations or spending elective time working with "under-served populations"; both categories included Indigenous people. The curriculum made no reference to the strength of our culture, the resiliency of our people, or the fact that embracing Indigenous people as whole people would support our healing as nations.

I remained in touch with some of the traditional knowledge keepers during my medical education and was learning more and more that within the traditional Onkwehonwe teachings were all the things the medical community identified as key components of chronic disease management, disease prevention, and health promotion. As I looked at the health programs being offered within the community, I wondered what *under-served* referred to, because what I saw happening in my community was an over-service of health programs and services designed in a way that placed the people in the role of "needy" and the health provider as the "helper/saviour/fixer." I saw traces of the traditional healing knowledge in the periphery but no centrality of that knowledge or practice within the health services. We were colonized in our own thinking and couldn't see for ourselves that within our own culture were the answers. To me, offering services from the "under-served" mentality was only perpetuating learned helplessness and did nothing to support us as Indigenous people to pick up those "original instructions" (referring to the teachings, ceremonies, and ways of being given to a people by the Creator) that nurtured our full expression as whole human beings.

In my first year of practice, I began working with the Six Nations Band Council (First Nations are the predominant Indigenous peoples in Canada south of the Arctic; those in the Arctic area are distinct and known as Inuit; the Métis, another distinct ethnicity, developed after European contact and relations primarily between First Nations people and Europeans) to establish a family health team. Community consultations demonstrated that the community was asking for inclusion of the traditional knowledge and medicine in a real way in their health care. Indeed, I had developed a strong sense that the Western physician supplanted the traditional medicine practitioner's role at the hub of health care sometime during the process of colonization. At Six Nations, this had occurred in 1924 when the RCMP entered the hereditary council chambers and arrested our chiefs, clan mothers, and healers at gunpoint and put in place the elected system of governance, and along with it Westernized medical practice. During the development of the family health team, a group of the traditional medicine practitioners asked to meet with me. During that meeting, they told me they had been watching me and wanted to work with me. For the first time at Six Nations, we would begin a respectful relationship between Traditional and Western ways of medicine in the way and spirit of the Two Row Wampum. The Two Row Wampum is an agreement from 1613 between the Rotinonshonni and the Dutch. Its two purple lines represented the two vessels of each nation travelling along the river of life, represented by three white lines said to indicate peace, respect, and friendship.

This book section examines a range of issues related to Indigenous health from the points of view of clinicians, academics, researchers, and policy people. Beginning with Bonnie Freeman, who explores historical institutionally mediated trauma by reviewing official policy, Acts of Parliament, and the attempts at assimilation with the residential school system and Indian Act, the stage is set for future chapters with the lasting impacts on families due to intergenerational trauma. Paul Tomascik, Barry Lavallée, and Thomas Dignan illustrate the need to push health care providers beyond the concept of culturally *competent* care to culturally *safe* care. Piotr Wilk and Martin Cooke explore the health status of Indigenous people living in urban environments, a disenfranchised and often forgotten majority among Indigenous peoples. Anna Banerji provides a clinician perspective on Indigenous children's health. Gwen Healey presents a health model of wellness from an Inuit perspective. To address the health of such populations, where the roots of ill health are political and social, it may be helpful to move away from a medical model. Residential schools pathologized the discourse of Indigenous health, with those in power judging, threatening, and correcting, often with the best of motives. This section focuses on trauma and resiliency, which may equally apply to other populations in this book overcoming adversity. Sometimes, the answer does indeed lie within, and Freeman addresses promoting resiliency through Indigenous means.

As you read this section, consider the following question: How would life for everyone in this country be different if all the Indigenous nations were unscathed, allowed to live in a Two Row Wampum kind of way with the newcomers to this country? In this way, I've come to understand that words like *cultural continuity* mean more than "allowing" Indigenous people to practise their culture. As is described in Chapter 4, cultural safety flows out of cultural continuity but extends this to the assurance that no person is assaulted, challenged, or denied their true identity of who they are or what they need. It means continuing life on this planet for everyone, every culture, every person. To me, that is the true meaning of *global health*. In a global health community, there is no place for "under-served" populations. We are all people, equally whole and valuable.

Timeline: Policies and Practices Influencing Indigenous Health

Bonnie M. Freeman

Time Immemorial-Present: Indigenous peoples in North America used the knowledge and ceremonies involving land, plants, the natural environment, and animals to treat and heal illnesses.

1701-1923: Treaties between British Crown and Indigenous peoples.

1763: The Royal Proclamation of 1763 recognized that Indigenous people were a sovereign people, and their lands and rights were to be protected.

1790-1876: Medical concerns regarding Indigenous peoples in Upper and/or Lower Canada were brought to Hudson's Bay Company physicians, military, police, missionaries, or fur traders, who provided medical aid.

1876: Tribes in central Saskatchewan and Alberta under Treaty 6 specified that a medical chest be placed in every Indian agent's home and Indians would not be required to pay for medical assistance.

1876-Present: The Indian Act. Indians became wards of the state; this policy controls almost every aspect of an Indian's life.

1880-1996: Residential schools. In 1920, it became mandatory for every Indian child to attend residential schools.

1904: Dr. Peter H. Bryce was the first federal official appointed by the Canadian government responsible for Indian health. In 1907, Dr. Bryce launched an investigation into the conditions and health of Indian children at residential schools.

1922: Nurses were placed in remote Indian communities to provide medical aid and treatment.

1927: Medical Branch of the Department of Indian Affairs was created to control the tuberculosis epidemic and to assume the Treaty 6 Medicine Chest clause.

1940s: Medical Branch became Indian and Northern Health Services Branch of Canada's National Health and Welfare.

1945: Federal government started universal health care in Canada, which included all Aboriginal people regardless of status and/or treaty rights.

1960: National Health and Welfare Department creates the Indian Medical Services Branch to improve health care and health services in Indian communities.

1966: The Hawthorn Report offered recommendations regarding the health conditions (poverty, poor housing, disease, etc.) of Indian reserves, as well reported on the varying abuses Indian children suffered in residential schools.

1979: Indian Health Policy was developed and consisted of three pillars of Indian health: community development, advocacy for Indian people, and Canadian Health systems.

1987: Health Transfer policy allowed the Canadian government to transfer health care funds to Aboriginal communities to provide their own health care and health services as determined by the community.

1996: The Royal Commission on Aboriginal People (RCAP) reports over three hundred recommendations to improve the health and well-being of Aboriginal people in Canada.

1998: Aboriginal Healing Foundation was created to understand what occurred at Indian residential schools and begin the healing process for Indian residential school survivors with community initiatives and programs.

2000: Medical Services Branch renamed the First Nations and Inuit Health Branch (FNIHB).

2000: National Aboriginal Health Organization—a not-for-profit and Aboriginal-controlled organization, designed to influence and advance the health and well-being of Aboriginal peoples—received funding from Health Canada.

June 11, 2008: Prime Minister Stephen Harper stood in the House of Commons and delivered an apology to Aboriginal people in Canada for the government's part in the residential schools.

2008: The Truth and Reconciliation Commission was established to begin resolving the residential school survivors' claims.

2012: National Aboriginal Health Organization funding was eliminated as part of the Canadian Federal Budget and ceased operations on June 30, 2012.

March 31, 2014: Federal government runs out of funds to support the Aboriginal Healing Foundation and is forced to close its doors.

Source: Mashford-Pringle (2011); Jacklin and Warry (2004); Stanhope et al. (2011); Lavoie et al. (2011); Shewell (2004).

REFERENCES

Jacklin, K. M., and W. Warry. 2004. "The Indian Health Transfer Policy in Canada: Toward Self-Determination or Cost Containment." In *Unhealthy Health Policy: A Critical Anthropological Examination*, edited by Arachu Castro And Merrill Singer, 215–34. Lanham, MD: Rowman & Littlefield.

Lavoie, L. G., J. Toner, O. Bergeron, and G. Thomas. 2011. *The Aboriginal Health Legislation and Policy Framework in Canada*. Prince George, BC: National Collaborating Centre for Aboriginal Health.

Mashford-Pringle, A. 2011. "How'd We Get Here from There? American Indians and Aboriginal Peoples of Canada Health Policy." *Pimatisiwin: A Journal of Aboriginal & Indigenous Community Health* 9 (1): 153–75.

Shewell, H. 2004. *"Enough to Keep Them Alive": Indian Welfare in Canada, 1873–1965*. Toronto: University of Toronto Press.

Stanhope, M., J. Lancaster, H. Jessup-Falcioni, and G. Viverais-Dresler. 2011. "Chapter 4: Health Promotion." In *Community Health Nursing in Canada*, 2nd ed., edited by Marcia Stanhope, Jeanette Lancaster, Heather Jessup-Falcioni, and Gloria Viverais-Dresler, 107–50. Toronto: Elsevier Health Sciences.

CHAPTER 3

The Impact of Intergenerational Trauma to Health: Policies, Relocation, Reserves, and Residential Schools

Bonnie M. Freeman

LEARNING OBJECTIVES

After reading this chapter, you should be able to:

1. Understand the roots of historical trauma and unresolved grief and appreciate how they impact Indigenous people's lives over generations.
2. Explain how colonization and government policies have contributed to the issues experienced by Indigenous people and lead to the inequalities and poor health of Indigenous peoples.
3. Articulate strategies used of assimilation and displacement of Indigenous peoples.

The health of Indigenous[1] families and communities is important to understand from a historical and social lens on how traumatic experiences over the generations have contributed to the poor health and well-being of Indigenous people in North America (Brave Heart-Jordan 1995; Lederman 1999). Lakota scholar Maria Brave Heart-Jordan (1995) coined the terms *historical trauma* and *historical unresolved grief*. Historical trauma is described as multiple emotional and psychological wounding experiences over a person's life. Yet, when traumatic experiences are focused on a particular group of people, the trauma transpires to close and extended family members, as well to whole communities and nations of people. Historical unresolved grief results from the unresolved experiences of trauma and grief, which an individual, family, and community have not had an opportunity to work through. Therefore, the unresolved trauma is impacted by new traumas and new experiences of grief, which the individual, family, or community are not able to mourn, process, or resolve. The trauma and grief then layers and builds internally within an individual or a family/community system and is unconsciously released through destructive behaviours to self and others, poor health, addictions, and so on (Brave Heart-Jordan 1995).

Indigenous peoples in Canada have experienced and continue to experience the Canadian government's intentional acts resulting in trauma through the structural oppression, paternalism, racism, and discrimination of legislation and policy; relocation to reserves; the enforcement of children to attend residential schools; discrimination against Native women; and the denial of Indigenous sovereignty as true nations (Frideres 1993). This chapter will examine how these policies and legislation have affected the overall health and well-being of Indigenous peoples in Canada, having forced them from their homelands, dismissed their cultural knowledge and practices, and attempted to dismantle their social systems by removing their women and children.

POLICIES

Prior to the development and implementation of Indian policies and laws in Canada, Indigenous people had agreements and treaties with the British Crown. One of the first formal policies by the British Crown was the Royal Proclamation of 1763. A consequence of this policy was the protection of First Nations lands from the encroachment and fraudulent dealings of early settlers prior to the formation of Canada and the United States (Tobias 1983; Prucha 1962). Therefore, many First Nations people have continued to refer to and interpret this policy as insisting that the Crown has judicial responsibility to work with First Nations people on a nation-to-nation basis.

This seemed to be reversed when, almost a century later, in 1857, the British Crown implemented the Gradual Civilization Act, which was a strategy to disenfranchise Indians in the context of their sovereign rights to the land and its resources. The purpose of the policy was to gradually civilize and assimilate Indians into colonial society by constructing and defining who was Indian, and what rights Indians did or did not have:

> The legislation proceeded to define who was Indian and then to state that such a person could not be accorded the rights and privileges accorded to European Canadians until the Indian could prove that he could read and write either French or English language, was free of debt, and of good moral character. (Tobias 1983, 42)

Ten years later with Confederation, the British North America (BNA) Act of 1867 failed to clearly define the political relationship between Indigenous people and early government systems. The underlying premise of the BNA Act was based on the Royal Proclamation of 1763. Section 91 (24) of the act recognized the "special status" of Indians in Canada and appointed the fiduciary responsibility and trusteeship to the federal government in overseeing Indians and their lands (Boldt 1993). The BNA Act also defined health services to Indian communities "as a provincial jurisdiction, and Indian Affairs as an area of federal jurisdiction, thus creating an ambiguity over Indian health that remains today" (Lavoie et al. 2011, 2). At the time of Confederation, the Canadian Constitution of 1867 "gave the federal government legislative authority over 'Indians and lands reserved for Indians'"

(Frideres 1993, 220) under section 91 (24) (Boldt 1993, 279). The newly formed government of Canada recognized the strong sovereignty that Native nations possessed within their communities and among other nations of Native people across Canada. Therefore, the federal government put in place the Enfranchisement Act of 1869, which disassembled their traditional systems of governance and replaced them with a system controlled and run by the Department of Indian Affairs (Milloy 1983). This legislation asserted federal power and jurisdiction over Indian lands; this policy also asserted authority over the resources and finances of Native people. The Enfranchisement Act is seen as the precursor of what is known today as the Indian Act (Milloy 1983, 2008). An all-male Band Council had the authority to make bylaws on reserve; however, any other decisions had to go through the Department of Indian Affairs and the federal government (Milloy 1983, 2008).

One of the first acknowledgements regarding the health and medical aid of Indigenous people was included in the making of Treaty 6. While this treaty seized the traditional territories of the Dene and Cree peoples in central Saskatchewan and Alberta, it also made promises of providing education and medical services. The Medical Chest clause in Treaty 6 specified that a medical chest be placed in every Indian agent's home, and that Indians would not be required to pay for medical assistance (Shewell 2004).

The official Indian Act was implemented in 1876, spelling out in detail the control of the federal government on almost every aspect of an Indian's life (Milloy 2008). The Indian Act clearly defined that Indian status and membership was determined by the primary male (father or husband) preceding over the household. Therefore, all Indian females would attain Indian status and membership from their father or husband. If an Indian female married a non-Indian, she and her children would forfeit their Indian status and membership. However, if an Indian male married a non-Indian woman, the non-Indian woman and her children would gain Indian status and membership.

In the 1960s, Native people exerted pressure for outstanding land claims (Frideres 1993), environmental concerns, and resource exploration. In the mid-1960s, the federal government commissioned Harry B. Hawthorn to investigate and advise policy-makers on the socioeconomic, political, and health conditions of status Indians (Frideres 1983; Cairns 2011). This investigation resulted in the "Hawthorn report," which described the poor social, economic, and health conditions (poverty, housing, disease, etc.) of Indian reserves and residential schools. The report argued that Indians deserved better treatment, equivalent to Canadian citizens, from the government, since constitutional title and treaty rights made Indians "citizens plus" (Cairns 2011). While the Hawthorn report attempted to support entitlements granted to Native people as outlined in treaties and other agreements, it also provided Indian Affairs Minister Jean Chrétien the basis to propose a new assimilation Indian policy, known as the 1969 White Paper (Frideres 1993; Smith 1996). The point of the 1969 White Paper was to terminate all special treatment, rights, and legal status of Indians; repeal the Indian Act; and phase out all federal responsibility for Indians and reserve lands (Macklem 2001; Smith 1996). However, "Aboriginal people were quick to denounce the White Paper" (Macklem 2001, 268). The National Indian Brotherhood

(NIB) responded to the government's "White Paper" with NIB's Red Paper or Brown Paper (Cardinal 1999). The NIB Red Paper called the government to task for the following: 1) to maintain Indian status and rights until Aboriginals were prepared and willing to renegotiate them; 2) to maintain Indian culture as Indian; 3) to recognize the rights and privileges established under the BNA Act, treaties, and governmental legislation; 4) to give resources and responsibility to only Aboriginals and Aboriginal organizations to determine priorities and development; 5) to allow Aboriginal people to control land that respects their historical and legal rights; 6) to review and not repeal the Indian Act with Aboriginal people, and, in addition, to disassemble the Department of Indian Affairs and create a federal agency that would be more attuned to Aboriginal peoples and their needs, aspirations, and sovereignty; 7) as Aboriginal people reject government-appointed commissioners, to recommend an independent, unbiased, and unprejudiced commission to have power to bring any witness or documents that it or Aboriginals wish to present (Indian Chiefs of Alberta [1970] 2011).

The last amendment to the Indian Act in 1985 was Bill C-31. This bill restored the status and rights of Indian women who had married a non-Indian man and their children (up to second generation) (Gehl 2000; Boldt 1993; Silman 1987; Jamieson 1986). While Bill C-31 was meant to redress the human rights of Indian women, the reality is that this legislation continues to oppress Canadian Indigenous women, men, and children, as the government continues to determine who is Native and who obtains or does not obtain Native membership/status through the Indian Act.

EFFECTS OF THE INDIAN ACT

The Indian Act of 1876 had a significant effect on many Aboriginal societies, particularly Native women and their children. By disengaging the social structures of Aboriginal societies and extracting the social, political, and economic rights of Aboriginal women through the Indian Act, the federal government was able to impose oppressive Eurocentric values and views of women onto Aboriginal societies (Gehl 2000), therefore undermining and stripping away the cultural importance of Aboriginal women and their roles, as mothers and grandmothers, within their nations. This has also had detrimental effects on Native youths' self-esteem, knowledge, and pride in who they are as Native persons.

Since the inception of the Indian Act in 1876, the federal government continued with various strategies to eradicate and assimilate Native people into Euro-Canadian society (Tobias 1983). Those Indians who tried to obtain a better life through post-secondary education involuntarily disenfranchised their rights and status as Indians with no knowledge that they participated in the process. The federal government also took advantage of the hardships Indians were experiencing, on and off reserves. The high rates of unemployment and poverty, poor and limited housing, and the lack of food and resources on Indian reserves made it hard for Native people to live and survive in this poor condition (Shewell 2004). Therefore, many Native men and women were forced to search for work off their reserves or to find other options to obtain money or buy food for their families (Shewell 2004).

RESERVE SYSTEM

While there is significant literature from both Canada and the United States regarding the relocation and reserve/reservation system of Native people in North America, Canada had a particular approach to developing the reserve system and residential schools and in encouraging Native people to move from Indian reserves to urban centres.

The reserve system in Canada developed as "laboratories of civilization" (St. Germain 2001; Tobias 1983), turning Indians into dark-skinned white men (Stanley 1983):

> In the 1830's the British initiated several experiments in civilization. Essentially, they entailed the establishment of Indian reserves in isolated areas. Indians were encouraged to gather and settle in large villages on these reserves, where they would be taught to farm and would receive religious instruction and an education. These endeavours became the basis of the reserve system in Canada. The reserve system, which was to be the keystone of Canada's Indian policy, was conceived as a social laboratory, where the Indian could be prepared for coping with the European. (Tobias 1983, 41)

Tobias (1983) articulates that reserves were Crown land, and settlers were forbidden by law to encroach or live on them: "By 1850, Indian lands were given special status by being protected from trespass by non-Indians and by being freed from seizure for non-payment of debt or taxes [by Indians]" (41). Eventually, reserves were defined in the Indian Act as a tract of land under the legal jurisdiction of the Crown: "in other words, reserves are legally controlled by the federal government, although Indians are permitted to 'use' the land" (York 1990, 58).

The literature indicates that the only endeavour the British undertook in the efforts of Indian removal was under the direction of Lieutenant-Governor Francis Bond Head in 1836. St. Germain (2001) explains that Bond Head was convinced that Indians in Upper Canada (Ontario) were doomed for extinction and devised a plan to ship all Indians to Manitoulin Island in Lake Huron: "This destination would serve as one large reserve where the Indians might live out their existence in peaceful and unfettered isolation" (81). While Bond Head was striving to free up as much land for white settlement, fortunately for Native people in Canada, the idea of total relocation and removal "was swiftly abandoned as an aberration" (81). However, various scholars indicate that the removal and relocation of Native communities within Canada continued to take place throughout history (Steckley and Cummins 2008; Surtees 1983). York (1990) explains that while "reserves were created to remove Indians from the path of white settlement," the government and many white settlers determined that Indian reserves continued to obstruct the growth of urban and industrial development (57). The land set aside for Indian reserves was one fifth the amount of land set aside in Canada for national parks: "Less than 0.2 percent of Canada's total area is reserved for Indians, while in the United States the proportion set aside for Indians is twenty times larger" (58).

Despite the attempt to civilize Native people, the British indicated that the goal of civilization through the reserve system was impractical and failing (Tobias 1983). Indians were not civilizing or assimilating into colonial society. The British concluded that because reserves were isolated from the colonies, Indians did not have the opportunity for socialization (Tobias 1983). Thus, "the Euro-Canadian would serve as an example of what the Indian should become, and the existence of the town, it was thought, would attract the Indian from the reserve and into the non-Indian community where the Indian's newly learned values would supplant his old values and allow him to be fully assimilated" (42).

RESIDENTIAL SCHOOLS

Today's Aboriginal youth carry the historical legacy, shame, and pain of their parents' and grandparents' psychological trauma, inflicted upon them through residential schools. At the time when these parents and grandparents were Aboriginal children as young as two years of age (Miller 2008), they were forcefully taken away or hesitantly given up by their families because of government policies indicating that Native children were to be civilized and assimilated into white culture (St. Germain 2001; Dippie 1982; Priest 1942). Deloria and Lytle (1983) have expressed that education was "one of the major weapons of forced assimilation since the establishment of colonies" (240).

The United States and Canada each developed a residential school system at the same time (Barker 1997; Smith 2005; Fournier and Crey 1997). In 1846 at a meeting in Orillia, Ontario, the early government of Canada committed itself to the residential school system for Indians, with responsibility shared and primarily administered by missionaries and religious denominations (Fournier and Crey 1997).

Native children who attended residential schools endured many levels of physical, mental, emotional, and spiritual abuse (Grant 1996; Chrisjohn, Young, and Maraun 2006; Smith 2005; Fournier and Crey 1997). One motto that was believed to justify and carry forward the efforts of assimilation and civilization, not only in the United States but in Canada as well, was the notion that the purpose of residential schools was "to kill the Indian and save the child" (Barker 1997; Fournier and Crey 1997). It was believed that residential schools could instill Christian beliefs, reading, and writing, and teach the skills of agriculture and domestic work. Native children were only taught to a Grade-3 level; the rest of their time was spent doing long hours of work, receiving very little food, and experiencing torturous acts that would cleanse the "savage" out of the beings of Native children (Chrisjohn, Young, and Maraun 2006; Fournier and Crey 1997).

McKenzie and Morrissette (2003) identify three forms of trauma in former students of residential schools associated with their adjustment as adults and parenting skills: first is the lack of love and the ability to establish relationships; a second form of trauma is the lack of cultural expression through language, clothing, hair, and ceremonies; and the third was the loss of family and the collective experience as a people.

Upon their return to their home communities, many of the Aboriginal youth lost their ability to communicate with their families in their Native language, and these Aboriginal youths also found it difficult to relate to their families. Tseng and Hsu (1991) eloquently articulate the impact that losing the vital components of culture has on a family:

> When the socio-cultural system of a group of people has been rapidly destroyed, families within the system will suffer from loss of their cultural roots, resulting in deterioration of the family as a whole. This is usually manifested by parents losing their cultural methods for organizing the family and subsequently experiencing confusion over how to perform properly their parental function. The children meanwhile often disassociate themselves from their parents both cognitively and emotionally and are unsure of their identity and direction in life. Such families have not only lost their own identity but have lost their cultural knowledge in functioning. (206)

Unfortunately, this loss of culture had great impact on not only Aboriginal families but also the whole community. First Nation communities that lost their children to residential schools also experienced a sense of loss when the children failed to fit back into the community fabric. Angus Grant (1996) explains:

> At sixteen the children were returned to their home communities—angry, contemptuous, superior, rebellious children. Healing attempts were almost impossible because the language of the children had been destroyed.... Bewilderment gripped the communities, but often before any resolution could be reached the returned children themselves became parents and their children were doomed to perpetrate the same cycle which worsened with every generation. (224–5)

As these young adults became parents, they transferred what was taught to them in residential school. Second and third generations of Aboriginal children were doomed to experience what their parents and grandparents experienced, not at the hands of nuns and clergy but from their own mothers and fathers. Aboriginal children had their spirits broken and their identities destroyed by those who were to love and care for them. The physical and psychological pains of those who attended residential schools still remain; however, as time and healing take place within Aboriginal communities, the horrific aftermath diminishes—but it is never forgotten. The last residential school closed in 1996.

INDIAN HEALTH SERVICES AND POLICIES

In 1904, Dr. Peter H. Bryce was appointed by the Canadian government as the first federal official to oversee the health of Indians. During Dr. Bryce's term, he launched an investigation into the conditions and health of Indian children at residential schools (FNCFCS

2016). The results revealed the extremely poor conditions and mistreatment of Indian children. This led to Dr. Bryce's continued advocacy for the improvement of conditions in residential schools until his forced retirement in 1921 (FNCFCS 2016): "His report was never released by the government but was published by Dr. Bryce in 1922 under the title *The Story of a National Crime: Being a Record of the Health Conditions of the Indians of Canada from 1904 to 1921*" (Wikipedia 2018).

In 1922, the federal government placed nurses in remote Indian communities to provide medical aid and treatment (Stanhope et al. 2011). With many illnesses rising to epidemic levels in Indian communities, the Department of Indian Affairs created the Medical Branch in 1927. This branch was to control the tuberculosis epidemic, as well as undertake the responsibility of the Medicine Chest clause of Treaty 6. Later in the 1940s, the Medical Branch was moved from the Department of Indian Affairs and became the Indian and Northern Health Services branch under Canada's National Health and Welfare Department (Mashford-Pringle 2011). In 1945, the federal government initiated the universal health care system in Canada, which included all Aboriginal people regardless of Indian status and/or treaty rights (Mashford-Pringle 2011).

In 1960, the National Health and Welfare Department created the Indian Medical Services Branch, with the primary goal of improving the health care and health services in Indian communities (Mashford-Pringle 2011). Almost 20 years later, in 1979, Minister of Health David Crombie introduced the Indian Health Policy, which consisted of three pillars focusing on Indian health: community development, advocacy for Indian people, and Canadian health systems (Lavoie et al. 2011). The policy also recognized that culture and tradition were important in Indian health and health care, and that Aboriginal people would generate and maintain their own system of health care (Lavoie et al. 2011). In 1987, the Canadian government introduced the Health Transfer Policy, which allows the government to transfer health care funds to Aboriginal communities to provide their own health care and health services as determined by the community (Jacklin and Warry 2004).

CONCLUSION

Several academics and Native scholars argue that the generations of injustices attributed to colonization, government policies, forced relocation, reservations systems, and residential/boarding schools have contributed to the determinants of health of Indigenous peoples in North America. While Indigenous peoples struggle to search or hold on to the cultural knowledge that has provided them with good health and well-being, the trauma and pain of colonization continues to have a detrimental and poor impact on the health and well-being of Indigenous peoples today. It appears that "many indigenous people stand on a ledge between historic cultural attachments on one side and persistent efforts to force them to abandon such attachments on the other" (Samson 2005, 2). Indigenous people have been forced to abandon their cultural attachments; additionally, they have not had the opportunity to overcome or heal from the generations of trauma (war, violence, prohibiting of ceremonies, massacres, starvation, relocation, assimilation, acculturation, and annihilation) inflicted on their lives. To gain a deeper understanding of the impact such traumatic experiences and policies have had on Indigenous people's health, cultural identity, and well-being, we must examine systemic barriers that continue to oppress and marginalize Indigenous people in Canadian society.

CRITICAL THINKING QUESTIONS

1. In 2008, Canada's Prime Minister Stephen Harper formally apologized to Canada's Indigenous people for the treatment of Indigenous children in residential schools. For some Indigenous survivors, this apology had a great meaning, while others could not accept it. Why do you think the prime minister's apology received mixed reactions from Indigenous people, and why did some not accept this apology?
2. How have historical events, colonization, and government policies contributed to the inequalities of health and social determinants of Indigenous peoples?
3. Looking at the many reports completed on the social and health conditions of Indigenous people in Canada, what can we learn from these reports, and what changes can we make to improve the health and well-being of Indigenous people?

RECOMMENDED READINGS

Berry, J. W. 1999. "Aboriginal Cultural Identity." *Canadian Journal of Native Studies* 19 (1): 1–36.

Boldt, M. 1993. *Surviving as Indians: The Challenge of Self-Government.* Toronto: University of Toronto Press.

Brave Heart, M. Y. H., and L. M. DeBruyn. 1998. "The American Indian Holocaust: Healing Historical Unresolved Grief." *American Indian and Alaska Native Mental Health Research* 8 (2): 60–82.

Dickason, O. P., and T. McNab. 2009. *Canada's First Nations: A History of Founding Peoples from Earliest Times.* 4th ed. Don Mills, ON: Oxford University Press.

Graham, E. 1997. *The Mush Hole: Life at Two Indian Residential Schools.* Waterloo, ON: Heffle.

Switlo, Janice G. A. E. 2002. "Modern Day Colonialism—Canada's Continuing Attempts to Conquer Aboriginal Peoples." *International Journal on Minority and Group Rights* 9: 103–41.

Waldram, J., D. A. Herring, and T. K. Young. 2000. *Aboriginal Health in Canada: Historical, Cultural and Epidemiological Perspectives.* Toronto: University of Toronto Press.

Warry, W. 2007. *Ending Denial: Understanding Aboriginal Issues.* Peterborough, ON: Broadview.

NOTE

1. First Nations Peoples within Canada generally refer to themselves as Native people or "Indians" when conversing among themselves. They also use terms within their own languages to identify themselves according to their "citizenship" with their nation, such as **Kenyen'keha** (Mohawk

Nation). When referring to ourselves as the original, Indigenous people of the land in North America, we use terms such as *Onkwehonwe* (Real People) or *Anishnaabe* (Original People). In this chapter, I have used the word *Aboriginal* sparingly due to the problems this term has in essentializing (Paradies 2006; Alfred 2005) the identity and nations of First Nations, Métis, and Inuit peoples under one defined governmental term and structure (Garroutte 2003; Lawrence 2010). I prefer to use the words *Indigenous*, *Native*, and/or *First Nations* throughout this chapter. I will also use the term *Indian* as it is referred to in academic and government documents.

REFERENCES

Alfred, T. 2005. *Wasase: Indigenous Pathways of Action and Freedom.* Peterborough, ON: Broadview.

Barker, D. 1997. "Kill the Indian, Save the Child: Cultural Genocide and the Boarding School." In *American Indian Studies: An Interdisciplinary Approach to Contemporary Issues*, edited by Dane Morrison, 47–68. Bern, Switzerland: Peter Lang.

Boldt, M. 1993. *Surviving as Indians: The Challenge of Self-Government.* Toronto: University of Toronto Press.

Brave Heart-Jordan, M. 1995. "The Return to the Sacred Path: Healing from Historical Trauma and Unresolved Grief among the Lakota." PhD diss., Smith College.

Cairns, A. 2011. *Citizens Plus: Aboriginal Peoples and the Canadian State.* Vancouver: UBC Press.

Cardinal, H. 1999. *The Unjust Society.* Vancouver: Douglas & McIntyre.

Chrisjohn, R., S. Young, and M. Maraun. 2006. *The Circle Game: Shadows and Substance in the Indian Residential School Experience in Canada.* Revised ed. Penticton, BC: Theytus.

Deloria, V., Jr., and C. M. Lytle. 1983. *American Indians, American Justice.* Austin: University of Texas Press.

Dippie, B. W. 1982. *The Vanishing American White Attitudes and U.S. Indian Policy.* Middletown, CT: Wesleyan University Press.

First Nations Child & Family Caring Society of Canada (FNCFCS). 2016. "Dr. Peter Henderson Bryce: A Story of Courage." https://fncaringsociety.com/peter-bryce.

Fournier, S., and E. Crey. 1997. *Stolen from Our Embrace: The Abductions of First Nations Children and the Restoration of Aboriginal Communities.* Vancouver: Douglas & McIntyre.

Frideres, J. S. 1983. *Native Peoples in Canada.* Scarborough, ON: Prentice Hall Canada.

Frideres, J. S. 1993. *Native Peoples in Canada: Contemporary Conflicts.* Scarborough ON: Prentice Hall Canada.

Garroutte, E. M. 2003. *Real Indians: Identity and the Survival of Native America.* Berkeley: University of California Press.

Gehl, L. 2000. "The Queen and I: Discrimination Against Women." *Canadian Woman Studies* 20 (2): 64–69.

Grant, A. 1996. *No End of Grief: Indian Residential Schools in Canada.* Winnipeg: Pemmican.

Indian Chiefs of Alberta. (1970) 2011. "Citizens Plus." Brief Presented to Federal Government. *Aboriginal Policy Studies* 1 (2): 188–281. https://journals.library.ualberta.ca/aps/index.php/aps/article/view/11690/8926.

Jacklin, K. M., and W. Warry. 2004. "The Indian Health Transfer Policy in Canada: Toward Self-Determination or Cost Containment." In *Unhealthy Health Policy: A Critical Anthropological Examination*, edited by Arachu Castro and Merrill Singer, 215–34. Lanham, MD: Rowman & Littlefield.

Jamieson, K. 1986. "Sex Discrimination and the Indian Act." In *Arduous Journey: Canadian Indians and Decolonization*, edited by J.R. Ponting, 112–36. Toronto: McClelland & Stewart.

Lavoie, L. G., J. Toner, O. Bergeron, and G. Thomas. 2011. *The Aboriginal Health Legislation and Policy Framework in Canada*. Prince George, BC: National Collaborating Centre for Aboriginal Health.

Lawrence, B. 2010. "Legislating Identity: Colonialism, Land and Indigenous Legacies." In *The SAGE Handbook of Identities*, edited by M. Wetherell and C. T. Mohanty, 508–29. London: Sage.

Lederman, J. 1999. "Trauma and Healing in Aboriginal Families and Communities." *Native Social Work Journal* 2 (1): 59–90.

Macklem, P. 2001. *Indigenous Difference and the Constitution of Canada*. Toronto: University of Toronto Press.

Mashford-Pringle, A. 2011. "How'd We Get Here from There? American Indians and Aboriginal Peoples of Canada Health Policy." *Pimatisiwin: A Journal of Aboriginal & Indigenous Community Health* 9 (1): 153–75.

McKenzie, B., and V. Morrissette. 2003. "Social Work Practice with Canadians of Aboriginal Background: Guidelines for Respectful Social Work." *Manitoba Journal of Child Welfare* 2 (1): 13–39.

Miller, R. G. 2008. "Residential School Survivor." Art Exhibit, November/December. Brantford: Woodland Cultural Centre.

Milloy, J. S. 1983. "The Early Indian Acts: Developmental Strategy and Constitutional Change." In *As Long as the Sun Shines and Water Flows: A Reader in Canadian Native Studies*, edited by Ian A. L. Getty and A. S. Lussier, 56–64. Vancouver: UBC Press.

Milloy, J. 2008. *Indian Act Colonialism: A Century of Dishonour 1869–1969*. Vancouver: National Centre for First Nations Governance.

Paradies, Y. 2006. "Beyond Black and White: Essentialism, Hybridity and Indigeneity." *Journal of Sociology* 42 (4): 355–67.

Priest, L. B. 1942. *Uncle Sam's Stepchildren: The Reformation of United States Indian Policy, 1865–1887*. Lincoln: University of Nebraska Press.

Prucha, F. P. 1962. *American Indian Policy in the Formative Years: The Indian Trade and Intercourse Acts, 1790–1834*. Boston: Harvard University Press.

Samson, C. 2005. "Burdened with Change: Land, Health and the Survival of Indigenous Peoples." Paper presented at the Problems and Possibilities in Multi-sited EthnographyWorkshop, Panel 2: Researching Rights on Land, Health and Life: The Survival of Indigenous Communities in the 21st Century, University of Sussex, June 27–28, 2005. https://www.ncrm.ac.uk/research/MIP/2005/multi-sitedethnography furtherinformation.php.

Shewell, H. 2004. *"Enough to Keep Them Alive": Indian Welfare in Canada, 1873–1965*. Toronto: University of Toronto Press.

Silman, J. 1987. *Enough Is Enough: Aboriginal Women Speak Out*. Toronto: Women's Press.

Smith, A. 2005. *Conquest: Sexual Violence and American Indian Genocide*. Cambridge, MA: South End.

Smith, M. H. 1996. *Our Home or Native Land? What Governments' Aboriginal Policy Is Doing to Canada*. Toronto: Stoddart.

Stanhope, M., J. Lancaster, H. Jessup-Falcioni, and G. Viverais-Dresler. 2011. "Chapter 4: Health Promotion." In *Community Health Nursing in Canada*, 2nd ed., 107–50. Toronto: Elsevier Health Sciences.

Stanley, G. F. G. 1983. "As Long as the Sun Shines and Water Flows: An Historical Comment." In *As Long as the Sun Shines and Water Flows: A Reader in Canadian Native Studies*, edited by Ian A. L. Getty and Antoine S. Lussier, 1–26. Vancouver: UBC Press.

Steckley, J., and B. Cummins. 2008. *Full Circle: Canada's First Nations*. Toronto: Pearson Prentice Hall.

St. Germain, J. 2001. *Indian Treaty-Making Policy in the United States and Canada, 1867–1877*. Lincoln: University of Nebraska Press.

Surtees, R. J. 1983. "Indian Land Cessions in Upper Canada, 1815–1830." In *As Long as the Sun Shines and Water Flows: A Reader in Canadian Native Studies*, edited by Ian A. L. Getty and A. S. Lussier, 65–84. Vancouver: UBC Press.

Tobias, J. L. 1983. "Protection, Civilization, Assimilation: An Outline History of Canada's Indian Policy." In *As Long as the Sun Shines and Water Flows: A Reader in Canadian Native Studies*, edited by Ian A. L. Getty and Antoine S. Lussier, 39–55. Vancouver: UBC Press.

Tseng, W. S., and J. Hsu. 1991. *Culture and Family Problems and Therapy*. Binghamton, NY: Haworth.

Wikipedia. 2018. s.v. "Peter Bryce." Last updated January 31. https://en.wikipedia.org/wiki/Peter_Bryce.

York, G. 1990. *The Dispossessed: Life and Death in Native Canada*. Toronto: Lester & Orpen Dennys.

CHAPTER 4

Intergenerational Trauma and Indigenous Health in Canada: How Racism Affects the Health of the Indigenous Patient

Paul Tomascik, Thomas Dignan, and Barry Lavallée

LEARNING OBJECTIVES

After reading this chapter, you should be able to:

1. Understand how intergenerational trauma and racism affect Indigenous health.
2. Know why Indigenous communities are unique from other populations at risk.
3. Learn the importance of cultural safety in Indigenous health care.

PROPERLY FRAMING THE MARGINALIZATION OF INDIGENOUS COMMUNITIES

The framing of Indigenous communities as marginalized suggests that the social determinants of health are not a haphazard occurrence but, indeed, are socially constructed. Employing the phrase *communities under threat*, however, draws attention to the relationship between racism and the oppression imposed upon Indigenous Peoples.

In this chapter, we will, for the most part, refer to Indigenous populations as *communities under threat*. This will distinguish the unique issues facing Indigenous peoples in the context of their health and healing. Additionally, this phrase separates Indigenous issues from those affecting other communities like immigrants and refugees. Further, this situates cultural safety much better in terms of an anti-racist and anti-colonial framework for the audience—an analytical framework necessary to employ a decolonized view of the current health status of Indigenous Peoples.

RACISM HARMS INDIGENOUS PEOPLES' HEALTH UNLIKE ANY OTHER POPULATION

Despite its profound impact, it is difficult for many health providers to fathom the extent that racism continues to damage Indigenous peoples' mental and physical health (Royal College of Physicians and Surgeons of Canada n.d.). Racism is shaped by the distribution of money, power, and resources in the hands of government authorities who control the social determinants of health, which result in disparity and inequity of care (Reading 2013).

Adelson (2005) differentiates between *disparity* and *inequity*: "Health disparities are those indicators that show a disproportionate burden of disease on a particular population. Health inequities point to the underlying causes of the disparities" (S45). Lasser, Himmelstein, and Woolhandler (2006) document that in Canada, inequities are frequently based on race.

A leading scholar at the Harvard School of Public Health, Krieger (2011) argues that a strong link exists between disease progression from ancient societies and their implications for improving population health and promoting health equity in current Indigenous communities. Krieger shows that the current health crisis facing Indigenous people in Canada is related to historical events spawned by colonial controls steeped in racism and still reflected in today's governmental policies.

Indifference, annoyance, negligence, and aggression are destructive manifestations of racism in interpersonal and systemic interactions leading to negative health effects in individuals, families, and communities. Many Indigenous people do not trust mainstream health care services; they do not feel safe using them (Health Council of Canada 2012). As a result, Indigenous patients are more likely to be diagnosed at a later stage of disease or to discontinue or avoid treatment altogether (National Collaborating Centre for Aboriginal Health 2011; Health Council of Canada 2012).

Racism drives the overarching belief that one's own race is superior to another's; it encourages discrimination that is declared as intolerance, ostracism, or outright hatred and is particularly virulent in the hands of those with power who practise it (Reading 2013).

Racism occurs in governments and public and private institutions to create regulatory, social, political, and economic favour over a "racialized" group of people (ERASE Racism 2015). Forcing people to conform to a system at the expense of their cultural values, interrogating Indigenous ways, or suppressing Indigenous issues into a romanticized world view are racist actions.

Physical, emotional, and sexual abuse; deprivation; humiliation; and social isolation were often employed to break the Indigenous pupil. Many children died in school custody. Trauma endured by these victims has led to tremendous suffering that is passed on to families and communities from one generation to the next. Post-traumatic stress response is common in Indigenous people who went through the residential school system and affects their relations, who endure the prevalence of complex co-morbidities from intergenerational trauma (Mitchell and Maracle 2005).

Beiser (2005) states that "it could be shown that whatever applies to majority culture Canadians also applies to new settlers. Research demonstrates that, although immigrant families are far more likely than families of native-born Canadians to be poor, immigrant children tend to have better health" (2).

Australia's Indigenous communities suffer tremendous health disparities brought on by social problems akin to people living in developing countries and are comparable to Indigenous people living in Canada. Comprising only 3 percent of the population (Australian Bureau of Statistics 2013), Australia's Indigenous people endure high rates of poverty, unemployment, imprisonment, infant mortality, drug abuse, alcoholism, diabetes, and heart disease (WHO 2008).

The government's response is to take control and force improvement measures on Australia's Indigenous people. Outcomes are poor; lack of consultation and cooperation in the

The Tragic Story of Brian Sinclair

Sometime in the waning hours of September 20, 2008, Mr. Brian Sinclair died in the waiting room of the emergency department of the Winnipeg Health Sciences Centre (WHSC). He was only 45 years old. The medical cause of Brian's death was a treatable condition known as acute peritonitis—an infection from a blocked catheter that spread into his bloodstream causing shock.

His death did not come quickly. He obediently waited for 34 hours in the hospital waiting room in pain and discomfort before succumbing to sepsis. This tragedy occurred after he was admitted, triaged for medical attention, and then subsequently forgotten about until it was too late. He died before any medical intervention or human comforts were considered. He did not have an advocate, and he passed away alone.

Brian did everything right in seeking medical attention. He entered a community health clinic in Winnipeg complaining of abdominal pain and being unable to relieve himself. An attending physician at the clinic immediately referred him to the WHSC for emergency treatment. Within a span of about 40 minutes, he arrived at the emergency department by taxi with a referral letter from the primary care physician. He was discovered dead in the waiting room, a day and half after being admitted.

Did it matter that Brian was a broken man when he entered the system? In this circumstance, it did. He was homeless, a double amputee, wheelchair-dependent, and he suffered from a range of chronic illnesses. Perhaps conclusions drawn from stereotyping, a form of racism, played a part in how he was treated. If anything, a man in this condition might warrant some compassion if not outright intervention. It did not. He was also an Indigenous man, which is what sealed his fate. An inquest into Brian Sinclair's death concluded that better health systems need to be in place to prevent such tragedies. Racism was not cited as a factor.

intervention undermines Indigenous communities' trust in the health system. Aggressive policies fuel fear and mistrust—hardly a good starting point for high-quality care.

Canada's Indigenous people fare no better. Forced assimilation in the former residential school system, preponderance of the Indian Act, racist policies, tightly controlled social determinants of health, and a health system designed around urbanized hospital-based care all conspire to contribute to Canada's poor record in nurturing healthy communities or helping Indigenous patients.

MEDICAL EDUCATION

Medical education is not immune to racism; its hidden curriculum reinforces traditional power structures that sometimes fit into definitions of racist behaviour. The *hidden curriculum* (also in Cooper et al., Chapter 24 in this volume) is defined as a set of influences that function at the level of organizational structure and culture that affect learning, teaching, and clinical practice (Association of Faculties of Medicine of Canada 2009).

In medical education, oppression is more obtuse but continues to be harmful to Indigenous patients, medical students, residents, and clinicians. This hidden curriculum continues to support oppressive power structures in medical schools (Association of Faculties of Medicine of Canada 2009). All forms of racism can appear in the hidden curriculum, which is buttressed by the dominant culture in charge of medical education. Additionally, the dominance of white/settler power and privilege in medical schools further expand the power differentials for those students who identify as Indigenous.

BREAKING THE WIDE SPECTRUM OF RACISM THROUGH CULTURALLY SAFE CARE

For culturally safe care to occur, it is critical that providers know that racism affects the Indigenous patient in daily life—even before he or she enters the clinic. In 2013, the Royal College of Physicians and Surgeons of Canada first released the *Indigenous Health Values and Principles Statement*, which is a blueprint for practising culturally safe care: it assesses health from the Indigenous patient perspective. In 2018 the Royal College released the second edition of the *Indigenous Health Values and Principles Statement*. Although the values and principles themselves remain largely unchanged from the original statement, several significant events precipitated the need to update the context in a second edition: the publication of the Truth and Reconciliation Commission's Calls to Action in 2015; Canada's full support in 2016 of the United Nations Declaration on the Rights of Indigenous Peoples; the Royal College's update of the CanMEDS framework (2015); the introduction of the Royal College's Competence by Design program to more effectively assess physician skills; and increasingly urgent calls by Indigenous leaders and their allies to address the gaps in Indigenous health. According to the Ontario Human Rights Commission (n.d.), racism occurs in several forms, including as prejudice and overt bias, stereotyping, racial profiling, racial discrimination, and oppression.

Solutions start with the understanding of historical (intergenerational) trauma, how the roots of racism are nourished, where racism takes place, and what harms racism causes.

Challenging racism's existence, no matter how benign or lethal its consequences appear for victims or perpetrators, takes courage and honest self-reflection. By applying principled interventions based on Indigenous health values, health care strives to become culturally safe.

To begin, it is essential to understand the historical, social, political, and ethical contexts of health disparities. By its own admission, Canada recognizes the extent of the disparities: the Public Health Agency of Canada contributed to a Federal/Provincial/Territorial Health Disparities Task Group (2004) that stated that one of the most important factors contributing to health disparities is the erosion of Indigenous identity.

Pathways to addressing health disparities and inequities are complex. Reading and Wien (2009) segmented the determinants of health into four categories: social (e.g., political, holistic, adequacy of public health data), proximal (e.g., health behaviours, education, food insecurity), intermediate (e.g., systems, infrastructure, cultural support), and distal (e.g., colonialism, racism, self-determination). As such, principles to foster Indigenous health must be interconnected and holistic, recognizing the stages of an Indigenous person's development from infancy to old age.

Health care providers are well positioned to nurture culturally safe care by being aware of personal, professional, ethical, and institutional transgressions that might be racist; they should recognize the patient's social, emotional, and spiritual boundaries, beyond just biomedical clues about the patient's health.

Cultural safety (also in Cooper et al., Chapter 24 in this volume) is the embodiment of two concepts: challenging privilege and addressing power imbalances. Culturally safe practice is predicated on critical self-reflection that seeks to interrupt racism and oppression. Reflecting on one's privilege and how this translates into the power differential within the patient-provider relationship is a first step. The health care provider then moves from reflection into active practices that challenge stereotypes, address inequities, and facilitate self-determination with Indigenous patients. While responsibility for ensuring cultural safety rests with the provider, evaluation of whether cultural safety is achieved lies with the Indigenous patient (IPAC, Royal College, and AFMC 2009).

Ensuring cultural safety by confronting racism and oppression is fraught with difficulties. Some non-Indigenous people view the dialogue about racial issues as an arena of conflict (DiAngelo and Sensoy 2014). Others view themselves as "racially innocent" and therefore unaccountable for racist behaviour of the dominant society (Dion 2009). Instead of challenging these transgressions, many people retreat from controversy into the refuge of privileged positions and excuse the manifestation of these events as remnants of history.

Partnering with Indigenous patients to interrupt racism in health care at all levels is central to cultural safety. In turn, providers come to see Indigenous people possessing strengths rather than deficits (Lavallée and Clearsky 2006).

Health care providers, educators, administrators, and policy-makers play critical roles in working towards a culturally safe health care system. Key aspects of becoming culturally safe include the following:

- Understanding the unique historical legacies affecting Indigenous peoples' health
- Recognizing one's privilege and how this impacts relationships
- Practising critical self-reflection
- Challenging stereotypes and incidents of racism
- Partnering with Indigenous people to influence system-level change

An Australian study (Freeman et al. 2014) examining a cultural "respect" framework on Indigenous health services points to several critical factors in a culturally respectful strategy, including,

- A "holistic" view that encourages understanding of the social determinants of health
- A strong complement of Indigenous health professionals
- Choice of access through outreach, home visits, and walk-in services
- Support for gender-specific services, Indigenous leadership, and cultural identity events

The study also emphasizes that barriers to achieving cultural respect include communications issues, racism, and the threat of externally developed programs in the absence of consultations with Indigenous communities.

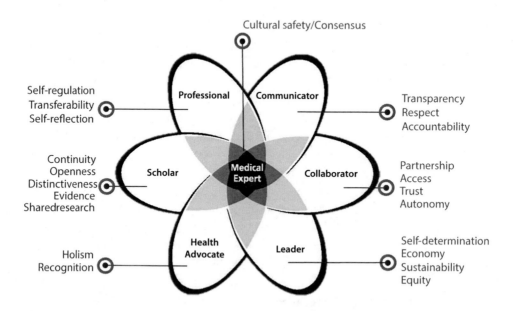

Figure 4.1: Indigenous Health Values and Principles for Culturally Safe Interventions

Source: Copyright © The Royal College of Physicians and Surgeons of Canada (2015). Reproduced with permission.

Table 4.1. Various Conceptualizations of the Social Determinants of Health

CanMEDS Roles	Indigenous Health Principles
Medical Expert	The culturally safe physician is a complete health care practitioner who embraces Indigenous knowledge/science, understands and accepts that racism exists and how historical/intergenerational trauma affects the health and well-being of the Indigenous patient, and takes steps to foster anti-racism interventions.
Communicator	The culturally safe physician communicates in clear, honest, and respectful dialogue about health matters and sees a mutual responsibility between him/her and the Indigenous patient/community for achieving shared health outcomes.
Collaborator	The culturally safe physician recognizes that the Indigenous patient-physician relationship is sacrosanct and without hierarchy or dominance; this partnership fosters access to health care and the resources necessary for health and wellness of the person, family, and community. It also facilitates the physician's ability to work effectively with community institutions to help the patient.
Leader	The culturally safe physician is equipped with the tools, knowledge, education, and experience to achieve the highest form of evidence-informed professional competencies, while practising with cultural humility, fostering an environment of cultural safety, and proactively pursuing anti-racism interventions.
Health Advocate	The culturally safe physician embraces Indigenous identity as the platform that promotes holistic health and encourages active participation of Indigenous people, in concert with physicians and other health care professionals, as "agents of change for health."
Scholar	The culturally safe physician understands that Indigenous health as an integral component of medical research, education, training, and practice and that this research is based on evidence from empirical sources, critical appraisal of relevant material beneficial to patients, leading Indigenous and non-Indigenous practices, and lifelong learning that can be adapted to serve Indigenous patients. Reflective practice grows a physician's skills in the collaborative patient-physician relationship.
Professional	The culturally safe physician is committed to the well-being of Indigenous patients, their families, communities, and cultures through ethical behaviours, compassion, integrity, respect, and a commitment to clinical competencies that engender health of Indigenous people.

Copyright © The Royal College of Physicians and Surgeons of Canada (2018). Reproduced with permission.

There are examples of Native-led and collaborative measures to address Indigenous health in Canada. The National Aboriginal Health Organization (2012) highlights a list of community-based leadership projects that reconcile health care disparities and inequities. Health Canada's First Nations and Inuit Health branch sponsors a number of innovative public health projects with positive results (Health Canada 2012). Successful projects subscribe to principles that resonate with Indigenous values.

Leadership platforms exist that could help stage culturally safe practices. The CanMEDS Physician Competency Framework describes the knowledge, skills, and abilities that specialist physicians require to deliver effective health care—although its principles can be adopted by other health care providers (Royal College of Physicians and Surgeons of Canada 2015). The framework is based on seven roles that all physicians need to be competent in. By mapping Indigenous health values against each role (see figure 4.1), providers can begin to reflect on their personal biases as well as the effects of their clinical skills on patient relationships. Providers who embrace these values do not interrogate or challenge Indigenous knowledge and ways of being, nor do they force patients into submitting to the health system, deliberately or through carelessness.

As shown in figure 4.1 and table 4.1, interpreting Indigenous health values through the CanMEDS framework results in seven principles to guide culturally safe interventions; patients can realize their full potential as Indigenous people without feeling threatened. The framework serves as a bridge from ideology to practice.

CONCLUSION

Altruistically, one might assume that health care equity is fairly and morally applied and that the health system treats each patient with respect and dignity on an equal footing. This, however, is not true for many Indigenous patients. The playing field is stacked against them before and after they enter the system because of constant exposure to racism, damage caused from intergenerational traumas, and a paternalistic health care system that lacks culturally safe interventions.

When health care providers begin to understand the values of their Indigenous patients and how damaging racism is, they will be better equipped to reflect on their behaviour and those of others. Only then can providers start to heal the damage caused by racism and truly help protect patients from harm.

CRITICAL THINKING QUESTIONS

1. Have you ever prescribed a treatment plan for a patient based on stereotypes or hidden assumptions?
2. What form of racism have you witnessed in practice or education?
3. Do you confront racism? How?
4. How do you behave when interacting with Indigenous patients?

5. Do you interrogate Indigenous knowledge and challenge Indigenous patients' traditional healing beliefs?

REFERENCES

Adelson, N. 2005. "The Embodiment of Inequity: Health Disparities in Aboriginal Canada." *Canadian Journal of Public Health* 96 (suppl 2): S45–61.

Association of Faculties of Medicine of Canada (AFMC). 2009. *The Future of Medical Education in Canada (FMEC): A Collective Vision for MD Education*. Ottawa: AFMC (with financial contribution from Health Canada). https://www.afmc.ca/future-of-medical-education-in-canada/medical-doctor-project/pdf/FMEC_CollectiveVisionMDEducation_EN.compressed.pdf.

Australian Bureau of Statistics. 2013. "Media Release: Aboriginal and Torres Strait Islander Population Nearing 700,000." 30 August. http://www.abs.gov.au/ausstats/abs@.nsf/latestProducts/3238.0.55.001Media%20Release1June%202011.

Beiser, M. 2005. "The Health of Immigrants and Refugees in Canada." *Canadian Journal of Public Health* 96 (2): S30–44.

DiAngelo, Robin, and Özlem Sensoy. 2014. "Getting Slammed: White Depictions of Race Discussions as Arenas of Violence." *Race Ethnicity and Education* 17 (1): 103–28.

Dion, S. D. 2009. "Historical Amnesia and the Discourse of the Romantic, Mythical Other." In *Braiding Histories: Learning from Aboriginal Peoples' Experiences and Perspectives*, by S. D. Dion, 3–13. Vancouver: UBC Press.

ERASE Racism. 2015. "Structural Racism Timeline." http://www.eraseracismny.org/structural-racism-timeline.

Freeman, T., T. Edwards, F. Baum, A. Lawless, G. Jolley, S. Javanparast, and T. Francis. 2014. "Cultural Respect Strategies in Australian Aboriginal Primary Health Care Services: Beyond Education and Training of Practitioners." *Australian and New Zealand Journal of Public Health* 38 (4): 355–61.

Health Canada. 2012. "First Nations, Inuit and Aboriginal Health." Last modified March 22, 2018. http://www.hc-sc.gc.ca/fniah-spnia/index-eng.php.

Health Council of Canada. 2012. *Empathy, Dignity, and Respect: Creating Cultural Safety for Aboriginal People in Urban Health Care*. Toronto: Health Council of Canada. http://www.healthcouncilcanada.ca/rpt_det.php?id=437.

Health Disparities Task Group of the Federal/Provincial/Territorial Advisory Committee on Population Health and Health Security. 2004. *Reducing Health Disparities—Roles of the Health Sector: Recommended Policy Directions and Activities*. Ottawa: Public Health Agency of Canada. http://www.phac-aspc.gc.ca/ph-sp/disparities/pdf06/disparities_discussion_paper_e.pdf.

Indigenous Physicians Association of Canada (IPAC), the Royal College of Physicians and Surgeons of Canada (Royal College), and the Association of Faculties of Medicine of Canada (AFMC). 2009. *First Nations, Inuit and Métis Health Core Competencies: A*

Curriculum Framework for Undergraduate Medical Education. Ottawa: IPAC and AFMC. https://www.afmc.ca/pdf/CoreCompetenciesEng.pdf.

Krieger, N. 2011. *Epidemiology and the People's Health: Theory and Context*. New York: Oxford University Press.

Lasser, K. E., D. U. Himmelstein, and S. Woolhandler. 2006. "Access to Care, Health Status and Health Disparities in the United States and Canada: Results of a Cross-National Population-Based Survey." *American Journal of Public Health* 96: 1300–7.

Lavallée, B., and L. Clearsky. 2006. "From Woundedness to Resilience: A Critical Review from an Aboriginal Perspective." *Journal of Aboriginal Health* 3 (1): 4–6.

Mitchell, Terry L., and Dawn T. Maracle. 2005. "Healing the Generations: Post-traumatic Stress and the Health Status of Aboriginal Populations in Canada." *Journal of Aboriginal Health* 2 (1): 14–25.

National Aboriginal Health Organization (NAHO). 2012. "NAHO Category Conferences." http://www.naho.ca/blog/category/conferences/ (URL no longer available).

National Collaborating Centre for Aboriginal Health. 2011. *Access to Health Services as a Social Determinant of First Nations, Inuit and Métis Health*. Prince George, BC: University of Northern British Columbia. https://www.ccnsa-nccah.ca/docs/determinants/FS-AccessHealthServicesSDOH-EN.pdf.

Ontario Human Rights Commission. n.d. "Examples of Racial Discrimination (Fact Sheet)." Accessed March 23, 2018. http://www.ohrc.on.ca/en/examples-racial-discrimination-fact-sheet.

Reading, Charlotte L. 2013. *Understanding Racism*. Prince George, BC: National Collaborating Centre for Aboriginal Health. http://www.nccah-ccnsa.ca/Publications/Lists/Publications/Attachments/103/understanding_racism_EN_web.pdf.

Reading, Charlotte L., and Fred Wien. 2009. *Health Inequalities and Social Determinants of Aboriginal Peoples' Health*. Prince George, BC: National Collaborating Centre for Aboriginal Health. https://www.ccnsa-nccah.ca/docs/determinants/RPT-HealthInequalities-Reading-Wien-EN.pdf.

Royal College of Physicians and Surgeons of Canada. n.d. "Indigenous Health Fact Sheet." Accessed March 23, 2018. http://www.royalcollege.ca/indigenoushealth.

Royal College of Physicians and Surgeons of Canada. 2015. CanMEDS 2015 Physician Competency Framework. Accessed March 23, 2018. http://canmeds.royalcollege.ca/uploads/en/framework/CanMEDS%202015%20Framework_EN_Reduced.pdf.

Royal College of Physicians and Surgeons of Canada. 2018. *Indigenous Health Values and Principles Statement*. Ottawa: Royal College of Physicians and Surgeons of Canada.

World Health Organization (WHO). 2008. "Australia's Disturbing Health Disparities Set Aboriginals Apart." *Bulletin of the World Health Organization* 86 (4): 245. http://www.who.int/bulletin/volumes/86/4/08-020408/en/.

CHAPTER 5

Health and Health Service Needs in Urban Indigenous Communities

Martin Cooke and Piotr Wilk

LEARNING OBJECTIVES

After reading this chapter, you should be able to:

1. Describe key aspects of urban Indigenous populations in Canada, including their relative size and cultural composition.
2. Identify key health issues facing urban Indigenous populations.
3. Identify some of the factors that affect health and health service delivery in urban Indigenous communities.

INTRODUCTION

As the other chapters in this section indicate, Indigenous peoples are at higher risk of a variety of poor health outcomes than are non-Indigenous citizens. This is true not only in Canada but in other former colonies as well. Australia, New Zealand, and the United States share broadly similar histories of European colonization with Canada and are therefore often compared. Life expectancy is frequently used as a summary indicator of population health status, and Indigenous populations in each of these countries have a five- to six-year lower life expectancy at birth than do other citizens (Statistics New Zealand 2015; Australian Institute of Health and Welfare 2018; Statistics Canada 2015; U.S. Department of Health and Human Services, Indian Health Service 2014).

The reasons for these health disparities and why they continue today are complex and involve a number of different pathways and mechanisms (Gracey and King 2009). Importantly, in all of these countries, the descendants of original inhabitants have poorer socioeconomic conditions than do the descendants of settlers or immigrants (Cooke et al. 2007; Mitrou et al. 2014). One common misconception is that these differences are due primarily to geography—to Indigenous people living primarily in rural or remote Indigenous communities. Although geography is important, and remote communities might be particularly under-served by health care and public health infrastructure, the fact is that a majority of the Indigenous populations in each of these countries lives in urban areas (figure 5.1). In Canada, more than half of the total Indigenous population lives alongside other Canadians in cities that are mainly well served by public health and

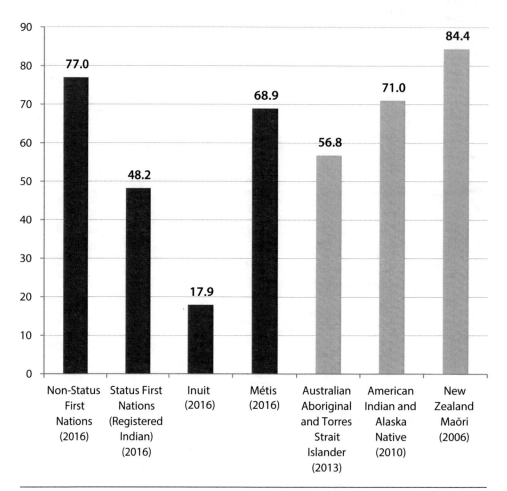

Figure 5.1: Percentage of Canadian, Australian, United States, and New Zealand Indigenous Populations Living in Urban Areas

Note: Canada: includes Census Metropolitan Areas (cities with a population of 100,000 or more) and Census Agglomerations (cities with 10,000 to 100,000); Australia: urban includes Major City areas and Inner-Regional Areas; New Zealand: urban includes Main Urban Areas, Satellite Urban Areas, and Independent Urban Areas; US: urban includes Urban Areas.

Sources: Statistics Canada (2018); Australian Bureau of Statistics (2013); Statistics New Zealand (n.d.); Urban Indian Health Institute (2013); author's calculations.

health care, including by physicians and allied health professionals. Understanding and reducing the health disparities faced by urban Indigenous populations should therefore be an important focus for policy and research.

The relative lack of research attention to urban Indigenous populations might be related to a tendency in both the academic and popular imaginations to construct Indigenous peoples and cultures as a static, unchanging, and exotic "other" (Browne and Varcoe 2006) and the stereotype that First Nations, Inuit, and Métis cultures are somehow incompatible with urban life. The reality, however, is that Canadian cities are also "Indigenous communities" (Newhouse 2003). The urban landscape is very much a part of many Indigenous peoples' lives, and Indigenous peoples, cultures, and institutions can be found in every Canadian city, large or small, north or south.

In this chapter, we discuss the health and health service needs of urban Indigenous populations. We begin with a description of Indigenous populations and their demographic and geographic characteristics and briefly present some of the evidence of the continuing high risk of poor health outcomes in this population. We then discuss some of the aspects of urban populations that make the delivery of services challenging in these contexts. Given the "upstream" social and economic factors that are at the root of most of these disparities, our concern is not only with clinical care but also the broader public health system, including health promotion, health education, and social services.

URBAN INDIGENOUS POPULATIONS IN CANADA

Although the best current estimates of the size of the urban population come from the 2016 Census of Canada, there are reasons to believe that these underestimate the number of Indigenous people in urban areas (Smylie et al. 2011). Nonetheless, the census numbers indicate that at least 51.8 percent (867,415 people) of the total Indigenous population of just under 1.7 million lived in cities with a total size of 30,000 people or more in 2016, compared with 68.6 percent of the total Canadian population (Statistics Canada 2017a, 2017b).

It is important to recognize the historical, cultural, and legal differences among the three Aboriginal populations that are identified in Section 35 of the Constitution Act of Canada, and how these are reflected in urban populations. Inuit, whose traditional territories are in the North, are the least urbanized. Of the 65,025 Canadians who identified themselves as Inuit in the 2016 census, 72.8 percent (about 47,000 people) lived in the four *Inuit Nunangat* or Inuit homelands of Nunatsiavut (northern coastal Labrador), Nunavik (northern Quebec), Inuvialuit (the western Arctic), and the Territory of Nunavut (Statistics Canada 2017a). Of the 27.8 percent of Inuit who lived outside of Inuit Nunangat, 56.2 percent (10,160 people) lived in cities of 30,000 or more, and most of those people (7,455) lived in Census Metropolitan Areas (CMAs)—cities with 100,000 people or more (Statistics Canada 2017a; Indigenous and Northern Affairs 2017). In particular, Ottawa, Edmonton, and Montreal have relatively large and growing urban Inuit populations (Statistics Canada 2009), both because these are centres of government and other employment but also because of the availability of health care services and the existing routes of air travel from the North.

For those identifying themselves as First Nations, area of residence is strongly related to legal "status" or registration under the Indian Act of Canada. In 2016, 744,855 First Nations people—roughly half of the total Indigenous population—identified themselves as "Registered Indians" or "treaty" or "Status" First Nations (Statistics Canada 2017a). Of these people, 40.4 percent lived on First Nations reserves, while 26.7 percent (about 220,000) lived in CMAs, and 18.6 percent (about 153,000) lived in smaller population centres with populations between 1,000 and 100,000 (Indigenous and Northern Affairs Canada 2017a).

Registration status is important for understanding health and health service delivery. Those registered under the Indian Act, as well as Inuit who are beneficiaries of an Inuit land settlement, are entitled to coverage by the federal government for a range of medically necessary items and services. Beneficiaries of these non-insured health benefits include Status First Nations and Inuit living in urban areas, who are therefore eligible for dental and vision care, drug coverage, some required medical equipment, mental health counselling, and transportation assistance beyond those available through provincial health programs or other plans such as private or employer insurance (Health Canada 2016).

"Non-Status" First Nations people, or people who identify themselves as First Nations but who are not registered under the Indian Act, account for 23.8 percent of the First Nations population, or 232,373 people (Statistics Canada 2017a). Métis are the descendants of a distinct Indigenous culture that developed from the blending of First Nations and European settlers before Confederation (Andersen 2014). In the 2016 census, more than half a million Canadians (587,545) identified themselves as Métis (Statistics Canada 2017a).

Many non-Status First Nations are the descendants of people who might have at one time had "status" or been members of a First Nation that had a treaty with the Crown, but lost registration rights due to the historical rules of the Indian Act. These have changed over time but include rules regarding the inheritance of status from parents (Guimond, Robitaille, and Senécal 2014). Other non-Status First Nations people are descendants of First Nations that had never been party to a treaty or otherwise recognized by the Canadian government. Before 1985, registration and membership in a recognized First Nation were essentially synonymous, meaning that people without status were generally not allowed to live in a First Nation reserve community.

The history of relations between Métis and Canadian governments has also been characterized by a lack of recognition. Unlike Inuit and many First Nations, Métis were often ignored as a distinct Aboriginal group until the passage of the Constitution Act of 1982, and the Supreme Court of Canada confirmed that Métis had constitutionally guaranteed Aboriginal rights in the 2003 *Powley* decision (Aboriginal Affairs and Northern Development Canada 2015). Métis have historically not had protected lands set aside for them, as is the case with First Nations and reserves (Andersen 2014).

Non-Status First Nations and Métis are therefore the most urbanized Canadian Indigenous populations (see figure 5.1). In 2016, 52.2 percent of non-status First Nations (121,265 people) and 44.7 percent of Métis (240,450 people) lived in CMAs (Indigenous and Northern Affairs Canada 2017a). Because they are not subject to the Indian Act, non-status First Nations and Métis are also not eligible for non-insured health benefits. In the 2016 *Daniels* decision, however, the Supreme Court of Canada ruled that Métis and non-Status First Nations are to be considered "Indians" under the Indian Act (*Daniels v. Canada* 2016). At the time of writing, it is not yet clear whether this will eventually include access to the same health benefits as those currently registered under the act.

The total Canadian Indigenous population has been growing, and this growth has taken place mainly in cities. The reasons for this growth are still often misunderstood, however (see the following box). Indigenous people are, on average, slightly more likely to move than are non-Indigenous Canadians, although people moving from First Nations or other Indigenous communities into the city is not the primary reason for the growth of urban populations. Nonetheless, migration does matter for service delivery. Population turnover or "churn" that results from people moving to and from cities and high residential mobility rates within cities present a challenge for the continuity of services and care (Clatworthy and Norris 2014; Place 2012). The motivations and needs of those moving into cities are also important. Educational or employment opportunities remain key motivations for moving, but access to health care services is also an important reason for migration, with people coming to cities temporarily to access treatment themselves or to support friends or family members (Place 2012). Overall, more women than men move from First Nations into cities, in part because of women leaving abusive or difficult family situations and to different employment opportunities for women and men in rural communities. This has resulted in Indigenous women predominating in urban populations (Clatworthy and Norris 2014).

Recent Growth in Urban Indigenous Populations Is Not Primarily Due to Migration

Over the early 2000s, the Indigenous population living in Census Metropolitan Areas (cities of 100,000 or more) grew at an average annual rate of more than 5 percent—much higher than that of the total Canadian population (Clatworthy and Norris 2014). It is often thought that much of this growth has been due to in-migration from First Nations reserves and other communities. On the contrary, in each census period since the 1970s, there has been more migration from cities to reserves than to cities from reserves (Clatworthy and Norris 2014). The main reason for urban growth is neither migration nor higher fertility, but instead more people identifying themselves as "Aboriginal" in the census; the majority of urban population growth has been among non-Status First Nations and Métis, who have generally not lived in reserve communities (Guimond, Robitaille, and Senécal 2014).

There are other aspects of the demography and geography of urban Indigenous populations that are important. As with the general Indigenous population, the urban Indigenous population is demographically young, with 26.5 percent aged 14 years and younger, compared with 16.5 percent of the non-Indigenous population. However, the size of the older adult population is also growing, and there is a sizable urban Indigenous baby boom population currently in their 50s and 60s (Statistics Canada 2018).

Unsurprisingly, the size and composition of urban Indigenous communities varies dramatically across the country. The 36,990 Indigenous people in the Toronto CMA represented only 0.8 percent of the total CMA population in 2011, whereas in the Winnipeg, Saskatoon, and Edmonton CMAs, Indigenous people represent 12.2, 10.9, and 5.9 percent of those cities' total populations, respectively (Statistics Canada 2018). Some cities, such as Hamilton, Vancouver, and Montreal, are very close to large First Nations, and some First Nations have reserve lands that are within city boundaries, with implications for migration and urban population composition (Indigenous and Northern Affairs Canada 2017b).

EVIDENCE OF HEALTH AND HEALTH SERVICE NEEDS IN URBAN INDIGENOUS POPULATIONS

Although Indigenous peoples in Canada have rightly complained of being "researched to death," the fact is that they are not well represented in Canadian health statistics (Place 2012, 11). Nonetheless, there is evidence that urban First Nations, Inuit, and Métis are at higher risk of a variety of poor health outcomes relative to other urban residents.

There is not sufficient space for a complete review here, but we recommend the excellent overview by Place (2012). Notable studies include the use of the 2000/2001 Canadian Community Health Survey (CCHS) by Tjepkema (2002) to examine health status and health care use by off-reserve Indigenous peoples. A study of mortality rates among urban Indigenous adults has found that urban Indigenous men and women lived an average of 4.7 and 6.5 fewer years after age 25 than non-Indigenous urban men and women, respectively (Tjepkema et al. 2010). Urban Indigenous adults' higher age-standardized rates of mortality were due to higher risk of infectious diseases, circulatory diseases, and most cancers. They were also at higher risk of death due to external causes, including suicide (Tjepkema et al. 2010).

Table 5.1 reports on some of the health differences between Indigenous people and other urban Canadians aged 25 to 44, from the 2014 CCHS. Non-Indigenous urban dwellers were more likely to report that their health was "excellent" or "very good" than were urban Indigenous people, and Indigenous people were more likely to report "fair" or "poor" overall health. Urban Indigenous people were also more likely to be obese than were non-Indigenous people, contributing to higher rates of diabetes mellitus (Katzmarzyk 2007). Urban Indigenous people were more likely to smoke than non-Indigenous people; however, there is also evidence that off-reserve Indigenous adults are less likely to be regular drinkers than are non-Indigenous adults (Tjepkema 2002), and they participate in more physical activity on average (Findlay 2011).

Table 5.1. Select Health-Related and Socioeconomic Characteristics of Urban Aboriginal and Non-Aboriginal Adults Aged 25 to 44, 2014

Characteristic	Urban Aboriginal (%)	Urban Non-Aboriginal (%)
Urban Geographic Residence		
CMA	71.4	87.2
CA	28.6	12.8
Body Mass Index		
Normal Weight	36.7	50.5
Overweight	33.3	30.6
Obese	30.0	18.9
Diagnosed with Diabetes	3.0	2.0
Current Smoker	45.5	20.7
Household Food Security Status		
Food Secure	69.6	91.8
Moderate or Severe Food Insecurity	30.4	8.2
Self-Perceived Health		
Excellent	15.6	25.4
Very Good	34.4	41.0
Good	31.3	26.8
Fair or Poor	18.7	6.8
Median Annual Household Income (2013)	$60,000	$80,000

Notes: CMA = Census Metropolitan Area; CA = Census Agglomeration. Percentages calculated using sample weights. Median income is rounded for disclosure.

Source: Data from the 2014 Canadian Community Health Survey, provided by Statistics Canada. Analysis and interpretation are the authors' alone.

Social factors play a key role in the excess mortality and morbidity of urban Indigenous people. On average, Indigenous people in urban areas have lower income (table 5.1) and educational attainment than other urban residents; this is related to higher unemployment rates and lower labour force participation (Mendelson 2004). Indigenous households are less likely to be food secure than are non-Indigenous ones (table 5.1). Housing is also an ongoing challenge, with high rates of homelessness among urban Indigenous people, as well as high prevalence of housing that is either crowded or in need of repair, contributing to high rates of residential mobility (Peters and Robillard 2013). Although Indigenous people are not as spatially concentrated as are other ethnic groups, they are disproportionately more likely to live in low-income areas in cities (Balakrishnan and Jurdi 2013). There is empirical evidence that these social determinants contribute to poor health outcomes. Controlling for education, household income, work status, and marital status attenuated, but did not eliminate, the Indigenous/non-Indigenous disparities in self-rated health, the presence of chronic conditions, activity limitation, and depression (Tjepkema 2002), or in all-cause mortality (Tjepkema et al. 2010).

Despite these poorer health outcomes and the presumed higher need, there is no evidence that Indigenous people are higher users of health care services. Although somewhat dated, evidence from the 2000/2001 CCHS finds no significant difference between Indigenous people and other Canadians in the percentage that had seen a physician or eye specialist in the previous year. However, fewer Indigenous people had seen a dentist, possibly because of a lack of dental coverage despite non-insured health benefits, and fewer reported having a regular doctor (Tjepkema 2002). More urban Indigenous than non-Indigenous people reported having unmet health care needs (19.8 percent vs. 12.7 percent), with a majority (56 percent) reporting "acceptability" as the reason their needs were unmet (Tjepkema 2002). Overt racism in the experience of health service delivery may be an underlying factor affecting urban Indigenous people's ability to find appropriate and acceptable treatment, as may a lack of "culturally safe" options (Allan and Smylie 2015).

CHALLENGES FOR SERVICE DELIVERY IN URBAN AREAS

Given the poorer health outcomes of urban Indigenous people, we are confident in saying that they are among Canada's "under-served" populations, in terms of their access to health care and clinical services, as well as the services that may affect the "upstream" determinants of health such as housing, employment support, and health education and health promotion. The reasons for this are complicated and ultimately rooted in colonialism and historical relations. Improving the services to urban Indigenous populations is complicated by the characteristics of these communities and the complexity of the institutions that serve them.

The first challenge that we will point out is the conception of *community*. It has become common to use the term to refer to any ethnoculturally defined population and sometimes to other groups. In the case of public health and health care service delivery, communities are often identified as targets of interventions or programming. In this case, it is worthwhile to consider how the complexity of urban Indigenous populations might affect attempts to improve services. Indeed, a city might not have a unified "Indigenous community" but instead have multiple communities with different cultures and health needs. Urban populations may include people from several major First Nations linguistic or cultural families, as well as people with connections to historical Métis communities in various parts of the country or to Inuit communities in the North. They include people who have come to the city recently, some of whom may have little experience or connection to urban areas. Some are members of First Nations that may be near to the city, or very distant. Others might have been urbanites their whole lives with deep roots in the urban environment. Many have mixed Indigenous or Indigenous and non-Indigenous heritage, and some may be newly discovering their Indigenous roots after the interruption of cultural transmission by residential schooling.

In addition to these cultural differences, legal definitions can create distinctions in service delivery between of those who have "status" or are beneficiaries of an Inuit land settlement and who are therefore entitled to services under the non-insured health benefits program, and those who are not (Allan and Smylie 2015, 25–26). In many cities, there is evidence of a growing urban Indigenous middle class, whose members may have different needs, experiences, and interests from those experiencing low income or housing instability (FitzMaurice, McCaskill, and Cidro 2012; Wotherspoon 2003).

If Indigenous urban populations and communities are complex, so is the system of organizations and institutions that serves them (Newhouse 2003). Whereas discrete First Nations can have clear jurisdiction with regard to the provision of health care and related services in their communities, urban Indigenous people live in much more complex service environments in which services may be provided by a range of providers, including clinicians, "universal" health and social service organizations, and Indigenous-specific providers. Some communities have Indigenous health centres, such as the Aboriginal Health Access Centres in some Ontario cities, that provide both Western and traditional health and wellness services to an urban clientele (Spence and White 2010). They might be clients of friendship centres, Métis organization offices, or other urban Indigenous organizations that provide health education or health promotion programs, among other services. Many of these programs and services are funded by provinces, such as the Aboriginal Healing and Wellness Strategy in Ontario, which seeks to improve the overall level of programming to Indigenous peoples (Ontario Ministry of Community and Social Services 2012). Others are provided by the federal government and may or may not be tied to a client's status. These distinctions might well become more complex with the implementation of the *Daniels* decision.

The cultural and legal complexity of urban Indigenous communities can make culturally sensitive or culturally informed service delivery difficult for both Indigenous and "universal" providers. Among Indigenous-specific providers, it can be difficult to be inclusive in such a diverse setting. Although many urban Indigenous organizations are formally status- and identity-blind, meaning that they provide services regardless of cultural identity or legal registration, this is difficult in practice, and organizations typically draw upon the cultural practices, teachings, and leaders they have at hand. While some urban residents will appreciate and benefit from the incorporation of Indigenous cultural symbols or practices into service delivery, whether or not they are of the clients' own cultural heritage (Peters, Maaka, and Laliberté 2014), others can be alienated by "pan-Aboriginal" cultural symbolism or language that does not speak to their own experiences (Ghosh and Spitzer 2014).

For universal service providers and clinicians who serve Indigenous people, there can be other challenges. Our own experience suggests that many would like to be better informed about the people they serve, and to either provide more appropriate services themselves or to be able to refer them to an Indigenous agency or healer. However, it can be difficult to know how to connect with and consult urban Indigenous communities in order to provide better services. Even for well-meaning health and social service agencies, identifying legitimate representatives of urban Indigenous communities, and the limits of that representation, can be daunting. Unlike First Nations or Inuit communities that have clear protocols for engagement, the lack of Indigenous governance frameworks in the city is a potential barrier to the establishment of relationships that would inform and improve service delivery (Morse 2010).

DISCUSSION

In this chapter, we have discussed key aspects of urban Indigenous populations and communities related to their health and health service needs. Urban Indigenous people are at higher risk of a number of health problems, including chronic and infectious diseases, as well as intentional injuries and mental illness. Indigenous populations in cities tend to be young and highly mobile, and this presents certain challenges to the provision of health and social services. However, the main characteristics that we think are important to consider are related to the diversity of these populations. The cultural, socioeconomic, and legal complexity of urban Indigenous communities presents challenges to providing culturally informed services.

Given this diversity in Indigenous communities and the institutions serving them, we propose that to achieve better service and health care for urban Indigenous peoples, we should not focus on individual programs or services for improvement but instead aim to improve the functioning of the overall urban health and social service system. We think that by strengthening the system, more general improvements in service delivery might be possible, including the provision of more culturally acceptable programs to serve urban Métis, First Nations, and Inuit residents, delivered by a mixed system of Indigenous and universal service providers (Wilk and Cooke 2015) (see the following box).

Improving the Health of First Nations and Métis Children in Our Communities: The Healthy Weights Connection

Indigenous children and youth living in urban areas are at higher risk of obesity than are other children, with implications for health later in life. Reducing this risk requires efforts from a number of actors in the community: schools, Indigenous organizations, public health units, city planners, and others.

Funded by the Public Health Agency of Canada, the Healthy Weights Connection project (http://www.healthyweightsconnection.ca) promotes inter-agency collaborations to improve the programming and services available to Indigenous children and their families, and to address the "upstream" determinants of poor diet and physical inactivity. Collaborative activities resulting from the project have included skate exchanges, educational grocery store tours, and distribution of Good Food Boxes to food-insecure families.

What we mean by these improvements in the functioning of local public health systems is fostering better connections between the agents in the system, including clinicians, Indigenous organizations, and others, that would allow for better coordination of services, sharing of information, referrals to culturally appropriate services where possible, and collaboration in the creation of new programs to meet specific local needs. Having institutionalized relationships between, for example, local hospitals and friendship centres, might improve a hospital's understanding of Indigenous patients' cultural needs and how to fill them, and this might give a friendship centre access to resources for programming they might not otherwise have (Spence and White 2010). Most importantly, ongoing relationships could help reduce the barriers between institutions and members of urban Indigenous communities, improving social capital and the capacity for community action (Hill and Cooke 2013).

Of course, some of these relationships already exist in some places, and it is important to recognize the diversity among Canadian cities with respect to their urban Indigenous populations and the institutions that serve them. Some cities have large urban Indigenous populations with well-functioning cultural, health, and social service institutions that are supported by and collaborate well with "universal" institutions (Newhouse 2003). Others have much more fragmented systems of service delivery, in which collaboration among service providers is an exception, rather than the rule (Spence and White 2010). Some cities have populations that are more culturally homogenous, perhaps including those that are immediately adjacent to First Nations, while others are very diverse, usually owing to their geography. As a result, no single approach for improving the service delivery to urban Indigenous people is likely to work in all cities. Instead, we expect that successful strategies will focus on the existing strengths of urban Indigenous communities and the institutions that serve them, and to be grounded in the histories, knowledge, and cultures of the people who live in them.

CRITICAL THINKING QUESTIONS

1. Imagine you are a Medical Officer for Health in charge of an urban public health unit. An important part of your mandate is reducing the health inequities between Indigenous peoples and other residents. What is the first thing you would do to address the problem?
2. What should be the role of clinicians and service providers in helping to address the systemic disparities in health between Indigenous and non-Indigenous urban residents?
3. If you live in a city, how visible are First Nations, Métis, or Inuit peoples or institutions in your area? If you knew someone was looking for culturally specific services, would you know where to refer them?

REFERENCES

Aboriginal Affairs and Northern Development Canada. 2015. "Frequently Asked Questions—Powley." Last modified June 4. http://www.aadnc-aandc.gc.ca/eng/1100100014419/1100100014420.

Allan, Billie, and Janet Smylie. 2015. *First Peoples, Second Class Treatment: The Role of Racism in the Health and Well-Being of Indigenous Peoples in Canada*. Toronto: Wellesley Institute.

Andersen, Chris. 2014. *"Métis": Race, Recognition and the Struggle for Indigenous Peoplehood*. Vancouver: UBC Press.

Australian Bureau of Statistics. 2013. "3238.0.55.001—Estimates of Aboriginal and Torres Strait Islander Australians, June 2011." August 30. http://www.abs.gov.au/ausstats/abs@.nsf/mf/3238.0.55.001#.

Australian Institute of Health and Welfare. 2018. "Life Expectancy and Deaths." Last updated January 16. https://www.aihw.gov.au/reports-statistics/health-conditions-disability-deaths/life-expectancy-deaths/overview.

Balakrishnan, T. R., and Rozzet Jurdi. 2013. "Spatial Residential Patterns of Aboriginals and their Socio-economic Integration in Selected Canadian Cities." In *Aboriginal Policy Research: Moving Forward, Making a Difference*, vol. 4, edited by Jerry P. White, Susan Wingert, Dan Beavon, and Paul Maxim, 263–73. Toronto: Thompson.

Browne, Annette J., and Colleen Varcoe. 2006. "Critical Cultural Perspectives and Health Care Involving Aboriginal Peoples." *Contemporary Nurse* 22 (2): 155–67.

Clatworthy, Stewart, and Mary Jane Norris. 2014. "Aboriginal Mobility and Migration in Canada: Patterns, Trends and Implications, 1971 to 2006." In *Aboriginal Populations: Social, Demographic and Epidemiological Perspectives*, edited by Frank Trovato and Anatole Romaniuk, 119–60. Vancouver: University of Alberta Press.

Cooke, Martin, Francis Mitrou, David Lawrence, Eric Guimond, and Dan Beavon. 2007. "Indigenous Well-Being in Four Countries: An Application of the UNDP'S Human Development Index to Indigenous Peoples in Australia, Canada, New Zealand, and the United States." *BMC International Health and Human Rights* 7 (1): 9.

Daniels v. Canada (Indian Affairs and Northern Development), [2016] 1 SCR 99, 2016 SCC 12 (CanLII). http://canlii.ca/t/gpfth.

Findlay, Leanne C. 2011. "Physical Activity among First Nations People Off Reserve, Métis and Inuit." *Health Reports* 22 (1): 47–54.

FitzMaurice, Kevin, Don McCaskill, and Jamie Cidro. 2012. "Urban Aboriginal People in Toronto: A Summary of the 2011 Toronto Aboriginal Research Project (TARP)." In *Well-Being in the Urban Aboriginal Community*, edited by David Newhouse, Kevin FitzMaurice, Tricia McGuire-Adams, and Daniel Jetté, 235–64. Toronto: Thompson.

Ghosh, Hasu, and Denise Spitzer. 2014. "Inequities in Diabetes Outcomes among Urban First Nation and Métis Communities: Can Addressing Diversities in Preventive Services Make a Difference?" *International Indigenous Policy Journal* 5 (1). https://doi.org/10.18584/iipj.2014.5.1.2.

Gracey, Michael, and Malcolm King. 2009. "Indigenous Health Part 1: Determinants and Disease Patterns." *Lancet* 374 (9683): 65–75.

Guimond, Eric, Norbert Robitaille, and Sasha Senécal. 2014. "Another Look at Definitions and Growth of Aboriginal Populations in Canada." In *Aboriginal Populations: Social, Demographic and Epidemiological Perspectives*, edited by Frank Trovato and Anatole Romaniuk, 97–118. Edmonton: University of Alberta Press.

Health Canada. 2016. "Non-insured Health Benefits (NIHB) Program—General Questions and Answers." Last updated August 29. https://www.canada.ca/en/health-canada/services/first-nations-inuit-health/non-insured-health-benefits/benefits-information/non-insured-health-benefits-nihb-program-general-information-questions-answers-first-nations-inuit-health-canada.html.

Hill, Gus, and Martin Cooke. 2013. "How Do You Build a Community? Developing Community Capacity and Social Capital in an Urban Aboriginal Setting." *Pimatisiwin: A Journal of Aboriginal and Indigenous Community Health* 11 (3): 421–32.

Indigenous and Northern Affairs Canada. 2017a. Custom tabulations from the 2016 Census of Canada. Ottawa: Statistics Canada.

Indigenous and Northern Affairs Canada. 2017b. "Urban Reserves." Accessed December 22, 2017. https://www.aadnc-aandc.gc.ca/eng/1100100016331/1100100016332.

Katzmarzyk, Peter T. 2007. "Obesity and Physical Activity among Aboriginal Canadians." *Obesity* 16 (1): 184–90.

Mendelson, Michael. 2004. *Aboriginal People in Canada's Labour Market: Work and Unemployment, Today and Tomorrow*. Ottawa: Caledon Institute.

Mitrou, Francis, Martin Cooke, David Lawrence, David Povah, Elena Mobilia, Eric Guimond, and Stephen R. Zubrick. 2014. "Gaps in Indigenous Disadvantage Not Closing: A Census Cohort Study of Social Determinants of Health in Australia, Canada, and New Zealand from 1981–2006." *BMC Public Health* 14 (1): 201.

Morse, Bradford. 2010. "Developing Frameworks for Urban Aboriginal Governance." In *Aboriginal Policy Research, Volume 8: Exploring the Urban Landscape*, edited by Jerry White and Jodi Bruhn, 3–30. Toronto: Thompson.

Newhouse, David. 2003. "The Invisible Infrastructure: Urban Aboriginal Institutions and Organizations." In *Not Strangers in These Parts: Urban Aboriginal Peoples*, edited by David Newhouse and Evelyn Peters, 243–55. Ottawa: Policy Research Initiative.

Ontario Ministry of Community and Social Services. 2012. "Goal of the Aboriginal Healing and Wellness Strategy." Last modified March 8. http://www.mcss.gov.on.ca/en/mcss/programs/community/ahws/goal_strategy.aspx.

Peters, Evelyn J., Roger C. A. Maaka, and Ron F. Laliberté. 2014. "'I'm Sweating with Cree Culture not Saulteaux Culture': Urban Aboriginal Identities." In *Aboriginal Populations: Social, Demographic, and Epidemiological Perspectives*, edited by Frank Trovato and Anatole Romaniuk, 285–302. Edmonton: University of Alberta Press.

Peters, Evelyn, and Vince Robillard. 2013. "Urban Hidden Homelessness and Reserve Housing." In *Aboriginal Policy Research: Moving Forward, Making a Difference*, vol. 4, edited by Jerry P. White, Susan Wingert, Dan Beavon, and Paul Maxim, 189–206. Toronto: Thompson.

Place, Jessica. 2012. *The Health of Aboriginal People Residing in Urban Areas*. Vancouver: National Collaborating Centre for Aboriginal Health.

Smylie, Janet, Michelle Firestone, Leslie Cochrane, Conrad Prince, Sylvia Maracle, Marilyn Morley, Sara Mayo, Trey Spiller, and Bella McPherson. 2011. *Our Health Counts: Urban Aboriginal Database Research Project Community Report*. Toronto: St. Michael's Hospital.

Spence, Nicholas, and Jerry White. 2010. "Thinking About Service Delivery: Aboriginal Providers, Universal Providers and Role of Friendship Centres." In *Aboriginal Policy Research, Volume 8: Exploring the Urban Landscape*, edited by Jerry P. White and Jodi Bruhn, 89–106. Toronto: Thompson.

Statistics Canada. 2009. *2006 Census: Aboriginal Peoples in Canada in 2006*. Ottawa: Statistics Canada. Last modified September 22. https://www12.statcan.gc.ca/census-recensement/2006/as-sa/97-558/index-eng.cfm.

Statistics Canada. 2015. *Aboriginal Statistics at a Glance*, 2nd ed. Ottawa: Statistics Canada.

Statistics Canada. 2017a. "Aboriginal Peoples in Canada: Key Results from the 2016 Census." *The Daily*, October 25. http://www.statcan.gc.ca/daily-quotidien/171025/dq171025a-eng.htm.

Statistics Canada. 2017b. "Dictionary, Census of Population, 2016: Population centre (POPCTR)." Last modified January 31. http://www12.statcan.gc.ca/census-recensement/2016/ref/dict/geo049a-eng.cfm.

Statistics Canada. 2018. "Aboriginal Identity (9), Age (20), Registered or Treaty Indian Status (3) and Sex (3) for the Population in Private Households of Canada, Provinces and Territories, Census Metropolitan Areas and Census Agglomerations, 2016 Census—25% Sample Data." Catalogue no. 98-400-x2016155. Last modified January 16. http://www12.statcan.gc.ca/census-recensement/2016/dp-pd/dt-td/Rp-eng.cfm?LANG=E&APATH=3&DETAIL=0&DIM=0&FL=A&FREE=0&GC=0&GID=0&GK=0&GRP=1&PID=110588&PRID=10&PTYPE=109445&S=0&SHOWALL=0&SUB=0&Temporal=2017&THEME=122&VID=0&VNAMEE=&VNAMEF=.

Statistics New Zealand. n.d. "New Zealand: An Urban/Rural Profile Update." Accessed December 22, 2017. http://archive.stats.govt.nz/browse_for_stats/Maps_and_geography/Geographic-areas/urban-rural-profile-update.aspx.

Statistics New Zealand. 2015. "New Zealand Period Life Tables: 2012–14." Wellington: Statistics New Zealand.

Tjepkema, Michael. 2002. "The Health of the Off-Reserve Aboriginal Population." *Health Reports* 13 (suppl): 1–17.

Tjepkema, Michael, Russell Wilkins, Sascha Senécal, Eric Guimond, and Christopher Penney. 2010. "Mortality of Urban Aboriginal Adults in Canada, 1991–2001." *Chronic Diseases in Canada* 31 (1): 4–21.

Urban Indian Health Institute. 2013. *US Census Marks Increase in Urban American Indians and Alaska Natives*. Seattle, WA: Urban Indian Health Institute.

U.S. Department of Health and Human Services, Indian Health Service. 2014. "Life Expectancy, American Indians and Alaska Natives, Data Years: 2007–2009." Washington, DC: Indian Health Service.

Wilk, Piotr, and Martin Cooke. 2015. "Collaborative Public Health System Interventions for Chronic Disease Prevention among Urban Aboriginal Peoples." *International Indigenous Policy Journal* 6 (4). https://doi.org/10.18584/iipj.2015.6.4.3.

Wotherspoon, Terry. 2003. "Prospects for a New Middle Class among Urban Aboriginal People." In *Not Strangers in These Parts: Urban Aboriginal Peoples*, edited by David Newhouse and Evelyn Peters, 147–66. Ottawa: Policy Research Initiative.

CHAPTER 6

Health for Canadian Indigenous Children

Anna Banerji

LEARNING OBJECTIVES

After reading this chapter, you should be able to:

1. Appreciate the disproportionate impact of health issues affecting Indigenous children and youth.
2. Illustrate some of the common health issues affecting Indigenous children and youth.
3. Understand how the social determinants of health and the impact of colonization have affected Indigenous child health.

OVERVIEW

This chapter highlights some of the important health issues for Indigenous children. Of 1.4 million Indigenous peoples, approximately 480,000 were under the age of 18 in 2011 (Statistics Canada 2015a). With a median age of 25 for First Nations (FN), 22 for Inuit, and 30 for Métis, compared to 40 years for non-Indigenous Canadians, Indigenous populations are young and comprise the most rapidly growing demography of any population in Canada (Statistics Canada 2011). Indigenous peoples experience both the lowest life expectancy and the highest infant mortality rate in Canada. For Inuit, the adjusted life expectancy is 64 years, 15 years below the Canadian average (Statistics Canada 2015b). Though Indigenous peoples are a heterogeneous mix, with each community having unique cultures, histories, and needs. One undeniable generalization exists: Indigenous peoples, on a population basis, have the worst health status and determinants on every measure of any Canadian demographic (Statistics Canada 2015b, 2018; Irvine, Kitty, and Pekeles 2012).

EXAMPLES OF HEALTH CONSEQUENCES IN INDIGENOUS CHILDREN

The health disparities that affect Indigenous peoples start before birth and continue throughout the life spectrum. In Nunavut, for example, the infant mortality rate was 26.3 per 1,000 live births in 2011, which is five times higher than the Canadian average (Statistics Canada 2018). Prenatal exposures or environments such as poor nutrition or exposure to toxins increase the risk of health issues later in life.

While Indigenous women are more likely than non-Indigenous women to abstain from alcohol use in pregnancy in general, a high rate of fetal alcohol spectrum disorders (FASD) exist in some Indigenous communities (Banerji and Shah 2017). The factors contributing to this are complex and include the legacy of residential schools compounded by the delays in pregnancy detection. These challenges are further exacerbated by a lack of diagnostic capacity for FASD, particularly for remote communities. As early diagnosis is one of the most important factors for reducing secondary disabilities and improving the long-term outcome of FASD, delays in diagnosis increase the risk of secondary disabilities such as poor school experiences, behavioural issues, and other long-term outcomes of FASD.

The greatest potential years of life lost in Indigenous children is due to injury (Allard, Wilkins, and Berthelot 2004), with Indigenous children three to four times more likely to die of unintentional injury compared to the Canadian average (Banerji, CPS, and First Nations, Inuit and Métis Health Committee 2012). Fires and motor vehicle collisions (MVCs) are the most common cause of death in children under 10 years of age, while MVCs and drownings are responsible for the most deaths in older children aged 10 to 19 (Banerji, CPS, and First Nations, Inuit and Métis Health Committee 2012). There are regional variations in the types of injury, impacted by climate, geography, and activities. Poor determinants of health, such as substandard housing, poverty, poor road conditions, and lack of fire prevention, contribute to this excess mortality. In general, Indigenous children who have sustained serious injuries do not have access to the same rehabilitation services as non-Indigenous children (Banerji, CPS, and First Nations, Inuit and Métis Health Committee 2012). There is almost no data for Inuit and Métis children, and Canada does not currently have any national injury surveillance or injury prevention strategy.

One of the most disconcerting outcomes of years of colonization is the high rates of intentional injury, including suicide, in youth. The suicide rates for First Nations youth are five to seven times higher than for non-Aboriginal youth. Inuit youth have among the highest suicide rates in the world at 11 times the national average.[1] The rates vary in different communities, over time, and can occur in epidemics. For example, Inuit males aged 15 to 40 had a suicide rate 40 times higher than the Canadian average for the same non-Indigenous demographic (Eggertson 2013). The reasons for the high rates are complex, but contributors may include poor determinants of health, poverty, isolation, substance abuse in the individual or family, and intergenerational trauma from residential schools and governmental policies. Suicide has a devastating impact on the family and the community, yet for most Indigenous communities, a lack of culturally safe suicide prevention and awareness programs has existed. Recently, however, the Inuit Tapiriit Kanatami (ITK 2016) has released the National Inuit Suicide Prevention Strategy, an exemplary community-driven strategy.

MALNUTRITION AND FOOD SECURITY

While Canada is a land of plenty, there is rampant food insecurity in many Indigenous communities. The price of food can be exorbitant while the quality is simultaneously poor. The barriers to achieving food security include the loss of traditional knowledge and skills for hunting or fishing and the cost of transportation and ammunition. The lack of ammunition to continue with traditional practices has stemmed from concerns about lead contamination in traditional foods (Hlimi et al. 2012; Dallaire et al. 2013). This has also led to a reduction in consuming these healthier traditional foods (Banerji, CPS, and Committee Métis Health, in press). Consequently, high-calorie foods with poor nutritional value that are easy to transport have replaced more nutritious foods. Furthermore, food security and quality are largely determined by the presence of poverty. In a cross-sectional study of Inuit children living in remote communities in Nunavut, nearly 70 percent of preschool children faced food insecurity (Egeland et al. 2010). The results of food insecurity include obesity, diabetes (Young et al. 2000), severe anemia (Christofides, Schauer, and Zlotkin 2005), rickets (Eggertson 2015b), and severe dental cavities, among other health issues. Non-insulin dependent (type 2) diabetes is a growing concern in Indigenous children and youth, especially for First Nations (Young et al. 2000).

Infectious diseases tend to be experienced at a significantly higher rate in Indigenous children than non-Indigenous children. Inuit infants in Nunavut and Nunavik have the highest rates of hospital admission for lower respiratory tract infections globally (Banerji et al. 2001; Banerji et al. 2016). When admitted, these infants have more severe disease with prolonged hospitalization, often requiring life support in intensive care units (Banerji et al. 2016). In 2014, the incidence of tuberculosis among First Nations was 19.3 per 100,000 people, 198.3 per 100,000 people among the Inuit, the latter 40 times the overall Canadian rate (Public Health Agency of Canada 2016).

HEALTH CARE ACCESS

All Canadian children have access to basic health care, such as a physician or hospital, as part of their provincial or territorial plans. Children identified as Status Indian (FN) and Inuit qualify for Health Canada's Non-insured Health Benefits (NIHB) program. In general, Métis do not qualify for extended benefits through NIHB except in the Northwest Territories. The NIHB program provides coverage for some medications, dental and vision care, some medical supplies and equipment, medical transportation, and short-term crisis intervention. Crisis intervention is monitored, and practitioners must reapply for funds to support this type of counselling. Furthermore, although the drug plan is limited, a physician can apply for exceptions; however, this can be an arduous process, thereby limiting access to medications that other Canadians have access to.

In addition, children living in remote or isolated locations may not have reliable access to health care providers, who often visit on a rotating basis. Furthermore, many rural Indigenous children do not have access to dental care, and many of the northern nursing stations suffer from chronic staff shortages. Even for many urban Indigenous children, poverty remains a major barrier for accessing services and paying for medications. Another major barrier is both real and perceived discrimination in the health care system (Allan and Smylie 2015).

Poverty continues to be a pervasive issue for many Indigenous communities and for urban Indigenous children, affecting all aspects of health including access to health care, medications, and food security. Homes on reserves often lack basic amenities, such as access to clean water (Eggertson 2008, 2015a), while also having insufficient infrastructure, including roads, water, sewers, and power (Assembly of First Nations 2013). To compound these harms, almost one quarter of FN adults on reserves live in overcrowded substandard homes (Assembly of First Nations 2013); in Nunavut, Inuit are ten times more likely than the Canadian average to live in overcrowded homes (Statistics Canada 2014). Lack of, and overcrowded, housing results in increased transmission of infectious diseases, such as tuberculosis and lower respiratory tract infections.

HISTORICAL ROOTS

To be a more culturally safe health care provider, one needs to first review the history of Indigenous peoples in this country and be prepared to address one's own positioning in settler society. The report by the Truth and Reconciliation Commission outlines the severe physical, emotional, and sexual violence perpetrated against children in residential schools over several generations (Sinclair, Wilson, and Littlechild 2015). During this period, the government and church forcefully removed children from their homes, as it was believed that FN were not capable of caring for their own children. The intent was to force assimilation—a way to eliminate the Indian from Canadian society. As outlined in the Truth and Reconciliation report (detailed in Chapter 3 by Freeman in this volume), these are now considered acts of "cultural genocide" (Sinclair, Wilson, and Littlechild 2015).

Why does this matter today? While many of the residential school survivors have shown much resiliency and some have gone on to be leaders in their communities, most have been traumatized. Some were severely traumatized and now as adults suffer from post-traumatic stress disorder, depression, and alcohol and substance dependence (Sinclair, Wilson, and Littlechild 2015). As children, they had limited contact with their parents and were taught to be ashamed of their Indigenous heritage. Many lost connections with their cultural roots, including the loss of language, customs, and family ties, and many did not have the opportunity to develop healthy parenting skills. These racially specific adverse childhood experiences led to poor health outcomes and challenged survivors during their adult years. Some of these individuals are the parents and grandparents of children we see today in our practices.

In addition, many of the colonialist policies continue today. Indigenous children receive less funding per capita for child welfare and education than other Canadian children (Office of the Auditor General of Canada 2011). Despite the auditor general's report, which continues to state concerns about the financial and educational barriers FN children encounter, very little has been done in amelioration (Office of the Auditor General of Canada 2011). Today, many of these families continue to live in poverty, facing food insecurity and lacking basic rights, such as access to safe housing and clean water. Additionally, many Indigenous families continue to endure systematic racism (Allan and Smylie 2015). The consequences of both the historical and contemporary treatment of Indigenous peoples and their families have led to a mistrust in the government and health care system; this often adversely affects their health-seeking behaviours.

CULTURALLY SAFE CARE

As a health care provider, knowledge of the history of Indigenous peoples in Canada is imperative for providing culturally safe care. The starting point, as suggested by most Indigenous leaders, includes an understanding of the historical aspects of Indigenous peoples in Canada and developing cultural competency. In 2013, the Royal College of Physicians and Surgeons (RCPSC) published the *Indigenous Health Values and Principles Statement*, which serves as an excellent resource for those working with Indigenous peoples or communities. The RCPSC has mandated that all medical schools include Indigenous health as part of their curriculum. In 2017, the RCPSC indicated that cultural safety training would be a mandatory part of the residency curriculum. In addition, the Canadian Nurses Association has developed several documents, including *Aboriginal Health Nursing and Aboriginal Health: Charting Policy Direction for Nursing in Canada* (Canadian Nurses Association and Aboriginal Nurses Association of Canada 2014). Likewise, other allied health programs are developing cultural safety initiatives.

Cultural safety courses are now being offered at many institutions, as well as at several academic conferences, including the University of Toronto's Indigenous Health Conference (http://www.cpd.utoronto.ca/indigenoushealth/). This conference has the specific goal of increasing cultural safety for working with Indigenous peoples. Another example is the International Meeting on Indigenous Child Health through the Canadian Paediatric Society and the American Academy of Pediatrics. Other clinical practice guidelines are listed at the end of this chapter.

While many of the challenges for Indigenous communities rely on political solutions, there are also many ways to advocate for improved health for Indigenous children, families, and communities.

AT THE INDIVIDUAL LEVEL

- Actively listen to your patient's family trajectory (cultural humility). Try to understand the differences in traditional concepts of health and incorporate them; allow room for traditional methods of healing. A common model used for health care encounters for health conditions is the LEARN Model (San'yas Indigenous Cultural Safety: http://www.sanyas.ca/):
    - **L**isten to the client's perspective
    - **E**xplain your perspective
    - **A**cknowledge the differences and similarities between these two perspectives
    - **R**ecommend a plan of action
    - **N**egotiate mutual agreement
- Increase your understanding of unique barriers the specific child and his/her family may face, while recognizing their resiliency.
- Be familiar with the Non-insured Health Benefits (NIHB) available in your region.
- Advocate for reinstating status for First Nations families where it has been lost.
- Advocate for medications that are not covered by NIHB when indicated.
- Think about anticipatory guidance for injury prevention (Banerji, CPS, and First Nations, Inuit and Métis Health Committee 2012), improved food security (Banerji, CPS, and Committee Métis Health, in press), and suicide prevention (ITK 2016).
- Take an Indigenous cultural safety course.

AT THE COMMUNITY LEVEL

- Work with Indigenous communities in your area or remote areas; get to know the communities you serve.
- Commit on a long-term basis to a few communities. This could build trust and have a great impact over time.
- Engage in community-based participatory research that could result in improved health outcomes.
- Advocate for rehabilitation and suicide prevention programs where indicated; suicidality is related to not seeing oneself in the systems that guide one's community.
- Advocate for poverty reduction strategies, including education and employment opportunities, with Indigenous communities.
- Advocate for Indigenous peoples' need for basic human rights, such as food security, safe affordable housing, and access to clean water.
- Engage with the politics of oppression; expose and challenge oppression.

CRITICAL THINKING QUESTIONS

1. When you see a sick Indigenous child in a health care setting, what are some of the factors that may have contributed to poor health?
2. If you have seen an Indigenous child where the treatment and/or outcomes were not optimal, can you think of some issues that may have affected the outcome?
3. What are ways that you can advocate for an Indigenous child or family?

CLINICAL PRACTICE GUIDELINES

Indigenous Physicians Association of Canada and the Association of Faculties of Medicine of Canada—*First Nations, Inuit, Métis Health: Core Competencies*: http://www.afmc.ca/pdf/CoreCompetenciesEng.pdf.

Society of Obstetricians and Gynaecologists of Canada—*Health Professionals Working with First Nations, Inuit, and Métis: Consensus Guideline. Journal of Obstetrics and Gynaecology Canada* 35 (6): https://sogc.org/files/HealthProfessionalsWorkingWithFirstNations,Inuit,andMetisConsensusGuideline2013.pdf.

Canadian Paediatric Society—*Health Research Involving First Nations, Inuit and Métis Children and Their Communities*: http://www.cps.ca/documents/position/health-research-first-nations-inuit-Métis-children.

Royal College of Physicians and Surgeons of Canada—*Indigenous Health Values and Principles Statement*: http://www.royalcollege.ca/portal/page/portal/rc/common/documents/policy/indigenous_health_values_principles_report_e.pdf.

RECOMMENDED READINGS

More information about health coverage for Indigenous populations in Canada can be found on the Health Canada, First Nations and Inuit Health website: https://www.canada.ca/en/health-canada/services/first-nations-inuit-health.html.

The Canadian Nurses Association, in collaboration with the Aboriginal Nurses Association of Canada, has developed two important resources for curricular uses in nursing education:

1. Canadian Nurses Association, and Aboriginal Nurses Association of Canada. 2009. *Cultural Competency Framework for Nursing Education*. Ottawa: Aboriginal Nurses Association of Canada. https://www.cna-aiic.ca/~/media/cna/page-content/pdf-en/first_nations_framework_e.pdf?la=en.
2. Canadian Nurses Association, and Aboriginal Nurses Association of Canada. 2014. *Aboriginal Health Nursing and Aboriginal Health: Charting Policy Direction for Nursing in Canada*. Ottawa: Canadian Nurses Association. https://cna-aiic.ca/~/media/cna/page-content/pdf-en/aboriginal-health-nursing-and-aboriginal-health_charting-policy-direction-for-nursing-in-canada.pdf?la=en.

NOTE

1. This data comes from various sources. Data for First Nations suicide rates (2000) come from unpublished data provided by the First Nations and Inuit Health Branch of Health Canada. Rates for all of Canada (2001) come from Statistics Canada (https://www.canada.ca/en/health-canada/services/first-nations-inuit-health/health-promotion/suicide-prevention.html). Rates for Inuit (1999–2003) are based on figures provided by the Nunavut Bureau of Statistics, Inuvialuit Regional Corporation, Nunavik Board of Health and Social Services, and Labrador Inuit Health Commission.

REFERENCES

Allan, B., and J. Smylie. 2015. *First Peoples, Second Class Treatment*. Toronto: Wellesley Institute.

Allard, Y. E., R. Wilkins, and J. M. Berthelot. 2004. "Premature Mortality in Health Regions with High Aboriginal Populations." *Health Rep* 15 (1): 51–60.

Assembly of First Nations. 2013. "Fact Sheet—First Nations Housing On-Reserve." June. https://www.afn.ca/uploads/files/housing/factsheet-housing.pdf.

Banerji, A., A. Bell, E. L. Mills, J. McDonald, K. Subbarao, G. Stark, N. Eynon, and V. G. Loo. 2001. "Lower Respiratory Tract Infections in Inuit Infants on Baffin Island." *CMAJ* 164 (13): 1847–50.

Banerji, A., Canadian Paediatric Society (CPS), and First Nations, Inuit and Métis Health Committee. 2012. "Preventing Unintentional Injuries in Indigenous Children and Youth in Canada." *Paediatrics & Child Health* 17 (7): 393–4.

Banerji, A., First Nations Inuit Canadian Paediatric Society (CPS), and Committee Métis Health. In press. *Food Security and Malnutrition in Indigenous Children and Youth in Canada*. Ottawa: CPS.

Banerji A., V. Panzov, M. Young, J. Robinson, B. Lee, T. Moraes, M. Mamdani, et al. 2016. "Hospital Admissions for Lower Respiratory Tract Infections among Infants in the Canadian Arctic: A Cohort Study." *CMAJ Open* 4 (4): E615–22. https://doi.org/10.9778/cmajo.20150051.

Banerji A., and C. Shah. 2017. "Ten-Year Experience of Fetal Alcohol Spectrum Disorder: Diagnostic and Resource Challenges in Indigenous Children." *Paediatrics & Child Health* 22 (3): 143–7.

Canadian Nurses Association, and Aboriginal Nurses Association of Canada. 2014. *Aboriginal Health Nursing and Aboriginal Health: Charting Policy Direction for Nursing in Canada*. Ottawa: Canadian Nursing Association. https://cna-aiic.ca/~/media/cna/page-content/pdf-en/aboriginal-health-nursing-and-aboriginal-health_charting-policy-direction-for-nursing-in-canada.pdf?la=en.

Christofides, A., C. Schauer, and S. H. Zlotkin. 2005. "Iron Deficiency and Anemia Prevalence and Associated Etiologic Risk Factors in First Nations and Inuit Communities in Northern Ontario and Nunavut." *Canadian Journal of Public Health* 96 (4): 304–7.

Dallaire, R., E. Dewailly, P. Ayotte, N. Forget-Dubois, S. W. Jacobson, J. L. Jacobson, and G. Muckle. 2013. "Exposure to Organochlorines and Mercury through Fish and Marine Mammal Consumption: Associations with Growth and Duration of Gestation among Inuit Newborns." *Environmental International* 54: 85–91. https://doi.org/10.1016/j.envint.2013.01.013.

Egeland, G. M., A. Pacey, Z. Cao, and I. Sobol. 2010. "Food Insecurity among Inuit Preschoolers: Nunavut Inuit Child Health Survey, 2007–2008." *CMAJ* 182 (3): 243–8. https://doi.org/10.1503/cmaj.091297.

Eggertson, L. 2008. "Despite Federal Promises, First Nations' Water Problems Persist." *CMAJ* 178 (8): 985. https://doi.org/10.1503/cmaj.080429.

Eggertson, L. 2013. "Risk of Suicide 40 Times Higher for Inuit Boys." *CMAJ* 185 (15): E701–2. https://doi.org/10.1503/cmaj.109-4594.

Eggertson, L. 2015a. "Canada Has 1838 Drinking-Water Advisories." *CMAJ* 187 (7): 488. https://doi.org/10.1503/cmaj.109-5018.

Eggertson, L. 2015b. "Rickets Re-emerges in Northern Aboriginal Children." *CMAJ* 187 (7): E213–4. https://doi.org/10.1503/cmaj.109-5027.

Hlimi, T., K. Skinner, R. M. Hanning, I. D. Martin, and L. J. Tsuji. 2012. "Traditional Food Consumption Behaviour and Concern with Environmental Contaminants among Cree Schoolchildren of the Mushkegowuk Territory." *International Journal of Circumpolar Health* 71: 17344. https://doi.org/10.3402/ijch.v71i0.17344.

Inuit Tapiriit Kanatami (ITK). 2016. *National Inuit Suicide Strategy*. Ottawa: ITK. https://www.itk.ca/wp-content/uploads/2016/07/ITK-National-Inuit-Suicide-Prevention-Strategy-2016.pdf.

Irvine, James, Darlene Kitty, and Gary Pekeles. 2012. "Healing Winds: Aboriginal Child and Youth Health in Canada." *Paediatrics & Child Health* 17 (7): 363–4.

Office of the Auditor General of Canada. 2011. "Chapter 4—Programs for First Nations on Reserves." In *2011 June Status Report of the Auditor General of Canada*. http://www.oag-bvg.gc.ca/internet/English/parl_oag_201106_04_e_35372.html.

Public Health Agency of Canada. 2016. "Tuberculosis in Canada 2014: Pre-release." Last modified March 15. https://www.canada.ca/en/public-health/services/publications/diseases-conditions/tuberculosis-canada-2014-pre-release.html.

Royal College of Physicians and Surgeons of Canada (RCPSC). 2013. *Indigenous Health Values and Principles Statement*. Ottawa: RCPSC. http://www.royalcollege.ca/portal/page/portal/rc/common/documents/policy/indigenous_health_values_principles_report_e.pdf.

Sinclair, M., M. Wilson, and W. Littlechild. 2015. *Truth and Reconciliation Commission Canada Executive Summary*. http://www.trc.ca/websites/trcinstitution/File/2015/Honouring_the_Truth_Reconciling_for_the_Future_July_23_2015.pdf.

Statistics Canada. 2011. "Census: Aboriginal Peoples in Canada in 2006." Last modified April 5. http://www12.statcan.gc.ca/census-recensement/2006/as-sa/97-558/p6-eng.cfm.

Statistics Canada. 2014. "Inuit in Canada: Selected Findings of the 2006 Census." Last Modified April 23. http://www.statcan.gc.ca/pub/11-008-x/2008002/article/10712-eng.htm.

Statistics Canada. 2015a. "Canada (Code 01) (Table). National Household Survey (NHS) Aboriginal Population Profile. 2011." Catalogue no. 99-011-XWE2011007. Last modified November 30. http://www12.statcan.gc.ca/nhs-enm/2011/dp-pd/aprof/index.cfm?Lang=E.

Statistics Canada. 2015b. "Chart 13: Projected Life Expectancy at Birth by Sex, by Aboriginal Identity, 2017." Last modified November 30. https://www.statcan.gc.ca/pub/89-645-x/2010001/c-g/c-g013-eng.htm.

Statistics Canada. 2018. "Infant Mortality Rates, by Province and Territory." Last modified February 23. http://www.statcan.gc.ca/tables-tableaux/sum-som/l01/cst01/health21a-eng.htm.

Young, T. Kue, Jeff Reading, Brenda Elias, and John D. O'Neil. 2000. "Type 2 Diabetes Mellitus in Canada's First Nations: Status of an Epidemic in Progress." *CMAJ* 163 (5): 561–6.

CHAPTER 7

Exploring the Development of a Health Care Model Based on Inuit Wellness Concepts as Part of Self-Determination and Improving Wellness in Northern Communities

Gwen K. Healey

LEARNING OBJECTIVES

After reading this chapter, you should be able to:

1. Appreciate variation in health determinants and health inequities between Indigenous and non-Indigenous populations in Canada.
2. Recognize differing world views on wellness, such as the biomedical world view and the Indigenous world view.
3. Understand the impact of Canada's colonial history in the North on Inuit communities.

Indigenous Canadians have historically had poorer health status than other Canadians, with higher rates of infectious diseases, injuries, suicide, heart disease, and diabetes within Indigenous populations (Reading and Wien 2009; Waldram, Herring, and Young 2007). While there have been improvements in the life expectancy and infant mortality rate among Indigenous communities in recent years, Indigenous peoples' overall health status remains far below that of the general population (Lavallée and Poole 2010; Health Canada 2003; King, Smith, and Gracey 2009). As a result, it continues to be an important focus for researchers and policy-makers.

Health care in Indigenous communities in Canada has largely focused on the application of Western or non-Indigenous approaches to understanding wellness. Indigenous communities have long promoted definitions of wellness that generally differ from conventional Western biomedical disease- and treatment-based definitions of health (King, Smith, and Gracey 2009). Many Indigenous wellness concepts share a common focus on the mental, emotional, spiritual, and physical aspects of being well and living well, and encapsulate a holistic belief in the importance of balance (King, Smith, and Gracey 2009). Recently, a growing body of literature has focused on articulating Indigenous knowledge perspectives on wellness, which has also contributed to a more meaningful understanding of the challenges experienced by Indigenous communities (Healey, Noah, and Mearns 2016; Chilisa 2012; Iseke and Moore 2012; Battiste 2000, 2002; Brady 1995).

In the Canadian North, the territorial governments administer most health services, except in Yukon, where some programs and services have been transferred to First Nations communities (Young and Chatwood 2011). Although the movement to self-determination for Indigenous peoples has advanced the most in Nunavut and Greenland, self-government and control of health services have not translated into better health outcomes (Young and Chatwood 2011; Galloway and Saudny 2012; NTI 2008).

In this chapter, I will first provide an overview of historic and contemporary events in Nunavut; I will then summarize the transition of this Arctic region over the last several decades and the context of Inuit community health and wellness concerns today. Lastly, I will share Inuit concepts, which can inform a model for health care that reflects the values of the people it serves.

HISTORICAL CONTEXT

Inuit are the Indigenous inhabitants of the North American Arctic; their homeland stretches from the Bering Strait to East Greenland—a distance of over six thousand kilometres. Inuit live in Russia, Alaska, Greenland, and the Canadian Arctic and, despite the distances between communities, share a common cultural heritage, language, and genetic ancestry. Inuit have occupied these Arctic regions for five thousand years (ITK 2005). Of the approximately 150,000 Inuit living in the circumpolar region today, 50,000 live in the four Canadian *Nunangat* (Inuit lands): Nunavut, Nunavik (Northern Quebec), Inuvialuit (northern Northwest Territories), and Nunatsiavut (northern Labrador); approximately 10,000 Inuit live in urban Canadian centres (Statistics Canada 2016). Nunavut, the largest region, became Canada's third territory in 1999.

(RE)SETTLEMENT

Before the arrival of other peoples, Inuit lived a nomadic lifestyle in *ilagiit nunagivaktangat*[1] or camps. Although the process of relocation to communities began as a response by Inuit to the presence of traders, explorers, and missionaries, it took new form with the systematic efforts of the government in the 1950s to "resettle" Canada's North. At that time, the Canadian government implemented resettlement programs in the eastern Arctic. Through these programs, Inuit were moved to more remote areas to protect Canada's sovereignty and trade and into centralized settlements to reduce relief costs. Documentation from that time indicates that resettlement programs facilitated the provision of supplies and supported policing efforts, and also assisted with the implementation of formal education and improved access to health care for remote populations (INAC 1996; Kirmayer, Brass, and Tait 2000). The *Report of the Royal Commission on Aboriginal Peoples* noted that in these years, government administrators were concerned with the reports of health and welfare coming out of the North, and they came to see the North as being in a state of crisis; this hastened the government initiative to form settlements (INAC 1996). Tuberculosis epidemics among Inuit people required immediate attention. Inuit children were also enveloped in the residential school system and separated from their families (King 2006). Early in this period, one high-ranking official wrote that his job was "to hasten the day when in every respect the Eskimos can take their own places in the new kind of civilization which we—and they—are building in their country" (Phillips 1957). This idealized view, which did not take into account the perspectives of Inuit, was never realized (QIA 2010). Kirmayer, Tait, and Simpson (2009) argued that over the past century, Canadian and American government policies have maintained the initial processes of colonization and have destroyed Indigenous cultures and ways of life through forced settlement, the creation of reserves, relocation to remote regions, residential schools, chronic underfunding, and poor resourcing of essential services such as health care, education, and bureaucratic control. In the process, opportunities have arisen in which Inuit advocated for and implemented adapted styles of leadership and coordination into the new situation, which resulted in the creation of several land claims agreements (QIA 2010).

The changes imposed on Inuit by the Canadian government were rapid—this was not a gradual progression from a traditional to a modern way of life, but a complete transformation (QIA 2010). Inuit were not consulted about these changes, and many never knew why they were imposed. For their part, the government agencies that were responsible for the transformation, primarily Indian and Northern Affairs Canada and the RCMP, are still not fully aware of their own history in the Arctic or the effects of their decisions and actions (QIA 2010). A few settlements had originated as trading posts, so they remained close to good hunting and harvesting areas. For the remaining posts, the single most important criterion for government was that they were accessible by sea or would fit into planned air routes; therefore, many of the settlements were not located near sufficient harvesting areas (INAC 1996; QIA 2010). For example, the community of Arviat, Nunavut,[2] was built on a coastal swamp, far from the inland caribou herds, which Inuit had followed for centuries and which are still harvested by the community today. The report of the Qikiqtani Truth Commission stated that Inuit have suffered and continue to suffer from this lack of attention to their hunting and harvesting needs, and this has played a critical role in wellness (QIA 2010; Kral et al. 2011).

CONTEMPORARY CONTEXT

Today, there are 25 communities in Nunavut ranging in population size from 150 to 7,100 (NBS 2013). All the communities are geographically isolated from each other and in winter are only accessible by air, water, or snowmobile. The population of Nunavut in 2016 was 35,944, of whom approximately 85 percent are Inuit (Statistics Canada

2017). Fifty-two percent of *Nunavummiut* speak the Inuit languages of Inuktitut or Inuinnaqtun at home (Statistics Canada 2013). Nunavut has a very young population compared to Canada as a whole. In 2011, 57.3 percent of its population comprised individuals aged 24 years and younger, compared to 29.2 percent in the whole of Canada (Statistics Canada 2013). Today, there is a chronic shortage of housing contributing to overcrowding among many families with young children in almost every community in Nunavut (Egeland, Faraj, and Osborne 2010; Statistics Canada 2010). Influences from media, television, the education system, and other sources (Condon 1987, 1990, 1995), as well as residential schooling (Kirmayer, Brass, and Tait 2000; Pauktuutit 2007), related traumas (Curtis, Kvernmo, and Bjerregaard 2005; Kirmayer, Tait, and Simpson 2009; Waldram, Herring, and Young 2007; Wolsko et al. 2007), and settlement into larger communities (Archibald 2004; Healey 2016), have contributed to a shift in traditional ways of life in contemporary communities.

Pervasive social determinants in Nunavut such as poverty, lack of adequate housing and overcrowding, food insecurity, and trauma are intermeshed with the quality of life for many Nunavummiut (NDH&SS 2005; Cameron 2011). Public health services and health promotion initiatives are largely the domain of the government of Nunavut's Department of Health. These programs consist of maternal-child health supports (e.g., well-baby clinics, immunization clinics, breastfeeding support, prenatal nutrition programs), chronic disease management, environmental health monitoring and supports, anti-tobacco use initiatives, sexual health surveillance and education, infectious disease control, oral health treatment and education, and nutrition and food security initiatives (Government of Nunavut Department of Health n.d.).

Nunavut has one hospital (in Iqaluit) and two large health centres in regional centres (Rankin Inlet and Cambridge Bay) staffed by physicians. Health centres staffed by community health nurses service the rest of Nunavut's communities, and physicians make visits throughout the year. Specialized services are accessed at tertiary care facilities in Yellowknife, Edmonton, Winnipeg, or Ottawa, if more advanced or complex care is required (Chatwood and Marchildon 2012).

The association between Indigenous self-government, community control of health services, and health equity is complex and is influenced by a multitude of political, social, and economic factors. Funds for health care in Nunavut originate from the federal government (NTI 2008). Even though the biomedical part of the system is core-funded, its funds are insufficient to pay for a system that is so widely spread out and so heavily dependent on hospitals and medical professionals based in southern Canada (NTI 2008). This unwieldy, fragmented, and logistically stretched biomedical system is not sustainable. Nunavut Tunngavik Incorporated (NTI 2008) has asserted that the health care system must evolve into a truly Nunavut-centred system. This can begin with a primary health care approach, which is based on Indigenous and Inuit philosophical concepts related to wellness. Such an approach would allow the healing and wellness strengths of Inuit culture and society to flourish as integral parts of the health system.

INDIGENOUS HEALTH CARE MODELS

Significant advances have been made to *engage* Indigenous communities in health care and research; however, there remains a need for health care models that are *born from* Indigenous perspectives on wellness, from the design to the implementation and delivery (Healey and Tagak 2014; Kovach 2009; Prior 2006; Wilson 2008). Current biomedical models operate under the assumption that illness is secondary to disease (Wade and Halligan 2004). The assumption that a specific disease underlies all illness has led to the medicalization[3] of some conditions that are simply part of the human experience, such as menopause or aging (Conrad 2007). It has also led to the disbelief of patients who present with illness without any demonstrable disease (Wade and Halligan 2004). Indigenous wellness perspectives are formulated on understandings of the world, which are based on interactions between people, as well as interactions with the land, animals, and spirit worlds (Chilisa 2012; Deloria 1995; Wilson 2008). Illness may originate from a place of disharmony rather than simply disease of the body, and wellness can be achieved by restoring emotional and spiritual balance, as well as by treatment of a physical ailment (Lavallée 2007). This differs from the common Western practice of focusing on the individual in isolation, outside of the individual's place in society or in connection to the land, animal, and spirit worlds. In an exploration of Indigenous healers in practice in the modern world, Solomon and Wane (2005) describe a Mi'kmaq healer who is able to determine a client's ailment and its cause and advise a remedy, and who is the keeper of the "shake-tent," through which he can directly intervene with the spirits and the Creator on behalf of the client(s). Requiring total darkness, the shake-tent lodge is known to be the highest of sacred ceremonies among Mi'kmaq, in which all types of healing is possible. The story of Zulu, an Indigenous healer of African ancestry, is also shared: she notes that Indigenous healing takes different forms depending on each situation (Solomon and Wane 2005). Zulu stated that in her experience, healers might prescribe a spiritual bath, which is a formal acknowledgment that something needs to be done about one's physical, mental, or emotional well-being. She also noted that traditional medicines are part of sacred practices that cannot be shared, discussed, or used without the respect and integrity passed down by the Ancestors. In a study of Inuit women's perceptions of pollution, Egan (1998) found that women identified pollution of the land to be linked to mental health and wellness in the community. From the perspective of participants, changing relationships with the land carried over into changing relationships in the community and substance use, ultimately affecting the health of the community overall (Egan 1998).

The concept of relationships is essential in the Indigenous world view, which is primarily "relational" (Thayer-Bacon 2003) and is something rarely discussed in the biomedical health care system. Supporting the relationships between the patient and his or her health care providers is as important in achieving wellness as supporting and understanding the relationship between the patient and their broader societal context. In Southcentral Alaska, for example, the "Nuka System of Care" is the name given to the health care system that was created, managed, and owned by Alaskan Native communities to achieve physical, mental, emotional, and spiritual wellness (Southcentral Foundation of Alaska n.d.). *Nuka* is an Alaskan Native word used for strong, giant structures and living things. The relationship-based Nuka System of Care is made up of organizational strategies and processes; medical, behavioural, dental, and traditional practices; and supportive infrastructure—all of which work together, in a relationship, to support wellness. By putting relationships at the forefront of what health care practitioners and administrators do and how they do it, the Nuka System was designed to continue to develop and improve for future generations (Southcentral Foundation of Alaska n.d.).

INUKTITUT CONCEPTS TO INFORM A HEALTH CARE MODEL IN NUNAVUT

Several concepts exist in Inuktitut, which convey the rich wellness perspective of Inuit. These include, but are not limited to, the Inuit concepts of *Inuuqatigiittiarniq* ("being respectful of all people"), *Unikkaaqatigiinniq* ("storytelling"), *Pittiarniq* ("being kind and good"), *Inuusiqatigiinniq* ("the way of being a person"), and *Piliriqatigiinniq* ("working together for the common good").

Inuuqatigiittiarniq

Inuuqatigiittiarniq is the Inuit concept of respecting others, building positive relationships, and caring for others. When each person considers their relationships to people and behaves in a way that fosters this relationship, they build strength in themselves and in others, and together as a community (Karetak 2013). This is foundational to Inuit ways of being (Karetak 2013). In the health context, part of building and fostering respectful relationships is clearly articulating one's intentions and motivations. Health care professionals need to be reflexive and ask themselves the questions that community members will inevitably ask them: Who are you? Where are you from? Who is your family? What are you doing here? What will happen to the knowledge that I share with you? How can we learn from each other? A commitment to an approach that values the relationships between system actors and users could help improve the efficacy of the system overall because it is based on the values of the people it is designed to serve.

Unikkaaqatigiinniq

Unikkaaqatigiinniq is the Inuit concept related to storytelling, the power of story, and the role of story in Inuit ways of being. In an Indigenous context, story is methodologically congruent with tribal knowledge (Wilson 2008). Inuit have a very strong oral history and oral culture. The telling of stories is a millennia-old tradition for the sharing of knowledge and the communicating of values, morals, skills, histories, legends, and artistry. Storytelling is a critical aspect of the Inuit way of life and ways of knowing (Bennet and Rowley 2004), and it allows respondents to share personal experiences without breaking cultural rules related to confidentiality, gossip, or humility. In a study of health determinants for Inuit women in Nunavut, participants drew upon examples and stories from the community to illustrate points about important health issues, such as teenage pregnancy and custom adoption, which further highlighted aspects of the health context involving the community, society, education, and cultural identity (Healey 2006; Healey and Meadows 2008). Although some Inuit knowledge or practices may be disappearing, the use of story to effectively communicate information remains part of life. It is for this reason that the recognition of the power of story is particularly important in the context of the health of Inuit.

Pittiarniq

Pittiarniq is the Inuit concept of "being good," which can be meant in a philosophical and moral sense but also in terms of action, such as "good behaviour" (e.g., in the case of children's behaviour). In Inuktitut, two terms have been discussed in the context of ethical conduct in a health or research setting. The first, shared by McGrath (2004), is *Pittiaq-*, which is related to "being good, kind, or well; doing good or rightly." McGrath argued that the term *Pittiaq-* refers to both technical and moral excellence. Without knowledge or experience of Inuit societal values, researchers from outside of the culture and epistemology interpret doing/being good (ethics) based on their own world views and assumptions about what "good" is. Although well-intended, those decisions can have a range of negative impacts on their particular research participants or even on Inuit society in general (McGrath 2004). The second term, shared by another community member who declined to be named, is *Inuuqatigiittiarniq*, which, as mentioned earlier, is related to the concept of being respectful of others. Both terms refer to behaviour—that one's actions are reflective of one's intention to "do good." As such, one will be respectful of other people and of the relationships between and among the facets of the interaction. Above all, everyone must be treated with respect, appreciation, and dignity (Beauchamp and Childress 2001; CIHR, NSERC, and SSHRC 2010; Flicker et al. 2007; McGrath 2004). A commitment to an approach that is mindful of and focuses on Inuit context, knowledge, questions, and perspectives is an integral part of demonstrating respect for the community at large.

Inuusiqatigiinniq

Inuusiqatiginniq is the Inuktitut concept of "the way of being a person." It can have different meanings in different contexts and, in general, is the term used to convey a holistic view of wellness. Holistic caring and healing models aim to treat the whole person—not just the illness in isolation—and take into account their environmental context, behaviours, and relationships, as well as multiple other factors, with the intent of offering a wide range of solutions to improve one's health (Montgomery Dossey and Keegan 2013). Holistic caring and healing practices have been promoted widely by Indigenous groups but have not featured prominently in practice (Montgomery Dossey and Keegan 2013). In 2014, the World Health Organization launched a strategy for improving the integration of traditional and Indigenous medical perspectives and medicines into health care approaches, including health services and systems, and traditional and complementary medicine products, practices, and practitioners (WHO 2014).

These concepts underscore the right of all Indigenous peoples to construct a health system in accordance with the self-determined definitions of what contributes to wellness and how we reach that goal over the life spectrum.

Piliriqatigiinniq

Piliriqatigiinniq is the concept for working in a collaborative way for the common good. Multidisciplinary collaboration strengthens programs, fosters greater sharing of knowledge, and promotes implementation of promising practices. The Qaujigiartiit[4] Health Research Centre developed a model for health research, which is based on a collaborative, multi-sectoral approach to developing and implementing projects. This model was developed in response to the community-identified need for health research that explores topics of concern to Nunavummiut and that is collected, analyzed, and disseminated in a holistic and collaborative way. The Piliriqatigiinniq model is a representation of the web of relationships individuals have with each other and is built upon the principle that anyone can be involved in advancing health in some capacity if all are working for the common good. The model serves as a reminder to look beyond the scope of what is commonly defined as *health* and *research* to include knowledge holders and stakeholders from multiple disciplines and walks of life.

CONCLUSION

Health care systems can and should mirror the values of the people they serve. In Nunavut, such systems should promote health care models that are grounded in Inuit ways of knowing and understanding wellness. Such models are a critical part of the ongoing self-determination processes for Indigenous communities. Truly understanding, and taking action of, the health challenges experienced in northern communities requires us to be critical of the models that are conventionally used; to challenge the dominant narratives of the origins of health inequities in our communities; and to design systems that reflect the world views of our communities.

CRITICAL THINKING QUESTIONS

1. Reflect upon your knowledge of Canada's North prior to reading the chapter. Did your knowledge of health determinants include the colonial history with Indigenous peoples? In what way will this knowledge influence your practice or work in the health field?
2. How does the content of this chapter differ from the narrative about Inuit communities that dominates national media coverage? Do you perceive a difference? If so, why do you think that difference exists?
3. Reflect upon whether or not the health care system you access emulates the values that are most important to you and the community you come from. Are they connected or disconnected? In what ways are they similar or different?

ADDITIONAL RESOURCES

Health NU App

In September 2017, the Qaujigiartiit Health Research Centre launched the "Health NU" orientation application (app) to bring forward the voices of our communities to welcome and orient new members of the health care workforce in Nunavut. Qaujigiartiit created the app in consultation with community members and health care providers to address a community-identified need for improved cultural and health systems orientation for health care providers. The app content was developed by Qaujigiartiit Health Research Centre and the technological and design aspects were developed by Pinnguaq Technology Inc (https://pinnguaq.com/). The app contains sections on the following: the ways we communicate and Inuktitut language resources; our history and settlement; the values of our families and communities; patient/client expectations in the health care setting; Nunavut's health care model and referral pathways; how to make mental health referrals for patients; preparing for your arrival; recommended readings, films, books, and websites; and an interactive map of Nunavut, with community-specific information including average weather, average cost of foods, maps, key phone numbers, and links to community Facebook pages. The app is available on both the Google Play store and the iOS App store free of charge: https://www.qhrc.ca/news/health-nu-launch.

NOTES

1. This is Inuktitut terminology, meaning "a place used regularly or seasonally by Inuit for hunting, harvesting and/or gathering" (QIA 2010).
2. Formerly known as Eskimo Point.
3. *Medicalization* refers to process by which non-medical problems become defined and treated as medical problems, usually in terms of illness and disorders (Conrad 2007).
4. *Qaujigiartiit* is the Inuktitut word for "looking for knowledge."

REFERENCES

Archibald, L. 2004. *Teenage Pregnancy in Inuit Communities: Issues and Perspectives*. Report prepared for the Pauktuutit Inuit Women's Association. Ottawa: Pauktuutit Inuit Women's Association.

Battiste, M. 2000. *Reclaiming Indigenous Voice and Vision*. Vancouver: UBC Press.

Battiste, M. 2002. *Indigenous Knowledge and Pedagogy in First Nations Education: A Literature Review with Recommendations*. Ottawa: Government of Canada, Department of Indian and Northern Affairs (INAC).

Beauchamp, T., and J. Childress. 2001. *Principles of Biomedical Ethics*. 5th ed. Oxford: Oxford University Press.

Bennet, J., and S. Rowley. 2004. *Uqalurait: An Oral History of Nunavut*. Montreal: McGill-Queen's University Press.

Brady, M. 1995. "Culture in Treatment, Culture as Treatment: A Critical Appraisal of Developments in Addictions Programs for Indigenous North Americans and Australians." *Social Science & Medicine* 41 (11): 1487-98.

Cameron, E. 2011. *State of the Knowledge: Inuit Public Health, 2011*. Prince George, BC: National Collaborating Centre for Aboriginal Health.

Canadian Institutes of Health Research (CIHR), Natural Sciences and Engineering Research Council (NSERC), and Social Sciences and Humanities Research Council of Canada (SSHRC). 2010. *Tri-Council Policy Statement: Ethical Conduct for Research Involving Humans*. Ottawa: Government of Canada.

Chatwood, S., and G. Marchildon. 2012. "Chapter 3: Northern Canada in *A Comparative Review of Circumpolar Health Systems* (Young & Marchildon, Eds.)." *International Journal of Circumpolar Health* 9 (suppl): 41-52.

Chilisa, B. 2012. "Postcolonial Indigenous Research Paradigms." In *Indigenous Research Methodologies*, edited by B. Chilisa, 98-127. Thousand Oaks, CA: Sage.

Condon, R. G. 1987. *Inuit Youth: Growth and Change in the Canadian Arctic*. London: Rutgers University Press.

Condon, R. G. 1990. "The Rise of Adolescence: Social Change and Life Stage Dilemmas in the Central Canadian Arctic." *Human Organization* 49: 266-79.

Condon, R. G. 1995. "The Rise of the Leisure Class: Adolescence and Recreational Acculturation in the Canadian Arctic." *Ethos* 23 (1): 47-68.

Conrad, P. 2007. *The Medicalization of Society: On the Transformation of Human Conditions into Treatable Disorders*. Baltimore, MD: Johns Hopkins University Press.

Curtis, T., S. Kvernmo, and P. Bjerregaard. 2005. "Changing Living Conditions, Life Style and Health." *International Journal of Circumpolar Health* 64 (5): 442-51.

Deloria, V. 1995. *Red Earth, White Lies: Native Americans and the Myth of Scientific Fact*. New York: Scribner.

Egan, C. 1998. "Points of View: Inuit Women's Perceptions of Pollution." *International Journal of Circumpolar Health* 57: 550-4.

Egeland, G.M., N. Faraj, and G. Osborne. 2010. "Cultural, Socioeconomic, and Health Indicators among Inuit Preschoolers: Nunavut Inuit Child Health Survey, 2007–2008." *Rural and Remote Health* 10 (2): 1365.

Flicker, S., R. Travers, A. Guta, S. McDonald, and A. Meagher. 2007. "Ethical Dilemmas in Community-Based Participatory Research: Recommendations for Institutional Review Boards." *Journal of Urban Health* 84 (4): 478–93.

Galloway, T., and H. Saudny. 2012. "Nunavut Community and Personal Wellness, Inuit Health Survey (2007–2008)." Montreal: Centre for Indigenous Peoples' Nutrition and the Environment, McGill University.

Government of Nunavut Department of Health. n.d. "Department of Health." Accessed June 17, 2014. http://www.gov.nu.ca/health.

Health Canada. 2003. "Closing the Gaps in Aboriginal Health." Last modified August 4, 2009. http://www.hc-sc.gc.ca/sr-sr/pubs/hpr-rpms/bull/2003-5-aboriginal-autochtone/index-eng.php.

Healey, G. 2006. "An Exploration of Determinants of Health for Inuit Women in Nunavut." MA thesis, University of Calgary.

Healey, G. 2016. "(Re)Settlement, Displacement, and Family Separation: Contributors to Health Inequity in Nunavut." *Northern Review* 42: 1–22.

Healey, G., and L. Meadows. 2008. "Tradition and Culture: An Important Determinant of Inuit Women's Health." *Journal of Aboriginal Health* 4 (1): 25–33.

Healey, G., J. Noah, and C. Mearns. 2016. "The Eight Ujarait (Rocks) Model: Supporting Inuit Adolescent Mental Health with an Intervention Model Based on Inuit Ways of Knowing." *International Journal of Indigenous Health* 11 (1): 92–110. https://doi.org/10.18357/ijih111201614394.

Healey, G., and A. Tagak, Sr. 2014. "Piliriqatigiinniq 'Working in a Collaborative Way for the Common Good': A Perspective on the Space Where Health Research Methodology and Inuit Epistemology Come Together." *International Journal of Critical Indigenous Studies* 7 (1): 1–14.

Indian and Northern Affairs Canada (INAC). 1996. "Relocation of Aboriginal Communities." In *Report of the Royal Commission on Aboriginal Peoples (Canada)*, vol. 1, edited by INAC, 395–522. Ottawa: Government of Canada.

Inuit Tapiriit Kanatami (ITK). 2005. *5000 Year Heritage*. Ottawa: ITK.

Iseke, J., and S. Moore. 2012. "Community-Based Indigenous Digital Storytelling with Elders and Youth." *American Indian Culture and Research* 35 (4): 19–38.

Karetak, J. 2013. *Conversations of Inuit Elders in Relation to the Maligait (Inuit Laws)*. Transcripts of dialogues with Inuit elders. Arviat, NU: Nunavut Department of Education, Curriculum Support Services.

King, D. 2006. *A Brief Report of The Federal Government of Canada's Residential School System for Inuit*. Prepared for the Aboriginal Healing Foundation. Ottawa: Aboriginal Healing Foundation.

King, M., A. Smith, and M. Gracey. 2009. "Indigenous Health Part 2: The Underlying Causes of the Health Gap." *Lancet* 374 (9683): 76–85.

Kirmayer, L. J., G. M. Brass, and C. L. Tait. 2000. "The Mental Health of Aboriginal Peoples: Transformations of Identity and Community." *Canadian Journal of Psychiatry* 45: 607–16.

Kirmayer, L. J., C. L. Tait, and C. Simpson. 2009. "Mental Health of Aboriginal Peoples in Canada: Transformations of Identity and Community." In *Healing Traditions: The Mental Health of Aboriginal Peoples in Canada*, edited by L. J. Kirmayer and G. G. Valaskis, 3–35. Vancouver: UBC Press.

Kovach, M. 2009. *Indigenous Methodologies: Characteristics, Conversations, and Contexts*. Toronto: University of Toronto Press.

Kral, M. J., L. Idlout, J. B. Minore, R. J. Dyck, and L. J. Kirmayer. 2011. "Unikkaartuit: Meanings of Well-Being, Happiness, Health, and Community Change among Inuit in Canada." *American Journal of Community Psychology* 48: 426–38.

Lavallée, L. 2007. "Physical Activity and Healing through the Medicine Wheel." *Pimatisiwin* 4: 127–53.

Lavallée, L., and J. Poole. 2010. "Beyond Recovery: Colonization, Health and Healing for Indigenous People in Canada." *International Journal of Mental Health and Addiction* 8: 271–81. https://doi.org/10.1007/s11469-009-9239-8.

McGrath, J. T. 2004. "Translating Ethics across the Cultural Divide in Arctic Research: Pittiarniq." Unpublished manuscript.

Montgomery Dossey, B., and L. Keegan. 2013. *Holistic Nursing: A Handbook for Practice*. Burlington, MA: Jones and Bartlett Learning.

Nunavut Bureau of Statistics (NBS). 2013. *Nunavut Population Estimates by Community*. Panniqtuuq, NU: Government of Nunavut.

Nunavut Department of Health and Social Services (NDH&SS). 2005. *Nunavut Department of Health and Social Services Social Determinants of Health in Nunavut. Workshop Report, March 8–10*. Iqaluit, NU: Government of Nunavut.

Nunavut Tunngavik Incorporated (NTI). 2008. *Annual Report on the State of Inuit Culture and Society: Nunavut's Health System*. Iqaluit, NU: Nunavut Tunngavik Inc.

Pauktuutit. 2007. *Sivumuapallianiq: National Inuit Residential Schools Healing Strategy; The Journey Forward*. Ottawa: Pauktuutit Inuit Women's Association of Canada.

Phillips, R. A. J. 1957. "Letter from R. A. J. Phillips, Chief of the Arctic Division, Canada to Bishop (Anglican) Donald Marsh, 16 December 1957." Northwest Territories Archives, Alexander Stevenson fonds, N-1992-023, box 17, file 7, Policy—Inuit 1935–1959.

Prior, D. 2006. "Decolonizing Research: A Shift toward Reconciliation." *Nursing Inquiry* 14 (2): 162–8.

Qikiqtani Inuit Association (QIA). 2010. *Qikiqtani Truth Commission Final Report: Achieving Saimaqatigiingniq*. Iqaluit, NU: Inhabit Media.

Reading, C., and F. Wien. 2009. *Health Inequalities and Social Determinants of Aboriginal Peoples' Health*. Prince George, BC: National Collaborating Centre for Aboriginal Peoples' Health. https://www.ccnsa-nccah.ca/docs/determinants/RPT-HealthInequalities-Reading-Wien-EN.pdf.

Solomon, A., and N. N. Wane. 2005. "Indigenous Healers and Healing in a Modern World." In *Integrating Traditional Healing Practices into Counseling and Psychotherapy*, edited by R. Moodley and W. West, 52–95. Thousand Oaks, CA: Sage.

Southcentral Foundation of Alaska. n.d. "Southcentral Foundation: Nuka System of Care." Accessed May 15, 2017. https://www.southcentralfoundation.com/nuka/.

Statistics Canada. 2010. *An Analysis of Housing Needs in Nunavut: Nunavut Housing Survey 2009–2010*. Edited by the Income Statistics Division. Iqaluit, NU: Statistics Canada.

Statistics Canada. 2013. "Population by Home Language, by Province and Territory (2011 Census) (Northwest Territories, Nunavut)." Last modified February 13. http://www.statcan.gc.ca/tables-tableaux/sum-som/l01/cst01/demo61d-eng.htm.

Statistics Canada. 2016. "Aboriginal Peoples in Canada: First Nations People, Métis and Inuit." Catalogue no. 99-011-X. Last modified September 15. http://www12.statcan.gc.ca/nhs-enm/2011/as-sa/99-011-x/99-011-x2011001-eng.cfm.

Statistics Canada. 2017. "Provincial/Territorial Profiles: Nunavut, 2016 Census." Catalogue no. 98-316-X2016001. Last modified November 16. http://www12.statcan.gc.ca/census-recensement/2016/dp-pd/prof/details/Page.cfm?Lang=E&Geo1=PR&Code1=62&Geo2=&Code2=&Data=Count&SearchText=Nunavut&SearchType=Begins&SearchPR=01&B1=All&GeoLevel=PR&GeoCode=62.

Thayer-Bacon, B. 2003. *Relational Epistemologies*. New York: Peter Lang.

Wade, D., and P. Halligan. 2004. "Do Biomedical Models of Illness Make for Good Health Care Systems?" *British Medical Journal* 329: (7479): 1398–401.

Waldram, J. B., A. Herring, and T. K. Young. 2007. *Aboriginal Health in Canada: Historical, Cultural, and Epidemiological Perspectives*. Toronto: University of Toronto Press.

Wilson, S. 2008. *Research Is Ceremony: Indigenous Research Methods*. Blackpoint, NS: Fernwood.

Wolsko, C., C. Lardon, G. V. Mohatt, and E. Orr. 2007. "Stress, Coping and Well-Being among the Yup'ik of the Yukon-Kuskokwim Delta: The Role of Enculturation and Acculturation." *International Journal of Circumpolar Health* 66 (1): 51–62.

World Health Organization (WHO). 2014. *WHO Traditional Medicine Strategy: 2014–2023*. Geneva: World Health Organization.

Young, K., and S. Chatwood. 2011. "Health Care in the North: What Canada Can Learn from its Circumpolar Neighbours." *Canadian Medical Association Journal* 183 (2): 209–14.

CHAPTER 8

Fostering Resilience with Indigenous Youth

Bonnie M. Freeman

LEARNING OBJECTIVES

After reading this chapter, you should be able to:

1. Explain how the holistic perspectives of health contributes the well-being of Indigenous people.
2. Appreciate how various Indigenous cultural initiatives foster and support Indigenous youth in enhancing health and social determinants.
3. Explain how Indigenous resilience is a protective factor in opposing inequalities of health and social determinants.

For many generations, First Nations people have experienced substantial oppression and social injustice resulting from policies of colonization and assimilation, leaving families and communities frustrated, depressed, full of anger, and hopeless (McKenzie and Morrissette 1993; Kirmayer, Simpson, and Cargo 2003; Reading and Wien 2009; Manson et al., 1996; Gagné 1998; Lederman 1999; Quinn 2007). According to *A Statistical Profile on the Health of First Nations in Canada: Report* (First Nations 2003), First Nations people under the age of 30 years make up over half (55 to 60 percent) of the total Aboriginal population. As the population of First Nations people continues to increase, so do many of the issues and problems Native youth are facing. The *Report of the Royal Commission on Aboriginal People* (Government of Canada 1996) describes how First Nations youth are enduring the loss of cultural identity, high rates of poverty, limited employment opportunities, overcrowding and inadequate living conditions, weakened social structures, racism, and a lack of recognition by mainstream society (Reading and Wien 2009).

For many Native youth, these demoralizing conditions have contributed to increased substance abuse, suicide and violence, and fatalities among Aboriginal children and youth

(Olson and Wahab 2006; Strickland, Walsh, and Cooper 2006; Chandler and Lalonde 1998). Various reports have indicated that suicides among Native youth are five to six times higher than the national average (White 2005; First Nations & Inuit Health 2003). Indigenous scholar Barbara Waterfall (2002) recognizes that the present-day conditions of Native people are "very grave" and are having a profound impact on children: "Addictions and violence are everyday occurrences. Many of our children do not want to live anymore. They do not see any hope" (150). What is very frightening is that the age at which Native youth are attempting suicide has become younger and younger.

Along with the high rates of trauma and violence in many First Nations communities, youth have limited outlets and services by which to express their frustrations and pain (First Nations & Inuit Health 2003). Communities such as Davis Inlet have witnessed gas/glue sniffing and addiction among their youth (Press 1995). In 2005, the school shootings that occurred in the Native community of Red Lake, Minnesota, had a tremendous impact on many people across the United States and Canada (*CBC News* 2005). Incidents such as these leave communities and social service organizations questioning the fragmentation of policies and services that are supposed to help Indigenous people.

There are many practitioners across North America incorporating cultural knowledge in an effort to bring positive changes to the demoralizing living and health conditions of Native communities, as well as to bring awareness to the historical injustices that have impacted these communities over generations. Indigenous people have struggled to preserve and maintain the long-existing cultural knowledge, beliefs, and values, which are firmly rooted within their communities. Gregory Cajete (1994) shares that regardless of the exhibited problems, Indigenous people's "cultural roots run deep":

> It is true that much has been lost in the wholesale assaults on Indian culture during the past 500 years. But, the cultural roots of Indian ways of life run deep. Even in communities where they seem to have totally disappeared, they merely lie dormant, waiting for the opportunity and the committed interest of Indian people to start sprouting again.... The tree may seem lifeless, but the roots still live in the hearts of many Indian people. (192)

Indigenous cultural roots are a part of healing, and healing begins with reconnecting to a system of cultural knowledge that honours the spirit of Indigenous people through the relationships with the land, ancestors, family, community, natural elements of the environment, and the animals. Cultural knowledge is conveyed through collectivity, ceremonies, and cultural practices upon the land, and connection with the natural environment; it produces a "good mind" and a bond to the "spirit-body-mind-self in relation to everything that is" (Voss et al. 1999, 86).

Health practitioners trying to understand and resolve Indigenous problems and issues from a Western perspective fail to consider the cultural knowledge that exists within Indigenous communities (Morrissette, McKenzie, and Morrissette 1993). Suzanne

Stewart (2008) found that several factors that are necessary for positive Indigenous health and wellness. Such positive factors include community, collectivity, cultural identity, a holistic approach, and spirituality. Stewart's *holistic approach* when working with Indigenous communities included food, ceremony, use of Elders or traditional healers, taking clients into nature, or attending community social events. An important component in Stewart's Indigenous mental health wellness model was *interdependence*—this refers to the establishment and maintenance of relationships and alliances throughout the client's life. Interdependence does not only include Indigenous associations; Indigenous clients have expressed that they want mainstream health care systems to connect with resources that are culturally appropriate and will assist them in their healing. A participant from Stewart's (2008) study expressed that she was hopeful that the mainstream health system would shift to a true health model of healing and well-being when caring for Indigenous communities: "I am hopeful that the mainstream [health system] and the funding will shift away from the illness/mainstream model and to incorporating cultural views and holistic view of mental health and healing that are about interdependence" (17).

Another area that was noted and lacking in a Western approach to health was *spirituality*: "Spirituality has been in Aboriginal culture for 12,000 [or more] years, has been a big part of life for Aboriginal people ... that's something that I believe, and I advocate for.... Spirituality is a big component of what clients need to heal" (Stewart 2008, 16). The Indigenous perspectives of interdependence and spirituality contribute and support the *cultural identity* of an Indigenous client. Therefore, the Indigenous client learns and experiences cultural practices, Native language, and spiritual ceremonies that increase an Indigenous person's self-esteem and pride. One of Stewart's participants shared the following experience:

> The reality is that if you don't have some iota or some speck [of understanding] of yourself as a person on the planet that has value and connectedness to who you are [culturally], it is very hard to change behaviour, build on behaviour, change thinking, build on different skills or abilities that will change your day-to-day experiences. (Stewart 2008, 15)

Marie Roué's (2006) work with the James Bay Cree demonstrates how a lack of culture and language integration into community programs and school initiatives can lead to an entire generation of youth with the inability to know themselves as Cree. Cree youth are "in the difficult situation of double social exclusion and marginalization" (Roué 2006, 18) from their community and mainstream society. There are some incidences where Indigenous youth find Western approaches and interventions helpful as a starting point in exploring their health and wellness. However, other Indigenous youth will simply appease their parents or the courts by attending treatment programs with no effort to really change (Morrissette, McKenzie, and Morrissette 1993; Kirmayer, Simpson, and Cargo 2003). Stewart (2008) and Duran (2006) caution health workers and practitioners against using a

Eurocentric perspective and/or intervention with Indigenous people, as this can perpetuate the oppression and colonization that already exists. Such an approach needs to change. Health practitioners need to broaden their views of health and well-being and take leadership from Indigenous communities. Kirmayer, Simpson, and Cargo (2003) note that many health programs and services lack the participation and leadership of Indigenous people and youth in creating such programs, thus failing to meet the needs of Indigenous youth or to benefit the overall community. In ancient traditional social structures, Indigenous "youth had a place in traditional decision-making processes, today they are largely excluded from community decision-making and are the passive recipients of mental health programs and services designed and delivered through centralized state decision-making processes" (Kirmayer, Simpson, and Cargo 2003, S21).

What we have learned from this is that by incorporating cultural knowledge and grassroots initiatives as they pertain to health and well-being, many individual and familial health elements such as depression, addictions, and low self-esteem experienced by Indigenous youth can be reduced and treated (Morrissette, McKenzie, and Morrissette 1993). Theresa O'Nell (1996), in her research with the Flathead Salishan tribes in Montana, for example, concluded that emotion and collectivity play an important role among Indigenous people and is the underlying construct of Indigenous well-being. Emotion connects and is expressed through culture, relationships, family/kinship, and the natural environment (O'Nell 1996; Thomas and Bellefeuille 2006). Therefore, emotion becomes a cultural prompter to positive behaviours and social action within Indigenous communities: "Emotion ... moves from being enveloped within the body to being situated in the dialogue between persons, their social circumstances, and cultural interpretations that organize the self-vis-à-vis those circumstances" (O'Nell 1996, 214).

Two studies (Morrissette, McKenzie, and Morrissette 1993; McKenzie and Morrissette 1993) highlight one of the earliest documented youth programs (1988), which evolved out of child care services in Winnipeg, Manitoba. An important aspect of this model was an acknowledgement of the generational impact of colonization, oppression, and marginalization experienced by urban Indigenous people. This acknowledgement recognizes the pain and trauma Indigenous people have endured over generations as a step to understanding and observing the healing process and resilience within individuals. The Winnipeg youth program incorporated the knowledge of Elders and cultural teachings, with an emphasis on the participation and leadership of Indigenous youth (Morrissette, McKenzie, and Morrissette 1993; McKenzie and Morrissette 1993).

Another example of initiatives that promote health and well-being among Native youth are the bush camp programs, which immerse youth in cultural knowledge and land-based activities with Elders. Roué (2006) shares the experience of Cree youth with bush camp programs while they overcome issues such as addictions, behavioural problems, violence, low self-esteem, and lack of connection to Cree identity. Through the joint efforts of the James Bay Cree community and Cree Health Board, bush camps were originally designed for youth who were not integrating well in school and suffered delinquency, alcohol/drug abuse, and/or suicide attempts (Roué 2006). Usually, youths facing such crisis situations were dangerous to themselves, their families, and their communities. Bush camp programs connected Cree youth with Elders who knew how to use their traditional Cree knowledge of the land and cultural practices to care for and build up a youth's self-esteem and identity (Roué 2006). Cree Elder Robbie Matthew, who was involved with the bush camp program for many years, explained that when young Indigenous men and women go on the land, they are "searching for knowledge and know-how, [and] they are also engaged in a spiritual quest":

> By going on the land of their ancestors, they receive from their elders the spiritual bond to the land that by accident their own parents were unable to transmit to them. Suffice it for me to describe how a very young man—a rebel in great suffering—lived through a spiritual experience with his great-uncle, which, according to his own family, radically transformed him. (Roué 2006, 20)

Therefore, it is of utmost importance for Elders and cultural knowledge holders to design and be involved with programs that encourage and promote health and well-being among Indigenous youth. Cultural knowledge, practices/know-how, and spirituality as it relates to the land and natural environment transform Indigenous youth and connect them back to their identity and collective lineage (Roué 2006), therefore healing Indigenous youths' spirit and providing them with a strength—a resilience central to their Indigenous nationhood and supported by their family and community. Heavy Runner and Marshall (2003) explain the importance of Indigenous resilience:

> [Resilience] … is the natural, human capacity to navigate life well. It is something every human being has—wisdom, common sense. It means coming to know how you think, who you are spiritually, where you come from, and where you are going. The key is learning how to utilize resilience, which is the birthright of every human being. It involves understanding our inner spirit and finding a sense of direction. (14)

As a cautionary note in understanding the concept of resilience, Hanewald (2011) describes resilience as a "positive adaptation in the face of severe adversities; vulnerability is a feature that renders a person more susceptible to a threat and risk is any factor that increases the chance of an undesirable outcome affecting a person" (22). However, critiques of youth resilience view the concept of resilience not as a quality or a characteristic that a person automatically possess. Rather, resilience fluctuates and varies throughout a person's development, depending on the environmental factors and resources that interact and impact at different points in an individual's life (Hanewald 2011). Howard, Dryden, and Johnson (1999) bring attention to practitioners labelling children and youth as resilient, as this could be dangerous, setting vulnerable youth up for failure. While youth may be able to face one sort of adversity, they may not be able to overcome broader societal risks or adversities such as poverty (Fergus and Zimmerman 2005). Risks and/or adversities also may differ between youth at varying socioeconomic levels, as well as between youth that live in urban or rural areas.

Keeping the cautionary notes in mind, a study by Dell, Dell, and Hopkins (2005; see also Dell et al. 2008) also explores the concept of Native resilience as it relates to Wolin's traits of resilience in two Indigenous youth treatment facilities. Both treatment facilities include a cultural and holistic (physical, mental, emotional, and spiritual) approach to treatment. However, the two facilities also had the goal of nurturing the resilience of the Indigenous youth they were working with and wanted to teach the connection between the inner spirit (strengths) and external spirit (family and community) through Indigenous cultural teachings and practices. As Indigenous youth went through this treatment process, they were able connect their sense of self-worth (inner spirit) to the value of collective support and belonging in their family and community (external spirit). As a result, Indigenous youth learned to balance their internal and external spirits and seek support from both in the healing and rebuilding of their lives through the means of culture, spirituality, and community resources (Dell, Dell, and Hopkins 2005). Table 8.1 illustrates how Dell and colleagues (2005, 2008) connected Wolins's seven resiliency traits to traditional Native teachings.

Table 8.1 provides the fundamental support for success in connecting a youth to their sense of purpose, which is at the core of resilience and improves the health and well-being of Indigenous youth through the context of Indigenous cultural knowledge, values, beliefs, and practices (e.g., sweat lodges, vision quests, fasting, horses) through the notion of resilience (Dell et al. 2008): "Personal wellness and improved health status for Native Americans is going to be one of the vehicles by which the strengthening of Nations can be achieved.... As so many of the elders and supporters ... say, 'it begins with the youth'" (Skye 2002, 133).

Table 8.1. Comparing Western and Indigenous Resilience Traits

Wolins's Resiliency Traits	Traditional Native Teachings
Morality	Interconnectedness, respect, humility, faith
Humour	Teasing as acceptance and welcome, balancing the seriousness of life, facilities learning
Creativity	Survival, tool making, continuance of life
Initiative	Personal courage, integrity, freedom, autonomy, promotion of wholeness and quality of life for all
Relationships	Kinship, sharing, unconditional love, generosity, community
Independence	Mastery, taking on of adult roles, courage, non-interference, reciprocity
Insight	Vision questing/fasting, strength, knowledge of self in relation to all else, identifying development in relation to gender, spirit name, and clan

Source: Wolins's Resiliency Traits in Dell, Dell, and Hopkins (2005, 6).

CULTURE AS A FOUNDATION FOR RESILIENCE AMONG INDIGENOUS YOUTH

Resilience within an Indigenous context encompasses purpose, cultural knowledge and practices, spirituality, connection to the land, ceremonies, Indigenous language, and the meaning of being Indigenous in the current day (identity and well-being). Michael Hart (2002) expresses that Indigenous people need "to recapture [their] peoples' language, history and understanding of the world, [and] take and live those teachings which will support [them] in this attempt to overcome oppression and reach *mino-pimatisiwin—the good life*" (32).

An underlying motivation for resilience is a sense of purpose through the means of culture. For Indigenous people, purpose may be in the form of awareness and taking a stand against the social injustice that their community or they as Indigenous people experience within society. Resilience, for some Indigenous youth, is an awakening to the spiritual and healing connection they have with their culture regarding their ancestral past and present and how it will affect future generations (Freeman 2015). For some Indigenous people, this spiritual awakening is delivered through dreams, prayers, or visions (Taylor 1996); for others, the awakening is not delivered until they become actively engaged with a ceremony or community initiative that awakens their spirit. Some examples of Indigenous youth experiencing this spiritual and cultural awakening is through their participation in the Oomaka Tokatakiya—the Future Generations Ride (Lakota youth), the Spirit of the Youth Unity Run, 2005–2008 and 2011 (Haudenosaunee youth), and the Protecting Our Mother Walk (Grassy Narrows youth). These journeys incorporated the Indigenous concept of *mino-pimatisiwin* (the good life) by connecting youth, Elders, and communities to their ancestral lands, history, languages, and cultural knowledge of health and well-being as a reformation back to the collectivity of their nation:

> This [walk] is a spiritual journey not a protest.... We walk to protect Mother Earth.... Every day brings another message. The idea for the walk came from a spiritual dream and it also came out of frustration of seeing all these people being arrested for trying to stand up for the land and their rights. (Martin 2008)

Indigenous resilience is a *holistic experience*. The physicality of such a collective journey awakens the mind and reaches down to the emotion and spirit of an individual. An Indigenous person can see their past, present, and future through this experience (Freeman 2015). The aunt of one of the youth expressed the following: "Our young people are experiencing a spiritual awakening.... I'm proud to see that warrior spirit coming out in them as we journey" (Martin 2008). A young man who recently became a father shared his realization while on the Protecting Our Mother Walk: "Becoming involved with my people has become a life-changing experience," he said. "I will probably miss my son's first steps, but I think of it as if I am taking them for him out here on the road" (Martin 2008).

There are many Indigenous community cultural initiatives assisting Indigenous youth, their families, and their communities to reclaim their resilience as a people. To do so is to heal from the generational traumas and reach deep down to the essence of the people through their culture and spirituality by connecting to their ways of knowing and being (Freeman 2015; Absolon 2011). This strengthens the cultural identity, health, and well-being of each individual member, as well as family and community members. Chandler and Lalonde (1998) revealed that Indigenous communities in British Columbia had lower rates of suicide due to a higher degree of social and cultural cohesion within the community. The authors referred to this community cohesion as *cultural continuity*, which relates to Indigenous communities having self-determination over land title, self-government, control of education, cultural-based facilities, and control over policies and practices of health and social programs (Chandler and Lalonde 1998). Cultural continuity also involves social connectedness, which is maintained through family and Elder engagement that passes cultural knowledge and practices to the next generations (Chandler and Lalonde 1998, 121). Reading and Wien (2009) have indicated through their study on health inequalities and social determinants that Indigenous self-determination is a vital determinant of health, influencing all other determinants, and that Indigenous communities need to be involved with "political decision making, control over lands, economies, education systems and social and health services" (23–24). However, the authors highlight the restrictive political environment in which Indigenous communities are challenged with exercising their self-determination over health policies and practices: "Equity requires authority and freedom, with authority involving material, psychosocial and political domains. Unfortunately, colonial governments and institutions do not act upon evidence, resulting in unequal participation of Aboriginal people in political institutions that govern their fate" (Reading and Wien 2009, 23–24).

CONCLUSION

The strength and resilience of Canadian Indigenous communities reside in the cultural knowledge, language, and epistemology of Indigenous people's health and well-being. Unfortunately, there is little empirical evidence and research from a Western perspective to substantiate that resilience is a determinate for good health and well-being. While there are cautionary perspectives to keep in mind as resilience is explored among youth, it is important to understand that resilience is not a characteristic trait and that resilience can vary depending on the geographical location and access to resources. However, from their perspective, Indigenous people have relied on their resilience and belief in their spirituality, cultural knowledge, and practices, as well as the connection to the land and natural environment, to support, preserve, and heal following generations of hardships and traumas. It is this kind of resilience that is central and foundational to the spirit and essence of Indigenous nations (Freeman 2015).

CRITICAL THINKING QUESTIONS

1. Reflect on the protective factors central to Indigenous resilience. How can Western models of health reconcile the inequalities of health and social determinants in Indigenous communities?
2. What structural changes need to happen on a political, economic, and social level to support Indigenous people's self-determination towards good health and well-being?
3. What kinds of Indigenous metrics can be used to support the notion of resilience as it relates to the impact of health and the improvement of social determinants?

RECOMMENDED READINGS

Dapice, A. N. 2006. "The Medicine Wheel." *Journal of Transcultural Nursing* 17 (3): 251–60.

Dillard, D. A., and S. M. Manson. 2000. "Assessing and Treating American Indians and Alaska Natives." In *Handbook of Multicultural Mental Health*, edited by Israel Cuéllar and Freddy A. Paniagua, 225–48. San Diego: Academic Press.

Fleming, J., and R. J. Ledogar. 2008. "Resilience and Indigenous Spirituality: A Literature Review." *Pimatisiwin: A Journal of Aboriginal and Indigenous Community Health* 6 (2): 47–64.

Fleming, J., and R. J. Ledogar. 2008. "Resilience, an Evolving Concept: A Review of Literature Relevant to Aboriginal Research." *Pimatisiwin: A Journal of Aboriginal and Indigenous Community Health* 6 (2): 7–23.

Hunter, L. M., J. Logan, J. Goulet, and S. Barton. 2006. "Aboriginal Healing: Regaining Balance and Culture." *Journal of Transcultural Nursing* 17 (1): 13–22.

LaFramboise, T. D., D. R. Hoyt, L. Oliver, and L. Whitebeck. 2006. "Family, Community, and School Influences on Resilience among Native American Adolescents in the Upper Midwest." *Journal of Community Psychology* 34 (2): 193–209.

Strickland, C. J., E. Walsh, and M. Cooper. 2006. "Healing Fractured Families: Parents' and Elders' Perspectives on the Impact of Colonization and Youth Suicide Prevention in a Pacific Northwest American Indian Tribe." *Journal of Transcultural Nursing* 17 (1): 5–12.

Whitebeck, L. B., G. W. Adams, D. R. Hoyt, and X. Chen. 2004. "Conceptualizing and Measuring Historical Trauma among American Indian People." *American Journal of Community Psychology* 33 (3/4): 119–30.

Wilson, K. 2003. "Therapeutic Landscapes and First Nations Peoples: An Exploration of Culture, Health and Place." *Health & Place* 9: 83–93.

Wilson, K., and M. W. Rosenberg. 2002. "Exploring the Determinants of Health for First Nations Peoples in Canada: Can Existing Frameworks Accommodate Traditional Activities?" *Social Science & Medicine* 55: 2017–31.

Wilson, W. A. "Indigenous Knowledge Recovery Is Indigenous Empowerment." *American Indian Quarterly* 28 (3/4): 359–72.

REFERENCES

Absolon, K. 2011. *Kaandossiwin: How We Come to Know*. Halifax: Fernwood.

Cajete, G. 1994. *Look to the Mountain: An Ecology of Indigenous Education*. Durango: Kivaki.

CBC News. 2005. "Teenage Killer Used Police Vest, Car." March 22. http://www.cbc.ca/news/world/teenage-killer-used-police-vest-car-1.547906.

Chandler, M. J., and C. Lalonde. 1998. "Cultural Continuity as a Hedge against Suicide in Canada's First Nations." *Transcultural Psychiatry* 35 (2): 191–219.

Dell, C. A., D. Chambers, D. Dell, E. Sauve, and T. MacKinnon. 2008. "Horse as Healer: An Examination of Equine Assisted Learning in the Healing of First Nations Youth from Solvent Abuse." *Pimatisiwin: A Journal of Aboriginal and Indigenous Community Health* 6 (1): 81–106.

Dell, C. A., D. Dell, and C. Hopkins. 2005. "Resiliency and Holistic Inhalant Abuse Treatment." *International Journal of Aboriginal Health* 2 (1): 4–12.

Duran, E. 2006. *Healing the Soul: Wound Counseling with American Indians and Other Native Peoples*. New York: Teachers College Press.

Fergus, S., and M. A. Zimmerman. 2005. "Adolescent Resilience: A Framework for Understanding Healthy Development in the Face of Risk." *Annual Review Public Health* 26: 399–419.

First Nations. 2003. *A Statistical Profile on the Health of First Nations in Canada: Report*. Ottawa: Health Canada.

First Nations & Inuit Health. 2003. *Acting on What We Know: Preventing Youth Suicides in First Nations*. Ottawa: Government of Canada.

Freeman, B. 2015. "The Spirit of Haudenosaunee Youth: The Transformation of Identity and Well-Being through Culture-Based Activism." PhD diss., Wilfrid Laurier University.

Gagné, M. 1998. "The Role of Dependency and Colonialism in Generating Trauma in First Nations Citizens: The James Bay Cree." In *International Handbook of Multigenerational Legacies of Trauma*, edited by Y. Danieli, 355–72. New York: Plenum.

Government of Canada. 1996. *Report of the Royal Commission on Aboriginal People*. Ottawa: Government of Canada.

Hanewald, R. 2011. "Reviewing the Literature on 'At-Risk' and Resilient Children and Young People." *Australian Journal of Teacher Education* 36 (2): 16–29.

Hart, M. A. 2002. *Seeking Mino-Pimatisiwin: An Aboriginal Approach to Helping*. Halifax: Fernwood.

Heavy Runner, I., and K. Marshall. 2003. "Miracle Survivors: Promoting Resilience in Indian Students." *Tribal College Journal* 14 (4): 14–19.

Howard, S., J. Dryden, and B. Johnson. 1999. "Childhood Resilience: Review and Critique of Literature." *Oxford Review of Education* 25 (3): 307–23.

Kirmayer, L., C. Simpson, and M. Cargo. 2003. "Healing Traditions: Culture, Community and Mental Health Promotion with Canadian Aboriginal Peoples." *Australasian Psychiatry* 11 (suppl): S15–23.

Lederman, J. 1999. "Trauma and Healing in Aboriginal Families and Communities." *Native Social Work Journal* 2 (1): 59–90.

Manson, S., J. Beals, T. O'Nell, J. Piasecki, D. Bechtold, E. Keane, and M. Jones. 1996. "Wounded Spirits, Ailing Hearts: PTSD and Related Disorders among American Indians." In *Ethnocultural Aspects of Posttraumatic Stress Disorder: Issues, Research and Clinical Applications*, edited by A. J. Marsella, M. J. Friedman, E. T. Gerrity, and R. M. Scurfield, 255–83. Washington, DC: American Psychological Association.

Martin, C. 2008. "Chrissy Takes a Walk. To Toronto. With Her friends." *SooToday.com*, May 14. http://www.sootoday.com/content/news/full_story.asp?StoryNumber=32042.

McKenzie, B., and V. Morrissette. 1993. "Cultural Empowerment and Healing for Aboriginal Youth in Winnipeg." In *Rebirth Political, Economic and Social Development in First Nations*, edited by Anne-Marie Mawhiney, 117–30. Toronto: Dundurn.

Morrissette, V., B. McKenzie, and L. Morrissette. 1993. "Towards an Aboriginal Model of Social Work Practice: Cultural Knowledge and Traditional Practices." *Canadian Social Work Review* 10 (1): 91–108.

Olson, L. M., and S. Wahab. 2006. "American Indians and Suicide: A Neglected Area of Research." *Trauma, Violence & Abuse* 7 (1): 19–33.

O'Nell, T. D. 1996. *Disciplined Hearts: History, Identity and Depression in an American Indian Community*. Berkeley: University of California Press.

Press, H. 1995. "Davis Inlet in Crisis: Will the Lessons Ever Be Learned?" *Canadian Journal of Native Studies* 15 (2): 187–209.

Quinn, A. 2007. "Reflections on Intergenerational Trauma: Healing as a Critical Intervention." *First Peoples Child & Family Review: A Journal on Innovation and Best Practices in Aboriginal Child Welfare Administration, Research, Policy & Practice* 3 (4): 72–82.

Reading, C. L., and F. Wien. 2009. *Health Inequalities and Social Determinants of Aboriginal Peoples Health*. Prince George, BC: National Collaborating Centre for Aboriginal Health.

Roué, M. 2006. "Healing the Wounds of School by Returning to the Land: Cree Elders Come to the Rescue of a Lost Generation." *International Social Science Journal* 58 (187): 15–24.

Skye, W. 2002. "E.L.D.E.R.S. Gathering for Native American Youth: Continuing Native American Traditions and Curbing Substance Abuse in Native American Youth." *Journal of Sociology and Social Welfare* 29 (1): 117–203.

Stewart, S. L. 2008. "Promoting Indigenous Mental Health: Cultural Perspectives on Healing: From Native Counsellors in Canada." *International Journal of Health Promotions & Education* 46 (2): 12–19.

Strickland, C. J., E. Walsh, and M. Cooper. 2006. "Healing Fractured Families: Parents' and Elders' Perspectives on the Impact of Colonization and Youth Suicide Prevention in a Pacific Northwest American Indian Tribe." *Journal of Transcultural Nursing* 17 (1): 5–12.

Taylor, J. 1996. "Mending the Sacred Hoop of the Lakota Nation: The Chief Big Foot Memorial Rides [*Si Tanka Wokiksuye Okolakiciy*]: A Teaching Case Study in Tribal Management for Oglala Lakota College." *Harvard Project on American Indian Economic Development*. Kyle, SD: Oglala Lakota College.

Thomas, W., and G. Bellefeuille. 2006. "An Evidence-Based Formative Evaluation of a Cross Cultural Aboriginal Mental Health Program in Canada." *Australian e-Journal for the Advancement of Mental Health* 5 (3): 1–14.

Voss, R. W, V. Douville, A. L. Soldier, and A. White Hat, Sr. 1999. "Wo'Lakol Kiciyapi: Traditional Philosophies of Helping and Healing Among the Lakotas: Toward a Lakota-Centric Practice of Social Work." *Journal of Multicultural Social Work* 7 (1/2): 73–93.

Waterfall, B. 2002. "Native People and the Social Work Profession: A Critical Exploration of Colonizing Problematics and the Development of Decolonized Thought." *Journal of Educational Thought* 36 (2): 149–66.

White, J. 2005. *Preventing Youth Suicide: Taking Action with Imperfect Knowledge. A Research Report Prepared for the British Columbia Ministry of Child and Family Development Children's Mental Health Policy Research Program.* Vancouver: University of British Columbia.

SECTION III

INNER-CITY AND OTHER SPECIAL POPULATIONS

SECTION INTRODUCTION BY S. LUCKETT-GATOPOULOS

Growing up, I spent many nights sleeping on couches, floors, and pullout couches. I shared beds with other kids or slept in sleeping bags. Sometimes I had a bedroom. Once I moved to the couch because a hole opened up in my bedroom ceiling, letting the snow in. I closed the door to that room and never opened it again. I was temporary, transient, often on the move.

The night before starting Grade 8, my father suddenly appeared. He had slunk off several months before, leaving me, with his ex-girlfriend and her children, and financial and emotional destruction in his wake. When my father showed up unannounced, I gathered together my belongings into a cardboard box and a plastic bag and packed them into his busted-up van, leaving yet another temporary family to move into a one-bedroom basement apartment. Just prior to my final year of high school, I was kicked out of my father's and new stepmother's home, and subsequently evicted from the place with the hole in the bedroom ceiling.

I reconnected with my mother, whom I hadn't seen since I was nine or ten years old, and moved in with her, my step-father, and my toddler half-brother. Soon we were joined by another half-brother, 18 years my junior, and, briefly, yet another of my younger brothers. Predictably, the house was steeped in conflict. I was grateful for the relative stability of that family unit and for my bed in the basement, but leaving for university was a relief.

Early in my undergraduate program, I floundered, nearly dropping out, first because of poor grades and later due to my inability to pay tuition. Eventually, with the generous and unexpected support of my aunt and uncle, I finished my undergraduate degree. A caring professor suggested I pursue medicine. Up to that time, my mind had been so occupied with survival that I hadn't seriously considered career aspirations.

I scraped together the money to write the MCAT, but it wasn't easy. Not only was there registration to pay, but I also had to buy a prep book. That summer, I worked in a research lab and studied in the library every day after work. From there, I would work out in the school gym and head home or to my serving job at a local restaurant. Maybe it was bad luck, maybe it was poor preparation, or maybe it was the stress of working hard for something I wasn't sure I deserved. That first time, I did very poorly on the MCAT.

I pursued a year-long college program in sign language, an avoidance strategy that allowed me to delay paying back my student loans. I applied to graduate school. I rewrote the MCAT. This time, I still worked while studying, but finding money for registration was less of a financial hardship with the graduate school stipend, work income, and support of my uncle and aunt. I did well and applied to medical school.

I soon learned that the MCAT was only the first financial hurdle to medical school. I applied to a limited number of schools because of the application fees, charges for transcripts, and all the other incidental expenses that come along with the process. But I did apply, and was offered interviews. I was accepted. I became a medical student and, eventually, an emergency medicine resident.

Since I started residency, I've told this story many times. It took me a long time to admit out loud that I was different than many of my peers, but I have come to accept that my story is not just unusual but also important in the way that it speaks about how we grow into ourselves as physicians, and implicitly about how we can make change within the medical education system, and within health care itself.

I often hear my colleagues joke about patients who come into the emergency department. Many are angry at the stupid decisions that bring patients to the point of poor health that we all pay for in a universal health care system. Sometimes I join in their frustration. I hear suggestions that we should limit access to the emergency department, that people should pay for their poor choices by being restricted from receiving ongoing high-cost care. The uneducated, poor, and socially disadvantaged are disproportionately the brunt of jokes and the carriers of the blame for the state of Canadian health care. It may be unfair, but I don't blame my colleagues.

Until you have slept on a park bench, it's hard to understand the series of non-choices that brings people there. Until you have fed yourself for a week on a 97-cent packet of plain spaghetti with margarine, it's hard to imagine why people can't just eat healthier food. Medical school is full of many wonderful people who strive to contribute in positive and meaningful ways. I've met students from a variety of cultural and religious backgrounds: some straight, others queer; some parents, others still living at home; some are from rural and remote communities, others from urban centres. Yet few have experienced the barriers to good health and education that come from very low socioeconomic status. Because of that, few can relate to the poor health and low socioeconomic status that many of our patients experience.

We have created a highly competitive system for admission to medical school that ensures that the most academically gifted students become physicians. This isn't a bad thing; medical school is difficult and requires smarts. But making change requires the compassion and empathy that come from experience. It demands perspective-taking. It calls upon us to be kind and non-judgmental, not just pleasant or nice.

As you ponder the evidence presented in these chapters, please remember my story and imagine how carers and providers like me, when admitted into the closed society of medicine, may develop into change-makers who can help inform and shape our shared vision of health care for all Canadians. Consider whether it might be easier to develop empathy if people from a variety of socioeconomic, ethnic, and other backgrounds were not merely patients but also valued colleagues. As you read through this section and the book, I urge you to consider how increasing diversity within our health care education system might also build a bridge, providing yet another link in a steadily growing chain, bringing us closer to the social and health equity that we seek.

Timeline: Minimal Supports for the Bottom of the Labour Market

Joe Mancini

1960s: Social policy in the 1960s benefited from the post-war economy that created average wages that allowed a family to own a house and a car and still have savings.

1980s: By the 1980s, the end of the Fordist period changed the nature of the economy. Wage growth was now stagnated and the number of unemployed climbed, while part-time, temporary jobs increased. A growing consumer economy gobbled up leftover wages. The federal government experimented with more generous forms of unemployment insurance. The *Transitions* report in Ontario called for an overhaul of social assistance.

1990s: Governments across Canada engaged in social policy retrenchment. In Ontario, the Harris government reversed labour reforms and reduced social assistance rates by 24 percent. In Alberta, the Klein government reduced public spending by 15 percent. The federal government clawed back unemployment insurance by making it increasingly difficult to gain eligibility. Drastic reductions in federal government provincial transfer payments resulted in provincial social spending cutbacks.

2000s: The temporary/part-time labour market continued to grow, representing 20 percent of the labour market by 2005. Self-employment grew to 15 percent of the labour market, but only half of this group earned a living wage.

2010s: Between 1980 and 2010, hundreds of thousands of workers lost jobs from the closing of large manufacturing factories. Only minimal job search assistance and re-training grants are offered to this group of workers.

CHAPTER 9

Historical Roots—Why in a Time of Unprecedented Wealth and Health Do We Have Homelessness and Ill Health?

Joe Mancini

LEARNING OBJECTIVES

After reading this chapter, you should be able to:

1. Recognize the relationship between unemployment and ill health.
2. Recognize economic trends that affect psychosocial integration.
3. Learn to recognize how economic conditions can directly impact the size of the population of people who are homeless.
4. Relate the issues and stories discussed in this chapter to your own family biography of work and compare your circumstances with Paul's (from the case study) to gain a wider understanding of the influence of socioeconomic conditions.

INTRODUCTION

This chapter reflects on the development of Canadian social policy in the post-war period, which I hope to show has been subordinate to the needs of the capitalist labour market. Even development of equitable social infrastructure in areas of income, health, and workers' rights may be subservient to the primary goal of ensuring job creation by the private sector. A line can be traced between longer bouts of unemployment and reduced stable employment to growing homelessness and dislocation, as between 1980 and 2010 those at the bottom of the labour market were left with temporary, part-time, and low-wage jobs. Table 9.1 addresses the origins of broader social trends impacting on precarious income and housing.

However, things are beginning to change. As 2018 began, Ontario, for example, launched a number of social policy initiatives including a substantial increase in minimum

Table 9.1. Historical Timeline of Economic Trends in North America

Period	Years	Characteristics
Fordist Period	1945–1975	This period refers to the long post-war economic boom that was typified by mass production and mass consumption, protected domestic markets, the rise of industrial unions, and the use of Keynesian economic policies. The Fordist era peaked with the oil shocks of 1973 and the resulting high inflation in Western countries.
Neo-liberalism and Globalization Period	1975–2008	Policies were enacted to reduce the power of labour unions, reduce social safety net benefits, and increase the use of temporary and contract labour. New trading rules allowed for increased offshoring using labour from low-wage countries. Technology changes included job automation, information network technology, financialization, and mobile communication.
The Great Recession Period	2009–Present	Governments try to deal with slow growth, high unemployment, and chronic deficits. Increased automation and new artificial intelligence (AI) applications threaten higher job loss in manufacturing and service employment. Unstable economic conditions continue.

Source: Adapted from Galbraith (2014).

wage, looser rules for navigating social assistance income, along with a pilot project to investigate basic income and universal drug coverage for those under age 25. Meanwhile, the Liberal federal government has rearranged the Canadian Child Tax Benefit to make it significantly more generous. Are these new social initiatives designed to lessen the impact of huge job losses that will result from robotic and artificial intelligence advances? Or are these economic initiatives more holistic, about building an economy of solidarity where the benefits of Canada's prosperous economy are shared? It is up to the reader to analyze the goal of Canadian social policy as the 2020s approach. This limited review of Canadian social policy gives the reader one perspective from which to judge.

THE PROCESS OF DEINDUSTRIALIZATION AND GROWING UNEMPLOYMENT

There are two streams of thought on how social policy is developed in Canada. The first line of thinking analyzes every policy initiative as an attempt to develop equitable social infrastructure in areas of income, health, and worker rights. The second stream is less optimistic: it views social policy as secondary to the needs of the capitalist economy. In this view, Canadian social policy between 1980 and 2010 can be summarized as policies designed to ensure those at the bottom of the labour market have little choice but to take low-wage jobs. The economy needs low-wage workers to choose work over social assistance to keep the economy humming along. This chapter takes the position that social policy during the past three decades has been unforgiving to those that have faced increased unemployment and reduced job opportunities. The exact history is less important than the actual resulting increases in joblessness, homelessness, and dislocation, which demonstrate declining social results.

In the period following the Second World War until the 1970s, full-time, long-term jobs were the norm, while the safety net of unemployment insurance supported workers when they were unemployed. In the early 1980s, the reduction in industrial jobs through automation, offshoring, and the use of temporary labour began a process which substantially disrupted both the labour market and the social income safety net. As part of the process of deindustrialization, under pressure from business leaders who questioned the social safety net, and reacting to growing deficits, politicians throughout Canada, federally and provincially, passed legislation in the 1990s making unemployment insurance and social assistance more difficult to access.

In the opinion of business and government bureaucrats, the labour market was a tough place, and too many workers were finding generous social income more satisfying than labour income. The result was that workers would have little choice but to rely on the labour market for income. An example of the tightening process across the country is the federal and Ontario provincial government changes regarding unemployment insurance. Employment Insurance, the new name for the Canada-wide worker's income insurance scheme, devised rules so that 70 percent of the unemployed in Ontario no longer qualified for benefits. Ontario Works, the new name for social assistance, was designed as workfare legislation with rules that could automatically close the file of a recipient who did not respond within a week to a computer-generated tracking letter. Such methods, combined with the 24 percent reduction in the amount of benefits people could receive, left people scrambling for the safety of the job market. There, they found part-time and temporary jobs that paid eight or ten dollars an hour.

Workers who competed against each other soon discovered a built-in system to keep wages in check. The growing use of temporary job placement agencies to hire part-time workers was a mechanism that served to reduce the wage and benefit costs of hiring workers. By 2015, the phrase *contingent labour force* was an accurate way to describe this growing group of workers made up of unemployed and temporary workers, often comprising over a third of the labour market (Lewchuck 2014; Vosko and Noack 2012).

Until the mid-1990s, the word *homeless* was not commonly used. For example, the group we worked with in downtown Kitchener that drifted through the workforce was not considered homeless, as they were still hopeful for their social prospects. However, that

Case Study: Paul

One of the first patrons to come to St. John's Kitchen (see the case study of St. John's Kitchen in Guenter, Oudshoorn, and Mancini, Chapter 15 in this volume) was a big, strapping 30-year-old labourer with a blonde flowing mullet, who often did not have work. His work boots signified that he came from a working-class family that had to fend for itself in a harsh world. Details of the challenges his family faced, whether alcohol abuse, mental health, violence, or abuse, were troubling. The sum of it is that Paul grew up in a world where either his family would rise above these realities or they would be overwhelmed in a downward spiral. Could his father keep his job? Could his mother keep the family together? Families that give way to alcohol abuse or experience mental health challenges often must deal with violence, frustration, and shame. Depression, anger, and alcohol-fuelled violence can leave a family's dignity tattered; they certainly did for Paul's family. Their sons and daughters scattered, trying to make sense of it all.

During those early years, we knew little about Paul's family. He would tell us about a trauma he experienced at his birth. He was sure the newspapers had covered it, and in later years, he would desperately ask us to help him find the article. But despite the compelling story, politicians and social service administrators weren't interested in stories—they wanted hard data. St. John's Kitchen had been open only six months, in June 1985, when a Social Resource Council survey found that Paul was typical of those who came to the Kitchen. He was an unemployed man under 35 who lived in the downtown area, mostly in rooming houses within 10 blocks of the Kitchen. The survey of 87 people showed that half were single, 72 percent had lived in Waterloo Region for two years or more, 17 percent had no income, while 70 percent lived on less than 400 dollars a month.

Paul's circumstances in life coincided with the 1980s labour market that developed a bias against surplus workers with a Grade 10 education. In the late 1970s, Paul and workers like him found work at the rubber plant, in pork production, at auto parts companies, and at shoe and boot manufacturers. By the 1980s, all these factories were under pressure as production moved offshore and new technology displaced workers. It was at this point that Paul started to see himself as a temporary worker. Many efforts were made to find him full-time work opportunities, but each work placement failed.

Full-time work soon became temporary work, and in Paul's mind, this fitted his lifestyle, as he was not altogether committed to being a full-time construction or factory worker. It is also true that no company came forward to champion Paul, to give him a chance to prove himself. Paul did not exactly fall through the cracks; he was way too big for that, and he could yell way too loud. But he was easy to ignore as he walked away when he could not meet societal expectations. After 20 years, the best job he could get was with the Working Centre's street cleaning team (see the description of the Working Centre in Chapter 15), and even then he constantly complained, but with his gargantuan stature and a broom, he exuded a dignity that made everyone know he was special.

> Street life took its toll on Paul, and he was rarely content in his last 10 years. He could threaten violence, give a big bear hug, and reminisce in a quick interaction. He would yell, "Why don't you help me? I can't live on the street anymore." He was known to break glass windows and doors when he pounded in frustration. The outreach program tried its best to find apartments that could accommodate Paul's larger-than-life personality. At his memorial service, his niece told the story of how sad she would feel when her mother would drive Paul to the House of Friendship hostel. "Why does he not want to live in a house?" she would wonder. Paul would visit his sister once a month, but he wanted no help from his family. One friend of his told of how tough he and Paul were. Before churches provided the Out of the Cold shelters, "they used to sleep under the back Working Centre porch covered in blankets and cardboard through rain, snow and ice. We would do anything to live free on the street."
>
> Paul was a member of the St. John's Kitchen community for almost 25 years before he passed away. Many like Paul live full lives on the edges of society, where they are never fully accepted, always scouting out a place to spend the night. Many cannot work because of the unresolved trauma or substance use that is circling through their head. They have a ready reason for their choices: "You may have been born into privilege, but I had no such luck." Several, by their actions, swear off work, finding acceptable excuses to refuse to become a cog in the working world. In Paul's case, he realized early on that he was at the bottom rung of society, with no chance of climbing. Instead, he developed strong friendships on the street and helped his fellow travellers through the good and the bad.

soon started to change. Jack Layton's (2000) landmark book on homelessness identified what social groups were already seeing on the ground, analyzing two decades of Canadian housing policy that failed to increase the supply of affordable housing. He also established the link between reduced affordable housing and increased job dislocation.

In retrospect, the period since 1980 has been a vicious cycle of dislocation, with workers quitting the labour market in frustration and a growing group of people who are chronically homeless in the downtowns of all Canadian cities. There is a direct correlation between loss of work and declining self-esteem. Many who become "dislocated from the integrated society in which they grew up ... turn[ed] to methamphetamine addiction, alcoholism, and other addictive habits to fill the voids in their lives" (Alexander 2011). Without work, those born into a fragmented social reality, often without parents or abused in their youth, have no leverage in their search for psychosocial integration. Increasingly, research demonstrates that mental health and addictions are intertwined symptoms of a crisis of meaning emanating from broken social bonds and exacerbated by limited work options (Alexander 2008).

The term *contingent labour force* recognizes that the unemployed are a diverse and wide-ranging group of workers who often go through long periods of job instability. The contingent labour force includes the 7 percent of unemployed along with the 20 percent of workers who are either part-time, temporary, or contract workers. Together with another group representing 7 percent of the labour force, those who are self-employed workers not earning a living wage, this amounts to a total of 34 percent of the labour market (Vosko, Cranford, and Zukewich 2003; Vosko and Noack 2012). This group finds themselves constantly securing income to meet basic needs such as rent and food. These figures do not include those on social assistance (OEDC 1998). For example, in the Waterloo Region in Ontario, over 19,000 individuals are on social assistance and not officially included in the labour force statistics (Desmond 2014). This level of insecurity contributes to mental health and addiction issues.

These statistics demonstrate that the employment market has evolved over the past 30 years to increasingly exclude large numbers of workers from regular participation in the labour market. In a winners-take-all society, the losers are those who cannot gain a regular income in the labour market. It is well documented that the process of exclusion is a major contributor to mental health breakdown. Together with the loss of income, the unemployed person is dealing with the sense of failure from losing their job. The inability to find new work leads to isolation, feelings of rejection, and declining self-esteem (Institute for Work and Health 2009; Standing 2011).

The casual acceptance of a temporary labour force for over a third of the workforce leads to a growing group who face a downward spiral of negative social outcomes. Will former workers be unemployed for progressively longer periods? Will they succumb to addictions without the distraction of regular work? Will they be able to retain their housing? Will they be able to keep their families together? Will they adopt homelessness as their new identity?

In the Canadian context, one can see a clear pattern: the rapid increase in rates of homelessness that occurred in the 1980s were subsequent to the freeze in development of new social housing and the growth of the contingent labour force. At the same time, there was a parallel growth in literature exploring the relationship of social conditions and health. In some cases, the focus has been on health challenges, both physical and mental, which put people at risk of being de-housed. On the ground, these realities have been increasingly present. When integrated social connections become frayed, they are worsened by joblessness and minimal housing options. With homelessness, mental and physical health declines and addictions become a recurring pattern stalking people's lives.

HOMELESSNESS AS A FIXTURE IN THE SYSTEM

The continuation of poor health once a person has obtained housing is a salient point that highlights some of the limitations of current responses to health and homelessness, but also begins to point to the potential of primary care (see Guenter, Oudshoorn, and Mancini, Chapter 15 in this volume). How then should housing be defined and identified in primary care? Housing status quickly becomes a cumbersome factor by which to define a population when considering the health care responses. This is because housing status is fluid, with the most frequent length of stay in all emergency shelters across Canada being only one night. Consider, then, a health outreach program that serves this target population: Is someone who is street-involved but has a place to stay refused care? Is someone who has been receiving services but has become housed then terminated from the program?

As homelessness has increased, so has the rigidity of systems imposing arbitrary structures. Questions about how services are delivered are important because they offer the opportunity to break the circle of dislocation where people abandoned by the labour market lose relationships, housing, and employment opportunities, while addictions and mental health issues fill the voids created by this loss of meaning. How can individuals be supported during this downward spiral?

Simply put, the only way to truly end homelessness is to provide individuals with a home—one that is safe, affordable, permanent, of quality, of one's choice, and having the appropriate supports. However, homelessness is a complex experience with complex interrelated factors that both lead people to be de-housed and make it difficult for people to find themselves a home. Health is one of these factors, and a significant one.

The approaches to addressing the social determinants of health in front-line medical care outlined above point to the potential for a shift towards meaningful health care action on these issues. It is hoped that the development and rigorous evaluation of tools for use in front-line care (see Goel and Bloch, Chapter 14 in this volume) will start to normalize health providers' actions on the social determinants of health. Through building capacity and awareness on the front lines, it is ultimately hoped that health providers will be motivated to engage in advocacy on a higher level, with the goal of systems change as a means to improve health on a large scale.

CRITICAL THINKING QUESTIONS

1. Thinking of the case study of Paul, what forces acted against him breaking his cycle of homelessness and unemployment? Think about forces at the individual, community, and population level.
2. It is clear that the health system operates independent of economic trends. How do economic factors result in new challenges for primary care providers?
3. When society leaves a proportion of its workers unemployed, those who languish in unemployment lose motivation for work and become isolated. What is the role of government to ensure unemployed workers have new work opportunities?
4. What are some other initiatives you can think of that would deliver effective primary care to the marginalized?

REFERENCES

Alexander, Bruce. 2008. *The Globalization of Addiction: A Study in Poverty of the Spirit*. Oxford: Oxford University Press.

Alexander, Bruce. 2011. "A Train Trip through Methland." *Bruce K. Alexander*, 2 February. http://www.brucekalexander.com/articles-speeches/248-a-train-trip-through-methland.

Desmond, Paige. 2014. "Waterloo Region Staff Still 'Not in a Good Place' with New Social Assistance Technology." *TheRecord.com*, December 2. http://www.therecord.com/news-story/5177678-waterloo-region-staff-still-not-in-a-good-place-with-new-social-assistance-technology/.

Galbraith, James K. 2014. *The End of Normal: The Great Crisis and the Future of Growth*. New York: Simon & Schuster.

Institute for Work and Health. 2009. "Unemployment and Mental Health." August. https://www.iwh.on.ca/briefings/unemployment-and-mental-health.

Layton, Jack. 2000. *Homelessness: The Making and Unmaking of a Crisis*. Toronto: Penguin Books Canada.

Lewchuck, Wayne. 2014. "Is Precarious Employment Low Income Employment? The Changing Labour Market in Southern Ontario." *Just Labour: A Canadian Journal of Work and Society* 22 (Autumn). https://justlabour.journals.yorku.ca/index.php/justlabour/article/view/5.

Ottawa Economic Development Corporation (OEDC). 1998. *Ottawa's Hidden Workforce*. Ottawa: OEDC Publications.

Standing, Guy. 2011. *The Precariat: The New Dangerous Class*. London: Bloomsbury Academic.

Vosko, Leah F., Cynthia J. Cranford, and Nancy Zukewich. 2003. "The Gender of Precarious Employment in Canada." *Industrial Relations* 58 (3): 454–82.

Vosko, Leah F., and Andrea M. Noack. 2012. *Precarious Jobs in Ontario: Mapping Dimensions of Labour Market Insecurity by Workers' Social Location and Context*. Toronto: Law Commission of Canada.

CHAPTER 10

Poverty, Homelessness, and Ill Health

Abe Oudshoorn

LEARNING OBJECTIVES

After reading this chapter, you should be able to:

1. Describe the logic behind differing definitions of poverty.
2. Understand different ways that poverty is measured.
3. Understand the rates of poverty in Canada.
4. Recognize how poverty is borne inequitably by different populations.
5. Understand the general relationship between poverty and ill health and the complex interactions among poverty, homelessness, and ill health.

DEFINING POVERTY IN CANADA

In Canada, the two most common measures of poverty are the Low-Income Cut-Off (LICO) and the Market Basket Measure (MBM). The LICO is used by Statistics Canada and represents an income under which a family would spend more than 70 percent of their money on food, clothing, and shelter.

This measure takes into consideration both family size and variation by community in cost of living. According to LICO, approximately 12.9 percent of Canadians were living in poverty in 2011 when calculated before tax, or 8.8 percent when calculated after tax (Statistics Canada 2013). This significant difference exists as the taxation system serves to redistribute income and, in particular, raise the income of those with the lowest incomes.

The other measure, the MBM, looks at the required costs of basic necessities, such as food, clothing, shelter, transportation, and footwear, for a family of four, and typically yields a poverty rate 1 to 3 percent higher than the LICO (Tamarack Institute 2005). What is lacking in both the LICO and MBM measures is a consideration of income distribution and relative poverty, which has an impact on social participation.

Relative poverty, meaning one's income in relation to others in society, is also linked to social participation. Where a family may be above absolute poverty and therefore able to meet basic necessities of life, participation in aspects of social life can be still out of reach if there is a high level of income inequality. This might include participation in recreation, political action, cultural communities, or other connections that require costs such as access to transportation.

While the rates of low income mentioned above represent all Canadians, it is worth noting that poverty is experienced significantly inequitably across populations in Canada. Consider the rates of individuals below the LICO calculated after tax from the most recently available statistics (see table 10.1). Particular populations, such as Indigenous people and racialized populations, are over-represented among those below the LICO.

Poverty, then, isn't simply about access to income; it is also inherently intertwined with both systemic and personal forms of discrimination, such as sexism, ageism, racism, colonialism, and ableism. Rates of persistent poverty in Canada, when those groups who are at higher risk are removed from the calculation, fall as low as 3.4 percent (Hatfield 2004).

Table 10.1. Low-Income Cut-Off Rates, 2013

Size of Family Unit	Community Size				
	Rural Areas Outside CMA or CA[1]	Census Agglomeration (CA)		Census Metropolitan Area (CMA)	
		Fewer than 30,000 Inhabitants[2]	Between 30,000 and 99,999 Inhabitants	Between 100,000 and 499,999 Inhabitants	500,000 Inhabitants or More
	Current Dollars ($)				
1 person	12,629	14,454	16,124	16,328	19,307
2 persons	15,371	17,592	19,625	19,872	23,498
3 persons	19,141	21,905	24,437	24,745	29,260
4 persons	23,879	27,329	30,487	30,871	36,504
5 persons	27,192	31,120	34,717	35,154	41,567
6 persons	30,156	34,513	38,502	38,986	46,099
7 or more persons	33,121	37,906	42,286	42,819	50,631

1. Can include some small population centres.
2. Includes population centres with fewer than 10,000 inhabitants.

Source: Statistics Canada (2013)

These complexities mean that poverty can be a surprisingly difficult term to define. *Merriam-Webster* (n.d.) defines being poor as "lacking material possessions." So how much of a "lack" is required to be deemed poor? And how do we account for the significant variation in "normal" amounts of material possessions from culture to culture and over time? Poverty has been further defined as a lack of the basic necessities required to sustain life. However, on this basis, most advanced societies are ruled out of having poverty by this definition: starvation in Canada today is exceedingly rare (Raphael 2011). Beckmann Murray et al. (2009) attempt to further differentiate poverty to improve its utility by distinguishing between *absolute poverty* as a lack of basic necessities and *relative poverty* as a degree of deprivation in relation to others.

Although rates of poverty can be measured based on economic indicators such as income, poverty is about more than money and involves factors such as inclusion and social participation. Therefore, it is suggested that an individual or family experiences poverty when they "lack or are denied the economic, social, or cultural resources to participate" in their community (Cassidy et al 2016, 10). The term *denied* in this definition is an important one as it indicates that social systems and public policy have a role to play in creating poverty.

Returning to consideration of the LICO and MBM presented above, the nuances of defining poverty are seen in the measurements of poverty in Canada. Incomes representative of poverty are defined differently, whether what is required are the basic necessities of life, broader necessities, or social participation. Measures may also be more or less attuned to variations in family size or differences in cost of living from community to community (see table 10.1). This can be significant, as both large urban areas and small remote communities can have significantly higher costs for food and housing than mid-sized communities in Canada's geographic south.

THE RELATIONSHIP BETWEEN POVERTY AND HEALTH

Poverty is highly correlated with ill health. Indeed, of all the determinants of health, the World Health Organization (WHO n.d.) highlights that poverty is the most important: "People in the lowest income category in Canada are ... five times more likely to report fair or poor health than in the highest income category" (Frohlich, Ross, and Richmond 2006, 134). This holds true internationally. As has been noted by Marmot (2010), people living in impoverished neighbourhoods face a 7-year shorter life expectancy than others, and 17 more years of illness. A study out of Hamilton, Ontario, found a 21-year difference in average age of death between low-income and high-income neighbourhoods (DeLuca, Buist, and Johnston 2012). Major causes of death in Canada, such as heart attack, as well as other indirect indicators of poor health, such as hospitalization, are inversely correlated with income quintile (Raphael 2011), meaning that as income increases, health risks decrease. For instance, the lowest income quintile in Canada has a 17 percent higher rate of cardiovascular disease than the average (Lightman, Mitchell, and Wilson 2008). In terms of mental health, even when controlling for geography and other social factors, the lower one's socioeconomic status is, the more likely one is to experience mental illness or psychiatric hospitalization (Hudson

2005). Depression rates for people living below the poverty line are 58 percent higher than the Canadian average (Smith et al. 2007). One causal component of these disparities is differences in access to health care based on income. For example, low-income women are less likely to access preventative health care measures such as pap smears and mammograms (Krzyzanowska et al. 2009). Roos and Mustard (1997), from their study of health disparities in Winnipeg, note that eliminating income-based disparities in health outcomes would more significantly increase life expectancy than eliminating all forms of cancer.

As with poverty in general, the health outcomes of poverty are borne disproportionately by particular populations such as female-led lone-parent families, racialized groups, and Indigenous people. The distinction of female-led lone-parent families is important due to the gendered nature of work in Canada, with lone-parent women less likely to be employed and, if they are employed, working fewer hours and earning a lower average wage than men (Statistics Canada 2015). Canadian research has demonstrated that while lone-parent status is very strongly related to low income, it also directly affects children's mental health and cognition measures when controlling for low income (Curtis et al. 2001). This means that children of lone-parent families are more likely to experience poorer mental health and lower cognitive ability. This outcome worsens as depth of poverty increases, and, as above, female-led lone-parent families are more likely to experience lower income (Statistics Canada 2015). For racialized groups in Canada, the trend is somewhat different, as variable health outcomes exist depending on ethnicity, length of time in Canada, and other demographic factors. However, Hyman and Wray (2013) note that for newcomers

Case Study: Camila

Camila is 27 years old. A mother to two boys aged five and three, she left their father a year ago because of his verbal abuse and insistence on controlling the family finances. Living in a mid-sized city in Canada, Camila had to leave her part-time employment at the time the family broke up. She hopes to get back to work if and when her younger son is accepted into a subsidized daycare spot, but for now she lives on a meagre social assistance income.

Camila has had a cough for over four weeks now, but with no primary health care provider, no transportation to get to a walk-in clinic, and no one to care for her toddler, she has been putting off treatment. However, when she becomes very feverish and experiences chest pain and nausea, she goes to an urgent care centre and is immediately admitted to hospital with pneumonia in both lungs.

After four days in hospital on IV antibiotics, Camila is able to return home to complete her treatment. Unfortunately, she needs to be readmitted three days later for a second round of IV antibiotics, involving another five days in the hospital. During this time, her children stay with an aunt, who herself is supporting three young kids.

The admitting physician notes that had Camila received treatment earlier, she could have avoided the hospital altogether.

to Canada, health declines over time, and this has been correlated with racialized status. Lastly, Indigenous people experience some of the poorest health outcomes of all population groups. Indigenous people are more likely to report poorer health than non-Indigenous people, are more likely to be experiencing a major mental illness, and are more likely to be living with a chronic health concern (Reading and Wien 2009). Importantly, in their review, Reading and Wien (2009) note that 37.9 percent of respondents also reported experiencing instances of racism within the 12 months prior to the survey. We will return to experiences of racism when we later address consideration of causation and poor health among particular populations.

THE RELATIONSHIP BETWEEN HOMELESSNESS AND HEALTH

As was described by Mancini in Chapter 9, homelessness can be perceived as a particularly devastating form of poverty. Being de-housed relates to both the economic component of poverty and the component of social exclusion. With housing being a foundational requirement for well-being, it is logical that people experiencing homelessness encounter even worse health outcomes than those generally experiencing poverty. The relationship between homelessness and health has been thoroughly explored within scholarly literature going back over 60 years (Jones, Roberts, and Brantner 1954). This has been particularly apparent for mental health challenges, with mental illness and poverty being deeply intertwined and together precipitating homelessness (Sullivan, Burnam, and Koegel 2000). A review of prevalence studies of mental illness in Western nations has found rates of psychotic illness as high as 42.3 percent among those experiencing homelessness (Fazel et al. 2008).

Other researchers have focused on the experience of homelessness as being bad for one's physical health, noting the high rates of acute and chronic medical conditions found within homeless populations (Burt et al. 1999). Rather more poignant are the high rates of mortality and the low average age of death, with mean age at death across studies with people experiencing homelessness ranging between 34 and 47 years (Podymow, Turnbull, and Coyle 2006). Canadian research has shown a probability of survival to 75 years of age is only 32 percent for homeless men and 60 percent for homeless women (Hwang et al. 2009). The same study found mortality rate ratios of 2.3 to 5.6 for suicide and rate differences (per 100,000) of 105 to 182 for ischemic heart disease. Ultimately, people experiencing homelessness face a 4.4 times higher risk of death than the general population (Morrison 2009). As can be seen in Jerry's case study (see case study below) not only can poor health precipitate homelessness and homelessness exacerbate poor health, but poor health can serve as a barrier to maintaining housing and can continue even after someone is re-housed (Gelberg and Leake 1993).

UNDERSTANDING CAUSATION

In exploring the trends and statistics presented in this chapter, there is a risk of concluding that particular populations are the cause of their own poverty, that low-income families make poor decisions about their health, or that people experiencing homelessness just

Case Study: Jerry

Jerry grew up in Eastern Canada as the eldest of six siblings born to a fisherman father and a full-time mother. Born in 1972, Jerry was 20 years old when the cod industry collapsed in Newfoundland and his father became unemployed. At this time, his father changed from being a weekend drinker to a daily drinker, and the children and Jerry's mother became targets of his violence. With no career plans of his own, an incomplete high school education, and the stresses of his home environment, Jerry began drinking at the age of 21. He began spending more time away from home with his drinking friends, and before long, he was no longer welcomed back home. He found himself homeless on the streets, and couches if lucky, of St. John's, Newfoundland.

Jerry's first winter of homelessness in St. John's was very difficult. The weather was very harsh, and because of his drinking, he was often refused entry to shelters and frequently found himself instead waking up in the hospital or a prison cell. Although Jerry's drinking contributed to his homelessness, it was also a barrier to him accessing services for people experiencing homelessness. By the spring of 1994, he decided to strike west across Canada to find a better climate. Following friends who had left during the winter, he headed for Vancouver. Hitchhiking away from St John's proved to be particularly challenging; he left behind acquaintances, his panhandling, and social assistance, among other sources of funding to support his drinking.

As alcohol withdrawal set in, he found himself turning to the only other option he saw available at the time: stealing mouthwash from pharmacies and variety stores. By the time he reached Ontario in the fall of 1994 after a variety of stops through Quebec, Jerry was very ill and very addicted to mouthwash. He was hospitalized in London, Ontario, for an esophageal bleed secondary to the drinking. Ultimately, Jerry decided to stay in London, as he had found a friend from Newfoundland there, and the hitchhiking had been too difficult.

Jerry became a constant presence within the community of people experiencing homelessness in London. He also frequented the local emergency services and the homeless-serving sector. With no managed alcohol program options in the area, Jerry again spent more time in the emergency room and in cells than he did in emergency shelters. Shelter staff managed to move Jerry into social housing a couple of times throughout the years, but in both cases, he was ultimately evicted due to damage to the residence and other people who were coming in and out to drink in his apartment. Jerry frequently expressed a desire to attain and maintain sobriety, but whether through medical withdrawal or through community-based addiction services, he was not able to maintain sobriety for more than a day or two in most cases. Although longer stays in provincial jail led to periods of sobriety and opportunities for social service staff to connect Jerry with housing and other supports, upon discharge, he always reconnected with his drinking friends.

With the advent of Housing First in London, Jerry, a very high user of emergency services, was considered a prime candidate for housing-based support. In the spring of 2016, Jerry was moved into an apartment of his choosing through a Housing First program. The apartment was on the private market, with a rent supplement provided directly to the landlord through the program, in addition to his housing portion of his social assistance cheque. Although there were challenges with his tenancy, similar to his previous experiences of housing, this time he had a housing support worker to provide him with in-home support and a housing selection worker to support the landlord. Through the summer of 2016, both Jerry and the broader system saw good outcomes from this arrangement. Jerry was much safer with stable housing, having a wound-care nurse know where to find him to provide dressing changes for a surgically repaired ankle that had become infected. He also encountered far fewer accidents and injuries, such as being struck by vehicles or assaulted while panhandling. He had exponentially fewer contacts with police, paramedics, the emergency room, and the justice system.

Unfortunately, just six months after having been re-housed and on the date of World Homeless Action Day, Jerry died. He had overdosed on alcohol while alone in his apartment, and when the housing stability worker was unable to make contact with Jerry, the police and landlord entered to find him dead. The community gathered for a memorial service at a local drop-in centre, with over one hundred people attending, including service providers and people with lived experience of homelessness. Although Jerry was housed at the time of his death, it was noted how his lifelong experience of homelessness led to his untimely death at the young age of 55.

need access to more health services. Rather, we need to look at the causal factors behind poverty, why populations are inequitably affected, and why this relates to poorer health outcomes. This invites a return to consideration of the social determinants of health and a population health lens that recognizes the structural components of society as playing a more important role in determining individual and family outcomes than personal choices around health behaviours (Marmot 2005). Indeed, even in considering health behaviours, we know that these are largely mediated by the determinants of health (Watt 2007). For example, we can track back from a health behaviour such as smoking to a person's experiences of poverty and conclude that addressing poverty is an important upstream approaching to changing health outcomes (Graham et al. 2006). While people experiencing homelessness often delay seeking treatment for health conditions (Khan et al. 2011), it is notable that the primary reported reason for this delay is negative past experience with health care providers (Ensign and Panke 2002). So, it's not that people are making poor choices about managing their health, but they are weighing the risks of experiencing prejudice and stigma with how bad they believe their health needs to be when seeking health care. Lastly, public policies, such as designs of health care, social services, and housing systems, have the potential to both create and perpetuate experiences of poverty and ill health.

HOW POLICY CREATES ILL HEALTH FOR THOSE EXPERIENCING POVERTY AND HOMELESSNESS

The policies listed in table 10.2 by no means comprise a comprehensive list of policies that interact with poverty and health, shape rates of poverty and homelessness, and impact health and well-being. Rather, the list serves as a brief illustration of the role that policy can play in both causing negative outcomes but also in potentially leading to positive outcomes. Further discussion of the role of policy for reform on health equity

Table 10.2. A Sample of Public Policies That Impact Poverty and Homelessness

Sector	Policies That May Serve as Barriers
Health	• Requirement to have a health card to access services • Requirement for a referral from a primary health care provider to access specialist support • Limited availability of medical detoxification • Fees to access physician notes for employment or to maintain a stay in shelter
Housing	• Limited availability of affordable housing stock • Limited affordable housing access for particular populations such as women leaving domestic violence • Pre-conditions to access affordable housing, such as sobriety • Clustered rather than distributed social housing development
Social Assistance	• Procedural delays in accessing assistance in cases of a rapid change in status, such as loss of housing or relationship breakdown • Limited availability of support for first and last month's rent when entering a new lease • Requirements in some provinces for homeless youth to demonstrate emancipation from parents before individually accessing social assistance
Justice	• Orders to reside in emergency shelter, thus forcing people into potentially long stays in shelter • Orders not to attend certain neighbourhoods, which might limit access to visit children, attend school, or obtain employment • Time and cost involved in expunging old criminal records, which serve as a barrier to employment
Child Welfare	• Definitions of neglect that disproportionately put families experiencing poverty at risk of child apprehension • Lack of cultural competence, leading to overrepresentation of Indigenous children in care

will continue in Andermann, Chapter 26. As well, those policies illustrated in table 10.2 are much more complex and interactive in reality and may not be problematic in and of themselves but play a role in a network of policies that frames the experiences of Canadians. These policies also shift over time: for example, two recent policy changes in the province of Ontario should improve the experience of people living in poverty. First, parents now receive ongoing social assistance rates consistent with having children when these children are temporarily taken into care. This prevents families from losing their housing and allows them also to meet the bedroom requirements of the child welfare system in order to regain custody of their children from care. Second, the adjudication process for those receiving a disability income through social assistance has been streamlined to reduce the process for those with a long-term disability of having to prove they still have the same disability. These examples demonstrate how simple policy changes can have a profound impact on poverty and the experience of poverty.

Ultimately, poverty can be considered a policy choice of advanced societies. When we in Canada set a social assistance rate that is below the LICOs, we are choosing to have those who require social assistance to live in poverty. When we have minimum wage set below the living wage, we are choosing to have individuals in certain types of employment live in poverty. These policy decisions, then, are deeply political and cultural. In a representative democracy, politics should relatively closely mirror the cultural considerations of the majority of the population. Therefore, it can be argued that we in Canada choose to have a certain degree of poverty in spite of an understanding of the negative health impacts that this poverty will have on families and individuals. Ultimately, an upstream approach to addressing the health effects of poverty necessitates a national conversation on poverty and policy in general.

CRITICAL THINKING QUESTIONS

1. This chapter has demonstrated that health and social systems work interactively in framing the experiences of poverty and health; however, in Canada, these services are delivered very separately with separate legislation, separate departments, and separate staff. How might health and social services work more collaboratively to achieve better outcomes for individuals and families experiencing poverty?
2. Thinking of the definitions of poverty presented in this chapter, is it possible to eradicate poverty in Canada? If no, why not? If yes, how?
3. What strategies can you think of to improve the quality of life and life expectancy of people experiencing homelessness in Canada?

REFERENCES

Beckmann Murray, R., Judith Proctor Zentner, Verna C. Pangman, and Clare Pangman. 2009. *Health Promotion Strategies through the Lifespan*. 2nd ed. Toronto: Pearson Prentice Hall.

Burt, Martha R., Laudan Y. Aron, Toby Douglas, Jesse Valente, Edgar Lee, and Britta Iwen. 1999. *Homelessness: Programs and the People They Serve: Summary Report*. Washington, DC: Urban Institute.

Cassidy, Maureen, Christopher Mackie, Vanessa Ambtman-Smith, Helene Berman, Dharshi Lacey, Andrew Lockie, Abe Oudshoorn, and Glen Pearson. 2016. *London For All: A Roadmap to End Poverty*. London, ON: Mayor's Advisory Panel on Poverty. http://www.abeoudshoorn.com/wp-content/uploads/2015/08/London-for-All.pdf.

Curtis, Lori J., Martin D. Dooley, Ellen L. Lipman, and David H. Feeny. 2001. "The Role of Permanent Income and Family Structure in the Determination of Child Health in Canada." *Health Economics* 10 (4): 287–302. https://doi.org/10.1002/hec.591.

DeLuca, Patrick F., Steve Buist, and Neil Johnston. 2012. "The Code Red Project: Engaging Communities in Health System Change in Hamilton, Canada." *Social Indicators Research* 108, (2): 317–27. https://doi.org/10.1007/s11205-012-0068-y.

Ensign, Josephine, and Aileen Panke. 2002. "Barriers and Bridges to Care: Voices of Homeless Female Adolescent Youth in Seattle, Washington, USA." *Journal of Advanced Nursing* 37 (2): 166–72. https://doi.org/10.1046/j.1365-2648.2002.02067.x.

Fazel, Seena, Vivek Khosla, Helen Doll, and John Geddes. 2008. "The Prevalence of Mental Disorders among the Homeless in Western Countries: Systematic Review and Meta-regression Analysis." *PLoS Medicine* 5 (12): e225. https://doi.org/10.1371/journal.pmed.0050225.

Frohlich, Katherine L., Nancy Ross, and Chantelle Richmond. 2006. "Health Disparities in Canada Today: Some Evidence and a Theoretical Framework." *Health Policy* 79 (2): 132–43. https://doi.org/10.1016/j.healthpol.2005.12.010.

Gelberg, Lillian, and Barbara D. Leake. 1993. "Substance Use among Impoverished Medical Patients: The Effect of Housing Status and Other Factors." *Medical Care* 31 (9): 757–66.

Graham, Hilary, Hazel M. Inskip, Brian Francis, and Juliet Harman. 2006. "Pathways of Disadvantage and Smoking Careers: Evidence and Policy Implications." *Journal of Epidemiology and Community Health* 60 (suppl 2): ii7–12. https://doi.org/10.1136/jech.2005.045583.

Hatfield, Michael. 2004. "Vulnerability to Persistent Low Income." *Horizons* 7 (2): 19–26.

Hudson, Christopher G. 2005. "Socioeconomic Status and Mental Illness: Tests of the Social Causation and Selection Hypotheses." *American Journal of Orthopsychiatry* 75 (1): 3–18. https://doi.org/10.1037/0002-9432.75.1.3.

Hwang, Stephen W., Russell Wilkins, Michael Tjepkema, Patricia J. O'Campo, and James R. Dunn. 2009. "Mortality among Residents of Shelters, Rooming Houses, and Hotels in Canada: 11 Year Follow-Up Study." *BMJ* 339: b4036. https://doi.org/10.1136/bmj.b4036.

Hyman, Ilene, and Ron Wray. 2013. *Health Inequalities and Racialized Groups: A Review of the Evidence*. Toronto. Prepared in collaboration with Toronto Public Health.

Jones, Herbert W., Jean Roberts, and John Brantner. 1954. "Incidence of Tuberculosis among Homeless Men." *Journal of the American Medical Association* 155(14): 1222–3.

Khan, Kamran, Elizabeth Rea, Cameron McDermaid, Rebecca Stuart, Catharine Chambers, Jun Wang, Angie Chan, et al. 2011. "Active Tuberculosis among Homeless Persons, Toronto, Ontario, Canada, 1998–2007." *Emerging Infectious Diseases* 17 (3): 357–65. https://doi.org/10.3201/eid1703.100833.

Krzyzanowska, Monika K., Lisa Barbera, Laurie Elit, Refik Saskin, Naira Yeritsyan, and Arlene S. Bierman. 2009. "Importance of Stratification When Measuring Quality of Care: Results from the Project for an Ontario Women's Health Evidence-Based Report Card (POWER) Study." *Journal of Clinical Oncology* 27 (15_suppl): 6573.

Lightman, Ernie, Andrew Mitchell, and Beth Wilson. 2008. *Poverty is Making Us Sick: A Comprehensive Survey of Income and Health in Canada*. Toronto: Wellesley Institute. http://www.wellesleyinstitute.com/wp-content/uploads/2011/11/povertyismakingussick.pdf.

Marmot, Michael. 2005. "Social Determinants of Health Inequalities." *Lancet* 365 (9464): 1099–104.

Marmot, Michael. 2010. *Fair Society, Healthy Lives*. London: Department of Health. http://www.ucl.ac.uk/gheg/marmotreview/Documents/finalreport/FairSocietyHealthyLives.

Merriam-Webster. n.d. s.v. "poor." Accessed April 11, 2017. https://www.merriam-webster.com/dictionary/poor?utm_campaign=sd&utm_medium=serp&utm_source=jsonld.

Morrison, David S. 2009. "Homelessness as an Independent Risk Factor for Mortality: Results from a Retrospective Cohort Study." *International Journal of Epidemiology* 38 (3): 877–83.

Podymow, Tiina, Jeffrey Turnbull, and Doug Coyle. 2006. "Shelter-Based Palliative Care for the Homeless Terminally Ill." *Palliative Medicine* 20 (2): 81–6. https://doi.org/10.1191/0269216306pm1103oa.

Raphael, Dennis. 2011. *Poverty in Canada: Implications for Health and Quality of Life*. 2nd ed. Toronto: Canadian Scholars' Press.

Reading, Charlotte Loppie, and Fred Wien. 2009. *Health Inequalities and Social Determinants of Aboriginal People's Health*. Prince George, BC: National Collaborating Centre for Aboriginal Health. http://www.nccah-ccnsa.ca/docs/social%20determinates/nccah-loppie-wien_report.pdf.

Roos, Noralou P., and Cameron A. Mustard. 1997. "Variation in Health and Health Care Use by Socioeconomic Status in Winnipeg, Canada: Does the System Work Well? Yes and No." *Milbank Quarterly* 75 (1): 89–111.

Smith, Katherine L. W., Flora I. Matheson, Rahim Moineddin, and Richard H. Glazier. 2007. "Gender, Income and Immigration Differences in Depression in Canadian Urban Centres." *Canadian Journal of Public Health* 98 (2): 149–53.

Statistics Canada. 2013. "Persons in Low Income Before Tax." Last modified June 27. http://www.statcan.gc.ca/tables-tableaux/sum-som/l01/cst01/famil41a-eng.htm?sdi=low%20income.

Statistics Canada. 2015. "Lone-Parent Families." Last modified November 27. http://www.statcan.gc.ca/pub/75-006-x/2015001/article/14202/parent-eng.htm.

Sullivan, Greer, Audrey Burnam, and Paul Koegel. 2000. "Pathways to Homelessness among the Mentally Ill." *Social Psychiatry and Psychiatric Epidemiology* 35 (10): 444–50.

Tamarack Institute. 2005. *Low Income ('Poverty') Lines.* Waterloo, ON: Tamarack Institute. http://vibrantcanada.ca/files/poverty_lines.pdf.

Watt, Richard Geddie. 2007. "From Victim Blaming to Upstream Action: Tackling the Social Determinants of Oral Health Inequalities." *Community Dentistry and Oral Epidemiology* 35 (1): 1–11. https://doi.org/10.1111/j.1600-0528.2007.00348.x.

World Health Organization (WHO). n.d. "Poverty and Social Determinants." Accessed March 21, 2018. http://www.euro.who.int/en/health-topics/environment-and-health/urban-health/activities/poverty-and-social-determinants.

CHAPTER 11

The Forgotten Victims: Impact of Parental Incarceration on the Psychological Health of the Innocent Children Left Behind

Jessica Reid

LEARNING OBJECTIVES

After reading this chapter, you should be able to:

1. Appreciate the multi-faceted impact of parental incarceration on children's mental health and well-being.
2. Identify factors that moderate and mitigate the short-term and long-term effects of having a parent behind bars.
3. Appreciate the role of supportive programs in reducing the impact of parental incarceration and the risk of problematic outcomes for children of prisoners.
4. Recognize the importance of research, education, and awareness in helping to reduce the societal stigma and isolation faced by children of incarcerated parents that serve to exacerbate the negative effects of parental incarceration on mental health and well-being.

In Canada, every year, over 350,000 children are separated from an incarcerated father (Withers and Folsom 2008) while an additional 20,000 children are separated from an incarcerated mother (Cunningham and Baker 2003). The mass incarceration movement in the United States has resulted in approximately 1 in 14 children losing a parent to prison (Murphey and Cooper 2015). Despite the growing prevalence, there has been and continues to be an overrepresentation of ethnic minority families who are impacted by the criminal justice system across North America.

In a recent report conducted in 2015/2016, Indigenous adults accounted for more than one quarter of admissions to provincial and territorial correctional services in Canada (Reitano 2017). However, Indigenous adults only comprise 3 percent of the adult population in Canada. Subsequently, the disparity in admissions was more prominent among Indigenous females compared to Indigenous males. Specifically, Indigenous females accounted for 38 percent of admissions into provincial and territorial correctional systems, while 26 percent of all male admissions identified as Indigenous. Furthermore, in the annual report for 2014–2015 from the Office of the Correctional Investigator, Sapers (2015) highlights that the overrepresentation in the number of inmates who identify as ethnic minorities in the Canadian federal correctional system has only exponentially increased over the past 10 years. Notably, results revealed that the number of Indigenous men and women in the federal system has grown more than 50 percent from 2005 to 2015. Similarly, the Black inmate population has increased by 69 percent.

Consistent with the discrimination in the criminal justice system, studies have shown that marginalized children in North America also have a greater risk of enduring the ripple effects of parental incarceration. In particular, the prevalence of experiencing separation from a parent behind bars is disproportionately with children of ethnic minorities, those who grow up in low socioeconomic households, and children with parents who have obtained only a high school education (Murphey and Cooper 2015). While children with incarcerated parents often experience several risk factors, the trauma of losing a parent to prison has been associated with short-term and long-term effects.

Based on the National Survey of Children's Health in the United States in 2011/2012, researchers identified parental incarceration as one of the eight adverse childhood experiences (ACEs) (Sacks, Murphey, and Moore 2014). ACEs are characterized by traumatic events that predict problematic long-term behavioural and health outcomes. In many cases, parental incarceration co-occurs with other adverse experiences (e.g., parental divorce). Exposure to multiple familial and environmental risk factors only elevates the vulnerability to poor health and well-being for children of incarcerated parents. For example, Phillips and Dettlaff (2009) found that children with caregivers who had been arrested were also more likely to experience parental substance abuse, domestic violence, and extreme poverty compared to children with caregivers who had never been arrested.

Generational familial trauma, substance abuse, and mental illness are frequently part of the personal histories of parents who become incarcerated. Markedly, 60 percent of imprisoned mothers and 16 percent of imprisoned fathers reported experiencing physical or sexual abuse during their childhood and adolescence (Glaze and Maruschak 2008). Subsequently, approximately 70 percent of imprisoned caregivers met the diagnostic threshold for substance dependence or abuse (Maruschak, Glaze, and Mumola 2010). Despite histories of neglect, abuse, and trauma among incarcerated parents, the majority of their children are not direct victims of maltreatment or their parent's crime. Findings from the National Survey for Child and Adolescent Well-Being in the United States revealed that one third of the cases of maltreatment (i.e., lack of supervision, failure to provide, emotional abuse, and sexual abuse) involved children with a caregiver who had a history of being arrested (Phillips and Dettlaff 2009). Although most victims did not have incarcerated parents, the history of generational trauma and exposure to multiple adverse events highlights the vulnerability of children of imprisoned parents.

To date, the effects of parental incarceration have predominantly been empirically examined in samples in the United States and Europe (e.g., Murray et al. 2009; Poehlmann et al. 2010). Potential differences in the effects across countries (e.g., Canadian samples), in cross-cultural comparisons (e.g., Indigenous populations), and among subpopulations of children with incarcerated parents, such as children with disabilities (e.g., fetal alcohol syndrome), have yet to be empirically explored. Future research is needed to expand our understanding of the impact of having a parent behind bars from a global and culturally diverse lens.

Several theoretical perspectives have been proposed to explain the effects of parental incarceration. However, in recent years, researchers (e.g., Poehlmann 2005) have suggested that Bowlby's theory of attachment is an ideal theoretical framework in understanding the impact of parental incarceration on mental health and behavioural outcomes. Specifically, Bowlby (1969, 1973) posited that attachment bonds are formed during early interactions between caregivers and infants and are proposed to be an evolutionary mechanism developed to protect children from danger, threat, and harm. Depending on the nature of early experiences with caregivers, children develop a positive or negative internal working model of the self and of others; this model has been argued to remain relatively stable throughout life. It has been proposed that these internal representations guide cognition, emotion regulation, and behaviours. To date, attachment theory has been used to explain a variety of behaviours and developmental outcomes including emotionality, social interaction, and coping behaviours (see, e.g., Kerns et al. 2007).

As parental incarceration results in a forced parent-child separation, researchers have argued that attachment theory may capture the impact of parental imprisonment and its association with problematic outcomes (Poehlmann 2005). Accordingly, Bowlby (1973) proposed that prolonged separation from an attachment figure is particularly distressing for children and can perpetuate the development of negative internal working models. Subsequent researchers have suggested that the links between parental incarceration, internalizing symptoms, and externalizing behaviours may be manifestations of attachment insecurity due to the disruption in the parent-child relationship (Poehlmann 2005; Poehlmann and Eddy 2013).

Although the focus of research on children with incarcerated parents centres on examining the impact during imprisonment, for many children, the effects often commence prior to experiencing prolonged separation from a parent. Notably, one in five children of incarcerated parents witnesses the arrest of a mother (Johnston 1991). According to a national US study, 67 percent of imprisoned parents reported being handcuffed in front of their children, while 27 percent reported that police officers employed weapons in the presence of their children (Harm and Phillips 1998). As a consequence, witnessing a parent's arrest in childhood is often a traumatic experience that has been linked to the development of post-traumatic stress (Bocknek, Sanderson, and Britner 2009; Phillips and Zhao 2010) and its common co-occurring symptoms of flashbacks and sleep disturbances, developmental regression, and depression (Bocknek, Sanderson, and Britner 2009; Foster and Hagan 2013; Lee, Fang, and Luo 2013; Poehlmann 2005).

While a parent's arrest often threatens the short-term mental health of children, parental incarceration has also been shown to have long-term effects on psychological health and well-being. In particular, experiencing parental abandonment often jeopardizes children's perceptions of self-worth and trust in their guardian's ability to attend to their emotional, physical, and social needs on a consistent basis. These ramifications, particularly when coupled with prolonged separation in the parent-child relationship, plagues children's psychological well-being and attachment security. Correspondingly, children of incarcerated parents frequently exhibit low self-esteem, experience internalizing symptoms (e.g., anxiety), and develop behavioural disorders (Murray and Farrington 2008). As these at-risk children mature to adolescents and adults, mental health issues typically become increasingly complex; substance abuse (Farrington 2000; Midgley and Lo 2013), delinquency (Huebner and Gustafson 2007; Murray and Farrington 2008), and long-term psychological disorders such as depression are particularly prevalent (Lee, Fang, and Luo 2013). In fact, over the course of the lifespan, it has been estimated that Canadian children of incarcerated parents are two to four times more likely to come in conflict with the law compared to peers with law-abiding parents (Withers and Folsom 2008).

Recently, researchers have suggested that child characteristics (e.g., gender, age) may influence the impact of parental incarceration on children's well-being and developmental outcomes. Specifically, some researchers have found support for gender differences in caregiver reports of children's internalizing symptoms and externalizing behaviours during early childhood (Haskins 2015; Wildeman 2010). Interestingly, as children age, results suggest that gender differences may be more pronounced, particularly when the effects are examined with contextual factors such as duration, frequency, and timing of parental incarceration (Swisher and Shaw-Smith 2015). For example, adolescent males who experienced shorter separations from their incarcerated father (i.e., less than a year) reported higher levels of depression compared to adolescent females. In contrast, longer separations from incarcerated fathers were more strongly associated with depression in adolescent females than their counterparts.

Differential effects between experiencing paternal incarceration and maternal incarceration have also been found. Although men have historically been disproportionately represented in the criminal justice system, many researchers argue that the collateral effects of maternal incarceration are more problematic for children's mental health and well-being (Cunningham and Baker 2003; Poehlmann 2005). In particular, most children live with their mothers prior to incarceration and, as a result, these children are more likely to be separated from their primary caregiver compared to children who endure paternal incarceration (Poehlmann 2005). Correspondingly, in Canada, 53 percent of federally sentenced mothers reported being the primary caregiver of children prior to incarceration (Shaw et al. 1991), and 80 percent of provincially sentenced mothers in Ontario were sole parents before the offence. Conversely, only 24 percent of federally sentenced fathers in Canada were sole custodial parents prior to incarceration.

Discrepancies in parental involvement prior to incarceration frequently yield differences in the impact of children being separated from an incarcerated mother compared to an incarcerated father. For example, Foster (2011) found that only 37 percent of American children resided with a father during their mother's incarceration, whereas 87 percent of American children lived with a mother while their father was serving a sentence. Consequently, almost half of incarcerated mothers reported that their children moved to live with their grandparents, about a quarter to a third each lived with fathers or other relatives, while 10 percent of children lived with friends, and 10 percent entered foster care (Hairston 2007). However, incarcerated fathers reported that 90 percent of their children lived with mothers, 10 percent lived with grandparents, 5 percent lived with other relatives or friends, and 2 percent entered foster care. It should be noted that the sum of these percentages exceeds 100 percent, as incarcerated parents reported on multiple children who lived with multiple caregivers. Similarly, in Canada, 80 percent of federally sentenced fathers reported that their children lived with their mothers during incarceration. Overall, children of imprisoned mothers are more likely to experience a change in caregivers (e.g., move to live with grandparents) (Kjellstrand et al. 2012), enter the foster care system, and become separated from siblings than children with imprisoned fathers (Glaze and Maruschak 2008).

Although maternal and paternal incarceration have both been associated with poor mental health and behavioural outcomes (see, e.g., Aaron and Dallaire 2010; Murphy and Cooper 2015; Murray et al. 2009), some evidence suggests that experiencing maternal incarceration is linked with greater mental health problems (Tasca et al. 2014) compared to paternal incarceration. Likewise, in a comparative meta-analysis, Foster and Hagan (2013) found that experiencing paternal incarceration during childhood was associated with substance use problems in late adolescence and adulthood while maternal incarceration predicted the presence of depressive symptoms. Factors such as number of sentences, length of incarceration, and type of offence also have been shown to play moderating roles on the impact of parental imprisonment.

Parental incarceration has consistently been found to have deleterious effects on offspring from birth to adulthood (Murray et al. 2009). However, researchers argue that timing and dose effects moderate the impact of parental incarceration (van de Rakt, Murray, and Nieuwbeerta 2012). Specifically, evidence suggests that children who experience parental incarceration during childhood, children who repeatedly experience parental imprisonment, and children who endure prolonged separations from an imprisoned parent have shown to have the most problematic trajectories. In fact, van de Rakt and colleagues (2012) found that children who were separated from their imprisoned fathers between birth and 12 years of age were more likely to have criminal convictions than children who had imprisoned fathers prior to birth and children with incarcerated fathers between the ages of 12 and 18 years of age. Furthermore, the number of parental offences predicted the frequency of sentences among juvenile offenders, while the seriousness of paternal criminality was associated with the seriousness of their children's crimes (Nijhof, de Kemp, and Engels 2009).

Researchers have begun to illuminate factors that may mitigate the effects of parental incarceration (see figure 11.1). As previously discussed, empirical evidence suggests that the characteristics of the child and the parent and exposure to trauma play a role in understanding the impact of parental incarceration on health. Moreover, the quality of the parent-child relationship and the stability of family home environment preceding, during, and following imprisonment have also shown to be influential factors (Poehlmann et al. 2010; Poehlmann and Eddy 2013). Studies have shown that experiencing consistent positive caregiving, having regular contact with the incarcerated parent, and undergoing minimal changes to home environments have been associated with better mental health outcomes (Poehlmann et al. 2010). Furthermore, it has been suggested that providing support for the child (e.g., peer support groups, mentoring programs, counselling) (Johnston 2012), the incarcerated parents and caregivers (e.g., parenting programs, support groups), and the whole family (e.g., visitation programs) may help to mitigate the effects of incarceration. Participation in after-school programs and mentoring programs in particular have been linked to improvements in children's self-esteem, educational attainment, and behavioural outcomes (Johnston 2012). Interestingly,

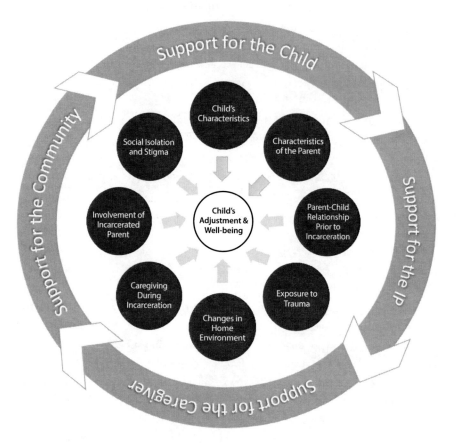

Figure 11.1: Factors Affecting the Impact of Parental Incarceration on Children's Adjustment and Well-Being

Note: IP = incarcerated parent.

supportive programs that involve the combination of parent training and support for the child, particularly when examining the impact of family visits on children's self-esteem, have shown to be most effective (Landreth and Lobaugh 1998).

Social support also has its role in reducing the impact of parental incarceration on children's self-esteem and mental health. Most children of incarcerated parents experience societal stigma and consequently are forced to cope with the challenges of parental incarceration in social isolation in addition to living in fear of judgment and ridicule (Poehlmann et al. 2010). To address the larger systemic issue of societal stigma surrounding parental incarceration, the San Francisco Children of Incarcerated Parents Partnerships developed a Bill of Rights (see box). This Bill of Rights is an example of the importance of educating, advocating, and supporting the community to recognize the needs of children affected by parental incarceration and working together to improve the outcomes of these at-risk children.

While children of imprisoned parents are at risk for a multitude of problematic outcomes, supporting these victims of crime remains an under-discussed, underfunded, and under-served societal issue in our health, education, and social service sectors. In 2018, there is a lack of supportive programs and services for children with a parent in prison across the globe. In comparison to Canada, there are a greater number of social service agencies and non-profit organizations in the United States, the UK, and Australia that provide specific supportive programming for children and families affected by incarceration. As a result, researchers suggest that the psychological, familial, social, and economic consequences of parental imprisonment coupled with the lack of supportive services contribute to deterioration in health and perpetuating the cycle of crime (Parke and Clarke-Stewart 2002; Poehlmann 2005). However, FEAT for Children, a registered charitable organization that I co-founded in Toronto, has been developed to address this need and provide supportive programming for children affected by parental incarceration (see box "FEAT for Children").

Children of Incarcerated Parents Bill of Rights (2003)

1. I have the right to be kept safe and informed at the time of my parent's arrest.
2. I have the right to be heard when decisions are made about me.
3. I have the right to be considered when decisions are made about my parent.
4. I have the right to be well cared for in my parent's absence.
5. I have the right to speak with, see, and touch my parent.
6. I have the right to support as I face my parent's incarceration.
7. I have the right not to be judged, blamed, or labelled because my parent is incarcerated.
8. I have the right to a lifelong relationship with my parent.

Reproduced with permission from San Francisco Children of Incarcerated Parents Partnership (SFCIPP 2003).

FEAT for Children

Fostering, Empowering, and Advocating Together (FEAT) for Children works to support children affected by parental incarceration. Currently, FEAT is the only organization in Canada providing supportive programming for children of prisoners. Since its inception in 2011, FEAT has improved the psychological, educational, and social well-being of over one thousand children and families in Ontario. It is anticipated that additional sites will develop to meet the growing needs of children impacted by parental incarceration across the country.

FEAT's Family Visitation Program enables children and family members to visit loved ones in prison every weekend. To optimize the impact of these visits, trained support staff guide children and guardians through the security procedures to reduce anxiety entering correctional institutions, facilitate peer group discussion on strategies to overcome the challenges associated with incarceration, and provide comfort following visits. Consistent with previous research that highlighted the rehabilitative quality of family visits for mental health and reducing recidivism (Bales and Mears 2008), participation in FEAT's Family Visitation Program has been associated with improvements in the mental health of the children, families, and incarcerated parents and a 50 percent reduction in recidivism rates two years after release, and it has served to promote successful reintegration into society. Moreover, children who visited their imprisoned fathers through FEAT's Family Visitation Program exhibited increases in self-esteem, improvement in security in their parental relationships, and a reduction in number and severity of depressive symptoms.

To further support the unique needs and psychological well-being of children of incarcerated parents, FEAT provides additional supportive programs (e.g., after-school program, peer mentorship program, empowerment retreats, peer support group for caregivers). These supportive programs are tailored to the unique needs of children of incarcerated parents and their families. The programs are designed to focus on building protective factors against criminality and improving their psychological, social, and emotional well-being. In particular, fostering the development of positive mentoring relationships, teaching healthy coping strategies, and providing leadership opportunities are core components of the support programs to help children overcome stigma and social isolation and develop prosocial attitudes and behaviours. To date, participation in these supportive programs have shown to improve children's mental health, increase social skills, and reduce delinquent behaviours.

Early intervention is fundamental to reducing the impact of parental incarceration and optimizing children's psychological, educational, and social outcomes. Although research is limited, evidence suggests that professionals across health, education, social service, child welfare, and justice systems need to work together to increase the success of early identification and improve access to vital supportive programs and services for children and families affected by the justice system. Specifically, developing a holistic system of care would help to support the complex needs of the vulnerable children and families affected by incarceration and improve outcomes. For example, the community hub support model has been effective in providing services tailored to the complex needs of other vulnerable populations (e.g., newly released men from correctional facilities) and may be an ideal framework for families impacted by incarceration. The collaboration of professionals across sectors to identify the needs of families, provide resources, and refer families to organizations that specialize in supporting the unique needs of this at-risk population would improve access to early intervention and support. Consistent with past research on the efficacy of similar support models, evidence suggests that the development of a holistic system of care for these at-risk children and families would optimize health, reduce the impact of parental imprisonment, and help to break the cycle of intergenerational crime.

CRITICAL THINKING QUESTIONS

1. Reflect upon your knowledge and assumptions of children of incarcerated parents prior to reading this chapter. When you thought of an adult being sentenced to jail or prison, did you consider the effects on the children left behind?
2. How were the human costs of incarceration and the negative impact on the health and well-being of the incarcerated individual as well as their families discussed in your previous studies?
3. San Francisco Children of Incarcerated Parents Partnership developed a Bill of Rights for children of incarcerated parents. Are there any additional rights that you would include to this bill to support children of incarcerated parents in Canada? What policy changes would you propose to support the rights of children of incarcerated parents and that may help to mitigate the impact of parental incarceration on health and well-being?
4. Review the recent stories in the national or local newspaper that discuss the health and well-being of at-risk children. How often are children of incarcerated parents included in this discussion? How might this angle mitigate and exacerbate the health and well-being of children affected by parental incarceration in Canada and worldwide?

REFERENCES

Aaron, L., and D. H. Dallaire. 2010. "Parental Incarceration and Multiple Risk Experiences: Effects on Family Processes and Children's Delinquency." *Journal of Youth and Adolescence* 39: 1471–84.

Bales, W. D., and D. P. Mears. 2008. "Inmate Social Ties and the Transition to Society: Does Visitation Reduce Recidivism?" *Journal of Research in Crime and Delinquency* 45: 287–321.

Bocknek, E., J. Sanderson, and P. Britner. 2009. "Ambiguous Loss and Posttraumatic Stress in School-Age Children of Prisoners." *Journal of Child and Family Studies* 18: 323–33.

Bowlby, J. 1969. *Attachment and Loss, Volume 1.* New York: Basic Books.

Bowlby, J. 1973. *Attachment and Loss, Volume 2: Separation.* New York: Basic Books.

Craigie, T. A. 2011. "The Effect of Paternal Incarceration on Early Child Behavioral Problems: A Racial Comparison." *Journal of Ethnicity in Criminal Justice* 9: 179–99.

Cunningham, A., and L. Baker. 2003. *Waiting for Mommy: Giving a Voice to the Hidden Victims of Imprisonment.* London, ON: Centre for Children and Families in the Justice System.

Farrington, D. P. 2000. "Psychosocial Predictors of Adult Antisocial Personality and Adult Convictions." *Behavioral Sciences and the Law* 18: 605–22.

Foster, H. 2011. "The Influence of Incarceration on Children at the Intersection of Parental Gender and Race/Ethnicity: A Focus on Child Living Arrangements." *Journal of Ethnicity in Criminal Justice* 9: 1–21.

Foster, H., and J. Hagan. 2013. "Maternal and Paternal Imprisonment in the Stress Process." *Social Science Research* 42 (3): 650–69.

Glaze, L., and L. M. Maruschak. 2008. *Bureau of Justice Statistics Special Report: Parents in Prison and Their Minor Children.* Washington, DC: U.S. Department of Justice. https://www.bjs.gov/content/pub/pdf/pptmc.pdf.

Hairston, C. F. 2007. "Focus on Children with Incarcerated Parents." Baltimore, MD: Annie E. Casey Foundation.

Harm, N. J., and S. Phillips. 1998. "Helping Children Cope with the Trauma of Parental Arrest." *Interdisciplinary Report on At-Risk Children and Families* 1: 35–37.

Haskins, A. 2015. "Paternal Incarceration and Child-Reported Behavioral Functioning at Age 9." *Social Science Research* 52: 18–33.

Huebner, B. M., and R. Gustafson. 2007. "The Effect of Maternal Incarceration on Adult Offspring Involvement in the Criminal Justice System." *Journal of Criminal Justice* 35 (3): 283–96. https://doi.org/10.1016/j.jcrimjus.2007.03.005.

Johnston, D. 1991. *Jailed Mothers.* Pasadena, CA: Pacific Oaks Center for Children of Incarcerated Parents.

Johnston, D. 2012. "Services for Children of Incarcerated Parents." *Family Court Review* 50 (1): 91–105. https://doi.org/10.1111/j.1744-1617.2011.01431.x.

Kerns, K., M. Abraham, A. Schlegelmilch, and T. Morgan. 2007. "Mother-Child Attachment in Later Middle Childhood: Assessment Approaches and Associations with Mood and Emotion Regulation." *Attachment and Human Development* 9 (1): 33–53.

Kjellstrand, J., J. Cearley, J. Eddy, D. Foney, and C. Martinez. 2012. "Characteristics of Incarcerated Fathers and Mothers: Implications for Preventive Interventions Targeting Children and Families." *Children and Youth Services Review* 34 (12): 2409–15.

Landreth, G. L., and A. F. Lobaugh. 1998. "Filial Therapy with Incarcerated Fathers: Effects on Parental Acceptance of Child, Parental Stress, and Child Adjustment." *Journal of Counseling & Development* 76 (2): 157–65. https://doi.org/10.1002/j.1556-6676.1998.tb02388.x.

Lee, R. D., X. Fang, and F. Luo. 2013. "The Impact of Parental Incarceration on Physical and Mental Health of Young Adults." *Pediatrics* 131 (4): 1188–95. https://doi.org/10.1542/peds.2012-0627.

Maruschak, L. M., L. E. Glaze, and C. J. Mumola. 2010. "Incarcerated Parents and Their Children." In *Children of Incarcerated Parents: A Handbook for Researchers and Practitioners*, edited by J. M. Eddy and J. Poehlmann, 33–51. Washington, DC: Urban Institute.

Midgley, E. K, and C. C. Lo. 2013. "The Role of a Parent's Incarceration in the Emotional Health and Problem Behaviors of At-Risk Adolescents." *Journal of Child & Adolescent Substance Abuse* 22 (2): 85–103. https://doi.org/10.1080/1067828X.2012.730350.

Murphey, D., and P. M. Cooper. 2015. *Parents behind Bars: What Happens to Their Children?* Bethesda, MD: Child Trends.

Murray, J., and D. P. Farrington. 2008. "The Effects of Parental Imprisonment on Children." In *Crime and Justice: A Review of Research*, vol. 37, edited by M. Tony, 133–206. Chicago: University of Chicago Press.

Murray, J., D. P. Farrington, I. Sekol, and R. F. Olsen. 2009. "Effects of Parental Imprisonment on Child Antisocial Behaviour and Mental Health: A Systematic Review." *Campbell Systematic Reviews* 4: 1–105. https://doi.org/10.4073/csr.2009.4.

Nijhof, K. S., R. A. T. de Kemp, and R. C. Engels. 2009. "Frequency and Seriousness of Parental Offending and Their Impact on Juvenile Offending." *Journal of Adolescence* 32 (4): 893–908. https://doi.org/10.1016/j.adolescence.2008.10.005.

Parke, R. D., and K. A. Clarke-Stewart. 2002. "Effects of Parental Incarceration on Young Children." Paper presented at the National Policy Conference: From Prison to Home: The Effect of Incarceration and Reentry on Children, Families and Communities, National Institutes of Health, Bethesda, MD, January.

Phillips, S. D., and A. J. Dettlaff. 2009. "More than Parents in Prison: The Broader Overlap between the Criminal Justice and Child Welfare Systems." *Journal of Public Child Welfare* 3 (1): 3–22. https://doi.org/10.1080/15548730802690718.

Phillips, S. D., and J. Zhao. 2010. "The Relationship between Witnessing Arrests and Elevated Symptoms of Posttraumatic Stress: Findings from a National Study of Children Involved in the Child Welfare System." *Children and Youth Services Review* 32 (10): 1246–54. https://doi.org/10.1016/j.childyouth.2010.04.015.

Poehlmann, J. 2005. "Representations of Attachment Relationships in Children of Incarcerated Mothers." *Child Development* 76 (3): 679–96. https://doi.org/10.1111/j.1467-8624.2005.00871.x.

Poehlmann, J., D. Dallaire, A. B. Loper, and L. D. Shear. 2010. "Children's Contact with Their Incarcerated Parents: Research Findings and Recommendations." *American Psychologist* 65 (6): 575–98. https://doi.org/10.1037/a0020279.

Poehlmann, J., and J. M. Eddy. 2013. "Relationship Processes and Resilience in Children with Incarcerated Parents: I. Introduction and Conceptual Framework." *Monographs of the Society for Research in Child Development* 78 (3): 1–6. https://doi.org/10.1111/mono.12017.

Reitano, J. 2017. "Adult Correctional Statistics in Canada 2015/2016." *Juristat* 85: 3–16.

Sacks, V. H., D. Murphey, and K. A. Moore. 2014. "Adverse Childhood Experiences: National and State-Level Prevalence." *Child Trends* 28: 1–11.

San Francisco Children of Incarcerated Parents Project (SFCIPP). 2003. "Children of Incarcerated Parents: A Bill of Rights." Berkeley, CA: SFCIPP.

Sapers, H. 2015. *Annual Report of the Office of the Correctional Investigator 2014–2015*. 42nd Annual Report. Ottawa: Correctional Investigator of Canada.

Shaw, M., K. Rodgers, J. Blanchette, T. Hattem, L. S. Thomas, and L. Tamarack. 1991. "Survey of Federally Sentenced Women: Report to the Task Force on Federally Sentenced Women on the Prison Survey." Ottawa: Correctional Service of Canada.

Swisher, R. R., and U. R. Shaw-Smith. 2015. "Paternal Incarceration and Adolescent Well-Being: Life Course Contingencies and Other Moderators." *Journal of Criminal Law & Criminology* 104 (4): 929–59.

Tasca, M., J. Turanovic, C. White, and N. Rodriguez. 2014. "Prisoners' Assessments of Mental Health Problems among Their Children." *International Journal of Offender Therapy and Comparative Criminology* 58 (2): 154–73. https://doi.org/10.1177/0306624X12469602.

van de Rakt, M., J. Murray, and P. Nieuwbeerta. 2012. "The Long-Term Effects of Paternal Imprisonment on Criminal Trajectories of Children." *Journal of Research in Crime and Delinquency* 49 (1): 81–108.

Wildeman, C. 2010. "Paternal Incarceration and Children's Physically Aggressive Behaviors: Evidence from the Fragile Families and Child Wellbeing Study." *Social Forces* 89 (1): 285–309. https://doi.org/10.1353/sof.2010.0055.

Withers, L., and J. Folsom. 2008. *Incarcerated Fathers: A Descriptive Analysis*. Research Report R-186. Ottawa: Correctional Service of Canada.

CHAPTER 12

Approaching the Health and Marginalization of People Who Use Opioids

Sharon Koivu and Thomas Piggott

LEARNING OBJECTIVES

After reading this chapter, you should be able to:

1. Appreciate the magnitude of the opioid crisis in Canada.
2. Examine the relationship between social determinants of health, such as homelessness, and addiction.
3. Consider strategies for responding to this crisis.

Marginalization can be insidious and systemic, its impact both simultaneously subtle and blatant—so glaring that we can't see it. Such is the case of people suffering from opioid-related substance-use disorder in Canada.

Addiction to opioids (sometimes referred to as narcotics) has become a health problem of unprecedented proportions, with overdose now a leading cause of death in many parts of the world. Gomes et al. (2014) found that in Canada, among those individuals between the ages of 25 and 34 years, approximately one out of every eight deaths was related to opioid overdoses.

Rates of opioid-related deaths in Ontario increased from 12 deaths per million in 1991 (127 deaths annually) to 42 deaths per million in 2010 (550 deaths annually) and to 62 deaths per million in 2017 (867 deaths annually)—an increase of 242 percent (Gomes et al. 2014; Public Health Ontario 2018). Rates in British Columbia have increased even higher as demonstrated in figure 12.1. In spite of increased awareness of the problem, the death toll keeps mounting. In 2016, the Public Health Agency of Canada found an estimated 2,800 people died of opioid overdoses, a national death rate of 77 per million people (Government of Canada 2017). The rates of overdose by Canadian province and

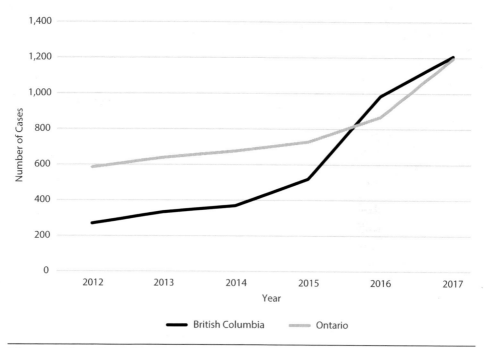

Figure 12.1: Trends in Opioid Overdose Deaths in British Columbia and Ontario, 2012–2017

Note: 2017 data for Ontario is based on preliminary reporting as of June 13, 2018.

Sources: BC Coroners Service (2018) and Public Health Ontario (2018).

territory are demonstrated in figure 12.2. Approximately 1 of every 170 deaths in Ontario is now related to opioid use (Gomes et al. 2014). By 2012, deaths in London, Ontario, due to drug overdose were three times more common than deaths due to motor vehicle crashes (Caldarelli, Skellet, and Locker 2014). Tragically, opioid-related deaths result in more than 20,000 potential life years lost annually in Ontario (Gomes et al. 2014). In addition to the tremendous toll on the families affected, this loss places a significant burden on society.

Infections caused by injection of prescription opioids, while not as likely to cause death in as rapid a manner as overdose, can be equally fatal. In addition to HIV and hepatitis C, people can develop numerous serious infections, including abscesses of the lung and spine; joint infections; sepsis; septic emboli to lungs, brain, and extremities; and endocarditis (heart valve infections), which can cause heart failure, stroke, loss of limbs, and death. At London Health Sciences Centre, we found that 33 percent of patients diagnosed with infective endocarditis had died within two years of diagnosis (Shetty et al. 2016). This population is the marginalized of the marginalized; their deaths are too frequently invisible.

To date, data on infectious complications of drug use are excluded from substance-use disorder deaths because these do not meet the current definition of "accidental death" and

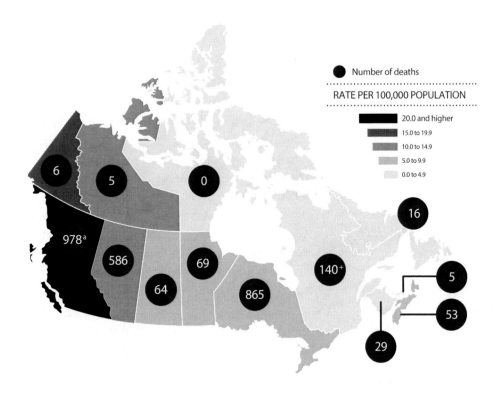

Figure 12.2: Number and Rate of Deaths Due to Opioid Overdose by Canadian Province or Territory

a British Columbia reports unintentional deaths related to all illicit drugs including, but not limited to, opiates

+ Expected to rise

Source: Reproduced with permission from the Government of Canada (2017).

are therefore overlooked by the Coroner's Office (Coroner's Act 1990). Thus, statistics on deaths from substance use, as overwhelming as they are, do not even come close to capturing the full extent of the problem.

Physician prescribing habits of opioids have been a central part of the problem, with deaths from accidental overdose directly related to rates of prescribing (Dhalla et al. 2009). In 2009, most opioids sold illegally on the street were obtained legally from physicians and then diverted, not stolen (Inciardi et al. 2009). The dramatic increase in the prescribing of opioids in the 2000s was due in part to myths and misunderstandings, some advanced by pharmaceutical marketing. Health care providers were misled into believing that pain prevented people from experiencing the euphoric effects of opioids, and, therefore, these individuals "could not get addicted."

The pharmaceutical marketing of opioids in North America was driven by one company over many others. Purdue Pharma of Stamford, Connecticut, brought the prescription opioid OxyContin to the market in 1995. It was heralded as revolutionary in treating severe pain, and although the evidence did not support it being less addictive, it was marketed as such due to its time-release delivery mechanism; in reality, its potential for abuse was greater than other opioids. The drug eventually made the Sackler family, who own the private company Purdue Pharma, over 35 billion dollars in revenue (Keefe 2017). Numerous states and the Canadian government have pursued legal action against Purdue, but it is too little too late; the damage is done (*Associated Press* 2017).

While prescription opioids such as OxyContin seem to have triggered the epidemic, the ripple effect is far-reaching. As prescribing practices begin to change, more people who use opioids are being forced to seek other sources of opioids for their addiction. Highly potent illicit synthetic opioids, such as fentanyl and carfentanil, are more commonly being found on the street. Samples obtained from law enforcement and submitted to Health Canada for testing have seen a 2,000 percent increase in fentanyl detection since 2012 (Government of Canada 2017). Deaths from highly potent opioids are rising as well: in 2016, half of opioid overdose deaths were associated with fentanyl or its analogues (Government of Canada 2017).

In the face of an overwhelming epidemic, hospitals have been slow to adapt to the needs of patients. People who are admitted to hospital with infectious complications of substance abuse are often pre-contemplative of addressing their disease, are admitted because they are acutely ill, and are not seeking addiction treatment or services. The health care providers offering direct care are not trained or skilled with this population, and, often, psychiatry will not offer support at this stage. Many are unrecognized victims of violence or physical or sexual abuse, with severe post-traumatic stress disorder. Gabor Maté (2008) has written that "not all addictions are rooted in abuse or trauma, but I do believe they can all be traced to painful experience. A hurt is at the centre of all addictive behaviours" (36). Countering this crisis requires an acknowledgement of this and the other determinants of addictions.

COUNTERING THE CRISIS

It is challenging to imagine an end in sight for the opioid crisis. But this must be our target, and as health care providers and policy-makers, we must do our best to serve the individuals and families affected by the crisis, who have for too long remained under-served. The first step is acknowledging the crisis. While it is something health care providers have witnessed for many years, it has only been in the past couple of years that society has paid increased attention to the crisis. While the former view of people who use drugs was a homogenous stereotype of the marginalized inner-city poor, the perspective has expanded, as opioid abuse has struck Canadians across geographical and income divisions. It is unfortunate that it has taken this expanded impact for the crisis to be recognized, but we must capitalize on the attention to mobilize action. Action must occur at every level in Canada, from the federal government's policy down to the pen of the provider.

POLICY RESPONSE

Governments have responded variably to the opioid crisis across Canada. In British Columbia, where opioid overdose was first identified as a crisis, Provincial Medical Health Officer Dr. Perry Kendall responded decisively, declaring a provincial emergency in order to mobilize resources to respond to the opioid crisis (BC Centre for Disease Control 2016). Other provinces have responded more slowly—in Ontario, the announcement of a public health emergency was proclaimed more covertly—but across the country, the opioids crisis is rising to the top of the political agenda (Ontario 2017). Intergenerational trauma, as discussed by Freeman in Chapter 3 of this volume, has exacerbated the opioid crisis in Indigenous communities. Based on data suggesting that opioid addictions affect 43 to 85 percent of individuals of certain First Nations, the Assembly of First Nations Special Chiefs Assembly (2016) adopted a resolution for the development of a First Nations Opioid Strategy.

At the federal government level, the opioid crisis is also gaining attention. While opioids were absent from Prime Minister Trudeau's Ministerial Mandate Letter to the Honourable Dr. Jane Philpott, upon election, as minister of health, she made the crisis a political priority (Trudeau 2015). Actions taken include Bill C-37 to facilitate the creation of safe injection sites and the approval of diacetylmorphine, or medical grade heroin, for use in treatment of addictions (Government of Canada 2016; Philpott 2017).

The government has recognized that tremendously more work is necessary to begin to address the opioid crisis. The federal government has published a four-pillar strategy for *Taking Action on Canada's Opioid Crisis*: 1) preventing problematic drug use; 2) supporting innovative approaches to treatment; 3) supporting a range of harm reduction tools and measures for individuals and communities; and 4) addressing enforcement, including of illegal drug production, supply, and distribution (Government of Canada 2013). Using the action plan's framework, we will now discuss interventions to respond to the opioids crisis.

TREATMENT OF ADDICTIONS

Without treatment, addiction is progressive and can result in disability or premature death (American Society of Addiction Medicine 2011). With treatment, recovery is possible. Treatment of addictions has therefore become integral in the response from health care providers to the opioid crisis. Opioid agonist therapy is the mainstay of treatment, providing a more stable alternative for people who use opioids. Two forms of opioid agonist therapy available are methadone and buprenorphine/naloxone; these are both becoming more accessible for people who use drugs. While methadone therapy has been available for many years as a harm reduction model to improve quality of life of people with opioid use disorder, special training and licensing is required for its prescription and has limited its availability. A safer alternative, buprenorphine/naloxone, is now the first-line opioid agonist therapy in Ontario and is covered by most drug benefit plans (CAMH 2016).

While training for its prescribing is available and recommended, no special licensing for physicians is necessary in Canada (Suboxone n.d.). It is hoped that this will enhance the availability of opioid agonist therapy.

Like other chronic diseases, addiction often involves cycles of relapse and remission. Providers should consider the Stages of Change Model (DiClemente and Prochaska 1998) and where their patient sits within the framework in order to tailor their efforts. People who use drugs are often under-served by health care providers because they are assumed to not be amenable to change; this assumption is dangerous and further marginalizes this population. There is evidence that even pre-contemplative patients can benefit from addiction counselling in hospital (DiClemente 1991).

HARM REDUCTION

Harm reduction has been integral to the response to the opioid crisis. *Harm reduction* refers to a focus on improvement of health and minimization of harms in people who use drugs, without a focus on stopping drug use. The aims of harm reduction have included preventing transmission of infectious diseases and the prevention of overdose from opioid use. The first aim, preventing transmission of infectious diseases, has been a long-standing public health priority through distribution of clean needles for people who use injection drugs. In Canada, needle distribution programs began in Toronto in 1987 (Canadian Centre on Substance Abuse n.d.).

While needle exchange programs reduce the harms of infectious disease transmission, the serious harm of overdose remains. Two harm reduction strategies have emerged to counter this harm for people who use drugs. The first is supervised injection sites (SIS) and the second is distribution of overdose prevention kits. SIS has been renamed to the preferred term *supervised consumption sites* to account for opioids consumed intranasally or orally, which may carry similar risk of overdose and may benefit from supervised consumption. SIS first started in Switzerland in 1986 as a strategy to both provide clean needles and reduce the harms of overdose (Hedrich 2004). Expansion in Europe ensued through the 1990s, with programs commencing in Germany, the Netherlands, and Spain. Outside of Europe, Australia's first SIS opened in Sydney in 2001. Vancouver's Insite, now globally renowned for the evidence in support of safe consumption facilities that has emerged, opened in June 2003 (Vancouver Coastal Health n.d.b).

Overdose prevention kits are distributed to people who use drugs, or their close family members or friends, to use in the event of a presumptive overdose. The kits contain a dose of naloxone and the materials for its administration. Traditionally this was a dose for intramuscular injection; however, now intranasal administration is becoming more widely available. Intranasal naloxone has the benefit of ease of administration and less training being required. Regardless of the administration route, proper instruction on procedures and when to use should be conducted alongside kit distribution. Depending on the jurisdiction these kits have been distributed by local public health authorities or pharmacists. Evidence collected to date demonstrates this is a lifesaving harm reduction strategy (Banjo et al. 2014).

A global model for addictions care centred on harm reduction has been developed at the supervised injection site Insite in Vancouver's Downtown Eastside (Marsh and Buchner 2015). Insite has operated as a supervised injection facility designed specifically to meet needs of people who have not been adequately served by pre-existing health services. Since opening, Insite has seen 3.4 million clients, and 6,440 overdose interventions by nursing staff have prevented countless deaths (Vancouver Coastal Health n.d.a).

In 2017, numerous other jurisdictions across Canada began turning to safe consumption sites in response to the opioid crisis. This has been facilitated by the harm reduction priorities set out in in the Government of Canada's Action Plan, including "support[ing] the establishment of safe consumption sites, facilitat[ing] access to naloxone, ensur[ing] timely laboratory drug analysis information is shared between partners, support[ing] legislation to protect individuals who seek emergency assistance for overdose, [and] reduc[ing] public health consequences of problematic drug use" (Government of Canada 2013).

ENFORCEMENT

Enforcement is one of the four pillars of Canada's Action Plan; however, it is likely the most controversial component within the health community. The strategies within enforcement include the following: "continu[ing] enforcement on the importation and trafficking of illegal opioids; pursu[ing] legislative, regulatory, policy and programmatic changes to better control substances and equipment; collect[ing], assess[ing] and shar[ing] information with law enforcement agencies domestically and internationally; [and] support[ing] education and training for law enforcement" (Government of Canada 2013).

For many in the health community, who have pushed for prioritization of harm reduction strategies, aspects of the law enforcement approach are counterproductive. Advocates for legislative reform in Canada point to evidence from other jurisdictions, such as Portugal, that have taken a progressive approach to drug use. In 2001, Portugal decriminalized all drug use, opting to treat addiction instead as a medical issue. The results of decriminalization in Portugal have shown no major increases in drug use, reduced adolescent drug use, a decrease in deaths, and reduced societal costs (Drug Policy Alliance 2015).

In the Canadian context, decriminalization of all drugs does not seem to be on the immediate political agenda, but many, including harm reduction worker Zoë Dodd, have advocated regardless (Tierney 2017). Progress has been made in conjunction with the increasing distribution of naloxone overdose prevention kits to protect those using the kits to save lives. The Good Samaritan Drug Overdose Act, passed in May 2017, protects people who experience or witness an overdose from charges for possession of controlled substances and breach of parole or probation orders—formerly barriers to the use of overdose prevention kits (Government of Canada 2018). Nonetheless, legal progress to protect people who use drugs and to endorse a prevention and harm reduction–oriented approach is still needed in Canada.

SURVEILLANCE AND EPIDEMIOLOGY

Greater knowledge of the evolving opioid crisis is necessary to drive the response. As with all surveillance on issues of public health concern, the data collection must drive action. In Canada, opioid surveillance has begun in a number of jurisdictions. Public Health Ontario (2018) has released an interactive opioid tool to provide public information on opioid morbidity and mortality, including by geography, age and sex, and type of drug. Local jurisdictions, such as Hamilton Public Health Services in Ontario, have also taken further initiative linking acute care data, including emergency room visits and paramedic response, with local public health interventions, such as the distribution of naloxone overdose prevention kits (Hamilton Public Health Services 2018). With this information, Hamilton was able to publicize that 1,700 naloxone distribution kits were distributed, resulting in 453 revivals (Hamilton Public Health Services 2018). Greater epidemiological data may improve our understanding of the determinants of opioid addictions and overdoses; however, data should drive evidence-based interventions.

EDUCATING HEALTH CARE PROFESSIONALS

While a healthy fear of opioids is increasingly being taught in undergraduate medical school, little training on addiction management or alternative strategies for pain control is provided (Goodair and Crome 2014). Furthermore, many physicians in practice received altogether no training in their education to manage the opioid crisis, despite increasing awareness of the issue. In a survey of practising family physicians in Canada, substance abuse was cited as the third most important area of competence for a newly practising family physician, ahead of ischemic heart disease, diabetes, and pregnancy (Hering et al. 2014). Awareness of the issue is rising; however, knowledge of the response remains limited.

Our curriculums need to adapt, and quickly. Postgraduate training in family medicine or psychiatry may variably address addictions prevention and treatment, but it is lacking from most other specialties—including for those who may be initiating opioids in hospital (e.g., following surgery). Education on the non-opioid strategies in our toolkit to treat pain are a critical need; multidisciplinary teams can manage pain more effectively. Education therefore needs to be integrated across medical education and within other health care professions as well.

Collectively as health care providers, we need to take ownership over the problem that has, in part, been our doing. Comprehensive education and training surrounding opioid prescribing is important, but this must also include training on harm reduction and a better understanding of the social determinants and upstream prevention of addictions.

PREVENTION AND WORKING UPSTREAM TO COUNTER THE OPIOID CRISIS

The Government of Canada's (2013) action plan puts forward prevention as a pillar in the opioid crisis response. The prevention strategies presented rely on education of the public and health care providers, and miss many "upstream" interventions as discussed by Meili and Piggott (Chapter 25 in this volume). Poverty and homelessness are significant contributors to addictions as discussed by Oudshoorn (Chapter 10 in this volume). Patients often cannot receive in-home services related to their addiction from publicly funded home care if they do not have a home. Without a home, and at times even a cellphone, patients leaving hospital are easily lost to follow-up. This further increases their risk of death. Homelessness enhances hopelessness; hopelessness drives addictions. A mutually reinforcing relationship is apparent between homelessness and mental illness and substance use (Echenberg and Jensen 2009).

The classical approach to homelessness was that individuals could not live stably in community-supported housing without having overcome their addiction. More recently, evidence from "housing-first" programs, such as At Home, Chez Soi, has supported a focus first on stable housing, showing that management of addiction will follow (Aubry, Nelson, and Tsemberis 2015). Addressing other social determinants such as employment and education level is also critical in responding to the opioid crisis in an upstream manner.

CONCLUSIONS

Substance-use disorder is a medical problem, but at its roots are the social determinants of health. Health care providers have contributed to the current epidemic. We need to understand our responsibility and accountability. If we respond with compassion, empathy, and understanding to this under-served population and engage in upstream work, we will find solutions to end this marginalization.

CRITICAL THINKING QUESTIONS

1. In what ways are people who use drugs marginalized?
2. What are the responsibilities of health care providers, public health practitioners, and policy-makers in the current opioid crisis?
3. What are solutions to the opioid crisis that address upstream factors and the social determinants of health? What are the challenges to adopting these solutions?

ADDITIONAL RESOURCES

1. For individuals interested in learning more about prescribing buprenorphine/naloxone, see the Suboxone Training Program: https://www.suboxonetrainingprogram.ca/.

2. The Centre for Addiction and Mental Health has numerous evidence-based resources for health care providers:
   http://camh.ca/.

3. The Canadian Society of Addiction Medicine has promoted awareness among health care professionals and the public more broadly:
   https://www.csam-smca.org/.

4. The Centers for Disease Control and Prevention (CDC) "Guidelines for Prescribing Opioids for Chronic Pain" (2016) provides guidance for practitioners:
   https://www.cdc.gov/drugoverdose/prescribing/guideline.html.

5. The 2017 Canadian "Guideline for Opioid Therapy and Chronic Noncancer Pain" is essential reading for all physicians prescribing opioids:
   Busse, Jason W., Samantha Craigie, David N. Juurlink, D. Norman Buckley, Li Wang, Rachel J. Couban, Thomas Agoritsas, et al. 2017. "Guideline for Opioid Therapy and Chronic Non-cancer Pain." *CMAJ* 189 (18): E659–66. https://doi.org/10.1503/cmaj.170363.

6. *In the Realm of Hungry Ghosts* by Dr. Gabor Maté is a stark yet inspiring portrait into the life and work of one physician working in Vancouver's Downtown Eastside with people who use drugs:
   Maté, Gabor. 2008. *In the Realm of Hungry Ghosts: Close Encounters with Addictions*. Toronto: Knopf Canada.

7. The Government of Canada website on opioids has numerous resources for care providers and the public, including the opioids toolkit (https://www.canada.ca/en/health-canada/services/substance-abuse/prescription-drug-abuse/opioids/resources-toolkit.html):
   https://www.canada.ca/en/health-canada/services/substance-abuse/prescription-drug-abuse/opioids.html.

REFERENCES

American Society of Addiction Medicine. 2011. "The Definition of Addiction." April 12. http://www.asam.org/advocacy/find-a-policy-statement/view-policy-statement/public-policy-statements/2011/12/15/the-definition-of-addiction.

Assembly of First Nations Special Chiefs Assembly. 2016. "Development of a First Nations Opioids Strategy." Resolution no. 82/2016. Assembly of First Nations 2016 Special Chiefs Assembly, Gatineau, QC, Final Resolutions. http://www.afn.ca/uploads/files/resolutions/sca-2016.pdf.

Associated Press. 2017. "New Jersey Becomes Latest State to Sue Purdue Pharma over OxyContin." *CBC News*, October 31. http://www.cbc.ca/news/health/new-jersey-lawsuit-purdue-pharma-oxycontin-1.4380376.

Aubry, T., G. Nelson, and S. Tsemberis. 2015. "Housing First for People with Severe Mental Illness Who Are Homeless: A Review of the Research and Findings from the At Home–Chez Soi Demonstration Project." *Canadian Journal of Psychiatry* 60 (11): 467–74. https://doi.org/10.1177/070674371506001102.

Banjo, Oluwajenyo, Despina Tzemis, Diana Al-Qutub, Ashraf Amlani, Sarah Kesselring, and Jane A. Buxton. 2014. "A Quantitative and Qualitative Evaluation of the British Columbia Take Home Naloxone Program." *CMAJ Open* 2 (3): E153–E161. https://doi.org/10.9778/cmajo.20140008.

BC Centre For Disease Control. 2016. "Provincial Health Officer Declares Public Health Emergency." *BC Gov News*, April 14. https://news.gov.bc.ca/releases/2016HLTH0026-000568.

BC Coroners Service. 2018. *Illicit Drug Overdose Deaths in BC*. Victoria, BC: BC Coroners Service. https://www2.gov.bc.ca/assets/gov/public-safety-and-emergency-services/death-investigation/statistical/illicit-drug.pdf.

Caldarelli, H., R. Skellet, and A. Locker. 2014. *Prescription and Non-prescription Drug Use and Their Impacts in Middlesex-London*. London, ON: Middlesex-London Health Unit. https://www.middlesex.ca/council/2014/july/22/C%2012%20-%20CW%20Info%20-%20July%2022%20-%20The%20Impact%20of%20Prescription%20and%20Non-Prescritpion%20Drug%20Use%20in%20Middlesex-London.pdf.

Canadian Centre on Substance Abuse. n.d. "Needle Exchange Programs FAQs," Ottawa: Canadian Centre on Substance Abuse. Accessed January 24, 2018. http://www.ccsa.ca/Resource%20Library/ccsa-010055-2004.pdf.

Centre for Addiction and Mental Health (CAMH). 2016. *Prescription Opioid Policy Framework*. Toronto: CAMH. https://www.camh.ca/en/hospital/about_camh/influencing_public_policy/Documents/CAMHopioidpolicyframework.pdf.

Coroners Act, R.S.O. 1990. Chapter C.37, Section 10. http://www.ontario.ca/laws/statute/90c37#BK19.

Dhalla, I., Muhammad M. Mamdani, Marco L. A. Sivilotti, Alex Kopp, Omar Qureshi, and David N. Juurlink. 2009. "Prescribing of Opioid Analgesics and Related Mortality before and after the Introduction of Long-Acting Oxycodone." *CMAJ* 181 (12) 891–6. https://doi.org/10.1503/cmaj.090784.

DiClemente, C. C. 1991. "Motivational Interviewing and the Stages of Change." In *Motivational Interviewing: Preparing People to Change Addictive Behaviour*, edited by W. R. Miller and S. Rollnick, 191–202. New York: Guildford.

DiClemente, C. C., and J. O. Prochaska. 1998. "Toward a Comprehensive, Transtheoretical Model of Change: Stages of Change and Addictive Behaviors." In *Applied Clinical Psychology: Treating Addictive Behaviors*, edited by W. R. Miller and N. Heather, 3–24). New York: Plenum Press. http://dx.doi.org/10.1007/978-1-4899-1934-2_1.

Drug Policy Alliance. 2015. *Drug Decriminalization in Portugal: A Health-Centred Approach*. New York: Drug Policy Alliance. https://www.drugpolicy.org/sites/default/files/DPA_Fact_Sheet_Portugal_Decriminalization_Feb2015.pdf.

Echenberg, Havi, and Hilary Jensen. 2009. "Risk Factors for Homelessness." Library of Parliament Background Papers. Publication no. PRB 08-51E. 2 February. Reviewed May 17, 2012. http://www.homelesshub.ca/sites/default/files/Risk%20Factors%20for%20Homelessness.pdf.

Gomes, Tara, Muhammad M. Mamdani, Irfan A. Dhalla, Stephen Cornish, J. Michael Paterson, and David N. Juurlink. 2014. "The Burden of Premature Opioid-Related Mortality." *Addiction* 109 (9): 1482–8. https://doi.org/10.1111/add.12598.

Goodair, Christine, and Ilana Crome. 2014. "Improving the Landscape of Substance Misuse Teaching in Undergraduate Medical Education in English Medical Schools from Concept to Implementation." *Canadian Journal of Addiction Medicine* 5 (3): 5–10.

Government of Canada. 2013. *Taking Action on Canada's Opioid Crisis*. Ottawa: Health Canada. Last modified April 3. http://publications.gc.ca/pub?id=9.848417&sl=0.

Government of Canada. 2016. "Regulations Amending Certain Regulations Made under the Controlled Drugs and Substances Act (Access to Diacetylmorphine for Emergency Treatment)." September 7. http://www.gazette.gc.ca/rp-pr/p2/2016/2016-09-07/html/sor-dors239-eng.html.

Government of Canada. 2017. *Actions on Opioids 2016 and 2017*. Ottawa: Health Canada. https://www.canada.ca/content/dam/hc-sc/documents/services/publications/healthy-living/actions-opioids-2016-2017/Opioids-Response-Report-EN-FINAL.pdf.

Government of Canada. 2018. "About the Good Samaritan Drug Overdose Act." Last modified March 6. https://www.canada.ca/en/health-canada/services/substance-abuse/prescription-drug-abuse/opioids/about-good-samaritan-drug-overdose-act.html.

Hamilton Public Health Services. 2018. "Hamilton Opioid Information System." Last modified March 21. https://www.hamilton.ca/public-health/reporting/hamilton-opioid-information-system.

Hedrich, Dagmar. 2004. *European Report on Drug Consumption Rooms*. Lisbon, Portugal: European Monitoring Centre for Drugs and Drug Addiction.

Hering, Ramm, Lisa Lefebvre, Pamela Stewart, and Peter Selby. 2014. "Increasing Addiction Medicine Capacity in Canada: The Case for Collaboration in Education and Research." *Canadian Journal of Addiction Medicine* 5 (3): 10–14.

Inciardi, James A., Hilary L. Surratt, Theodore J. Cicero, and Ronald A. Beard. 2009. "Prescription Opioid Abuse and Diversion in an Urban Community: The Results of an *Ultra*-rapid Assessment." *Pain Medicine* 10 (3): 537–48. https://doi.org/10.1111/j.1526-4637.2009.00603.x.

Keefe, P. R. 2017. "The Family That Built an Empire of Pain." *New Yorker*, October 30. https://www.newyorker.com/magazine/2017/10/30/the-family-that-built-an-empire-of-pain.

Marsh, David, and Chris Buchner. 2015. "Insite: Treatment and Care for People with Chronic Addiction and Complex Health Issues." Vancouver: Vancouver Coastal Health.

Maté, Gabor. 2008. *In the Realm of Hungry Ghosts: Close Encounters with Addictions*. Toronto: Knopf Canada.

Ontario. 2017. "Ontario Expanding Opioid Response as Crisis Grows." December 7. https://news.ontario.ca/mohltc/en/2017/12/ontario-expanding-opioid-response-as-crisis-grows.html.

Philpott, Jane. 2017. "Bill C-37: An Act to Amend the Controlled Drugs and Substances Act and to Make Related Amendments to Other Acts." 42nd Parliament, 1st Session, December 3. https://openparliament.ca/bills/42-1/C-37/.

Public Health Ontario. 2018. "Opioid-Related Morbidity and Mortality in Ontario." Last updated March 7. http://www.publichealthontario.ca/en/dataandanalytics/pages/opioid.aspx.

Shetty, N., D. Nagpal, S. Koivu, and M. Mrkobrada. 2016. "Surgical and Medical Management of Isolated Tricuspid Valve Endocarditis in Intravenous Drug Users." *Journal of Cardiac Surgery* 31 (2): 83–8. https://doi.org/10.1111/jocs.12682.

Suboxone. n.d. "SUBOXONE® Training Program." Accessed January 21, 2018. https://www.suboxonetrainingprogram.ca/.

Tierney, A. 2017. "Meet the Harm Reduction Worker Who Called Out Trudeau on the Opioid Crisis." *Vice News*, April 25. https://www.vice.com/en_ca/article/ez3m5a/meet-the-harm-reduction-worker-who-called-out-trudeau-on-the-opioid-crisis.

Trudeau, J. 2015. "Minister of Health Mandate Letter." Ottawa: Government of Canada. https://pm.gc.ca/eng/minister-health-mandate-letter_2015.

Vancouver Coastal Health. n.d.a. "From the Ground Up: Vancouver's Supervised Injection Site's Role in Accessing Treatment and Care." Accessed August 30, 2015. http://www.vch.ca/public-health/harm-reduction/supervised-injection-sites.

Vancouver Coastal Health. n.d.b. "Insite User Statistics." Accessed January 24, 2018. http://www.vch.ca/public-health/harm-reduction/supervised-injection-sites/insite-user-statistics.

CHAPTER 13

Pathways to Health Equity for LGBTQ Populations

Nathan Lachowsky, Jacqueline Gahagan, and Kelly Anderson

LEARNING OBJECTIVES:

After reading this chapter, you should be able to:

1. Distinguish between sexual orientation and gender identity.
2. Appreciate the diversity within LGBTQ populations and the intersections with other marginalized populations.
3. Identify health disparities and resiliencies among LGBTQ populations in Canada.
4. Recognize how structural determinants of health such as heteronormativity negatively impact the health of LGBTQ populations.

A PREFACE: LGBTQ TERMINOLOGY

LGBTQ is an acronym intended to capture the dominant Western self-identity labels (not practices) that individuals share as sexual orientation and gender identity (SOGI) minorities. In this case, *LGBTQ* refers to lesbian, gay, bisexual, transgender, and queer. However, there is a wide variety of terminology related to sexual orientation, gender, sexuality, and queer cultures. *Lesbian*, *gay*, and *bisexual* are sexual orientation identity labels, which can be understood as one's preference for sexual and romantic partners. In terms of sexual orientation, the 2014 Canadian Community Health Survey found that 3 percent of Canadians identified themselves to be gay, lesbian, or bisexual (Statistics Canada 2015). *Transgender* or *trans* people are those whose gender identity differs from their physical sex characteristics, as determined by social norms and expectations. *Queer* is a catchall term used proudly by some individuals to defy gender or sexual restrictions; however, given the negative historical use of the term, it is not reclaimed by everyone and may be hurtful for some.

The history of language is an important one to consider in relation to LGBTQ populations. For example, the term *homosexual* was used in law and medicine to describe a perversion or pathology (O'Neill 2013). Homosexual acts between consenting adults was decriminalized in Canada in 1969. However, the term was not removed from the American Psychiatric Association's *Diagnostics and Statistical Manual of Mental Disorders* until 1986. Further, the term *homosexual* is not considered community-based, and while some individuals may choose this label or descriptor for themselves, it is generally considered an offensive and discriminatory term, and many advocate for the abandonment of its use. We emphasize the importance of using language that individuals and communities adopt to describe themselves, either in terms of sexual orientation or gender identity, as one way to demonstrate cultural competency. However, it is always better to ask than assume, and to remember that individuals may have their own history and comfort with different terminology. As such, it should be kept in mind that no "one size fits all" solution exists in the use of terminology in describing LGBTQ populations.

LGBTQ as a population label is homogenizing of and reductionist towards a diverse population of people, even with a label such as *queer* included. Although there are shared experiences in terms of discrimination and health inequities, the LGBTQ label does not capture the full spectrum of people within these communities; as such, it often fails to fully animate the diversity of lived experiences within health care systems and practices. Practically speaking, such attempts to use homogenizing labels will inevitably ignore and erase other marginalized sexual orientations, gender identities and expressions, and sexual practices. From a health promotion perspective, we must question and interrogate the utility of LGBTQ as a macro-category as a helpful framework for the provision of culturally competent, population-specific approaches to advancing and improving health equity. By cultural competence, we mean the capacity to effectively work with and provide care for LGBTQ people to address their needs.

What makes LGBTQ populations different from other populations, and why they are an important group to include and consider within this book, is largely based on societal norms and expectations of heteronormativity and cis-genderism, also known as cisheterosexism. The social privilege afforded by mainstream society to those who are heterosexual and those whose gender identity and expression are congruent with their biological sex and society's norm of a gender binary is important to acknowledge and understand as health care practitioners. By *social privilege*, we mean the advantages and rights that certain groups of people have in society as a product of their social location (e.g., gender, age, race or ethnicity, class, religion, sexuality, ability). When considering upstream determinants of health, dismantling this cisheteronormative framing and the systems that perpetuate it are perhaps the most critical ways in which to improve the health and well-being of people across the gender spectrum and of all sexual orientations.

LGBTQ HEALTH IN CANADA

There are persistent examples of health inequities experienced among sexual and gender minoritized communities across Canada. For example, enduring high rates of HIV infection among gay men in urban Canadian centres (PHAC 2013) and low rates of preventative screening such as breast and cervical cancer screening among lesbians, bisexual women, and trans people are noteworthy in advancing health outcomes (Quinn et al. 2015). Men who have sex with men are 71 times more likely to be diagnosed with HIV than other men, and they comprise half the people living with HIV in Canada: an estimated 35,490 of 71,300 in 2014 (PHAC 2014). In addition, there is a growing body of literature that demonstrates significantly higher rates of mental health disorders, suicide, and self-harm among both LGBTQ youth and adults (Brennan et al. 2010; King et al. 2008). For example, suicide attempts were twice as likely and mental health disorders (e.g., depression, anxiety, substance dependence) were 1.5 times as likely among lesbian, gay, and bisexual people compared with heterosexual people (King et al. 2008). These higher rates of poor health outcomes may be, in part, attributable to minority stress and social isolation. Perhaps less known is that pelvic exam and screening rates for cervical cancer are lower among trans men (Taylor and Bryson 2016; Quinn et al. 2015). These examples of health inequities offer a focus on negative health outcomes currently enumerated in our Canadian population, rather than on how health systems themselves may be inaccessible or unwelcoming for many LGBTQ individuals. The long-standing deficit-focused approach to understanding and measuring LGBTQ health suggests the need to shift our thinking to address what issues and which LGBTQ populations are not being captured or rendered visible in our public health research, surveillance, or clinical data sets (Colpitts and Gahagan 2016a; Gahagan and Colpitts 2017). How do we investigate both health inequities and resilience among these populations? How do we meaningfully engage and learn from community voices and lived experiences regarding the health outcomes that are most important and/or relevant to them in balance with public health and governmental priorities? Case 1 is a first-person account of a trans patient and the culturally competent care, support, and allyship demonstrated by their social worker and doctor.

Beyond this chapter, this book has focused on several key populations in terms of health equity in Canada: inner-city homeless people, Indigenous people, and immigrants. Within each of these categories, LGBTQ individuals are either overrepresented or commonly rendered invisible (known as erasure). Queer youth are disproportionately represented in homeless populations, present with complex needs, yet are often systemically excluded from shelters and related health and social care (Abramovich 2012). Within Indigenous populations, *Two-Spirit* is a term meant to (re)capture the inclusive or strength-based lens used by certain tribes to understand those who we as English

Case 1

"I grew up in Northern Africa, within a very orthodox religious family, and came here as a refugee with my family when I was twelve. I have sisters, and I knew from when I was small that I wanted to be like them, and not like my brothers. Any interest in my sisters' clothes, or how they played, was scorned from an early age. In the refugee camp, I was not allowed to spend time with the girls. I had to be part of a gang of boys and men responsible for haggling, stealing food, and making sure we had supplies. We also protected our camps. When we came to Canada, it was the first time I saw that not all men were forced to behave in the masculine, aggressive, and often violent ways that I'd been taught. I started to, in private, experiment with wearing some women's clothing and makeup. I made female friends at school and they could understand me in a way that no man could. I felt I was one of them. I realized I was attracted to men. All of this would have been foreign, shameful, and unsafe physically to reveal to my family, so I hid—never vocalizing any of these thoughts, never letting anyone see me dressed in a feminine way, trying to not even think those thoughts. In my early twenties, I started going out and meeting some trans women that I met online. I knew in my heart that I had found a place I belonged, that I needed to be female. Soon after I left the home of my family and started living alone. I decided I would wear clothes that felt right to me, and grew my hair. I got electrolysis for my facial and chest hair, and wore makeup to make me feel more confident. I am naturally lean and have a feminine voice, which helped my social transition. I was lucky to be referred to a doctor that helped me start hormones with some counselling around my transition. I felt confident enough to change my name, even on my driver's license and health card, with the help of a social worker and my doctor. I'm now applying for top surgery, and I feel that fully completing my physical transition will be a turning point for me in my life. I'm no longer able to be integrated with my family because of the stigma and taboo associated with my choices. But I finally feel that I'm able to live an external life that is congruent with who I am inside."

settlers/colonizers label as LGBTQ, and to reimagine an Indigenous lens on Western concepts of SOGI (Greensmith and Giwa 2013). Finally, LGBTQ refugees have unique experiences of migration and immigration applications (and hearings) and, if successful, experiences within Canadian communities and society (Lee and Brotman 2011). We want to emphasize the prominence and inclusion of an LGBTQ subpopulation within and across all other populations of interest. We recommend a health approach known as intersectionality to examine these health disparities, which includes SOGI along with other aspects of social location (e.g., race, class, gender) (Crenshaw 1991; Hankivsky 2014; Mink and Weinstein 2014; Mulé and Smith 2014), as these help reveal the critical junctures associated with the resultant health disparities.

LGBTQ STATUS AND THE SOCIAL DETERMINANTS OF HEALTH

As has been discussed in this book previously, gender is a well-acknowledged determinant of health. Although sexual orientation is a critical upstream driver of health equity for LGBTQ populations, it is not officially recognized as a key determinant of health by the Public Health Agency of Canada (1999). This has been recognized in the United States, however, where SOGI has been integrated into data collection and policy spheres (Cahill and Makadon 2014). Canada is nonetheless lagging behind in formally acknowledging and including the needs of SOGI populations in mainstream health and social care policies and programs. An individual's SOGI affects not only health outcomes and susceptibility to disease and infection; perhaps more importantly, access to and use of culturally safe health education and care services are also impacted. The Fenway Institute (2014), for example, outlines the case of LGBTQ populations as under-served in health care and continues to push to address related health inequities that can lead to poor health outcomes.

The preponderance of sexual health literature on LGBTQ populations provides a powerful example to think through some of these health equity issues. However, a challenge in doing so is to not reify the current synonymous equation of LGBTQ with sexually transmitted infections (STIs). Historically, health research has focused on the greater burden of STIs among LGBTQ populations, ignoring the resilience demonstrated by these communities in terms of pioneering sexual health education and prevention approaches (e.g., the widespread adoption of condom use) despite system-wide oppression. Nonetheless, gay, bisexual, and queer men in Canada are commonly reported as having enduring STI disparities compared with heterosexual men (Brennan et al. 2010). However, gay, bisexual, and queer men are not routinely provided with appropriate STI testing (pharyngeal and rectal swabs), despite recommendations for such being in place; this then contributes in part to the ongoing propagation of these epidemics. Part of this challenge relates to the lack of physicians' awareness regarding their patients' sexual orientation. A 2014 national survey of over eight thousand gay, bisexual, and other men who have sex with men found that 37.5 percent had not revealed their sexual orientation to their primary care provider, with those who were bisexual-identified and younger less likely to disclose (Trussler and Ham 2016). Not establishing rapport and open communication with patients may create a barrier to appropriate care, as well as decreased adherence to physician advice and treatment plans (Dean et al. 2000). Homophobic experiences from health care providers (intentional or otherwise) can lead to patients' unwillingness to reveal their sexual orientation or their gender identity, or to discuss certain sexual practices that might "out" them to their health care providers. Health research has documented gay and bisexual men's experiences with health care providers, which has included embarrassment, anxiety, inappropriate reactions, patient rejection, hostility, harassment, excessive curiosity, pity, condescension, ostracism, refusal of treatment, detachment, avoidance of physical contact, or breach of confidentiality (Brotman, Ryan, and Cormier 2003). In Case 2 a patient living with HIV and other

Case 2

"I have recently been faced with my own mortality at age 63, and only now understand the importance of having to put end-of-life plans in place. Having been HIV+ since 1980 and diagnosed with cancer for the third time, and potentially facing the challenges of ALS, I was faced with very frank and necessary conversations with two close friends.... I found myself living in Oshawa, and now Toronto, alone and, quite frankly, scared out of my wits. What now? What needs to be taken care of so I am prepared for the final journey of my life? But it had to be placed on the table for all to see, understand, question—and for me to crystalize exactly how and who are to act upon my final wishes. For me, this process presented a clear and concise picture of how my final days and after my death are to be fulfilled. In the LGBT community, we have been challenged all our lives—perceived and realized. We spent a good deal of our lives feeling rejected, different, alone, and lonely, distant from family and friends—often living several different lifestyles in order to mask who we really are. Not only do we often spend our lives in guilt, fearing rejection, recipients of bullying, derogatory comments and slurs, physical and emotional abuse, but now facing the reality that as we are viewed as being "different," how we can find a safe place for the older days of our lives. Are we going to be ostracized or abused in a senior's residence? Can we be ourselves or do we have to go back "into the closet"—a lifestyle many of us endured throughout our lives? Not only are we facing our end-of-life issues and concerns; we are facing how we can live out the remaining years of our lives as who we are—trying to be true to ourselves and to those we love and cherish. By taking the reins and putting these necessary documents and wishes into action, we secure who we are/were as we chose to live. This is the time to face these concerns and issues head on while we are still strong and focused—and in control of our faculties. I can't impress upon you how important it is to proceed as quickly as possible."

intersecting health issues describes the social challenges he faces as he ages as a member of the LGBTQ community.

Relatedly, some health care providers administer inadequate sexual health screening and care to lesbian and bisexual women, including lack of referral for pap smears, working under the faulty assumption that these women are at low risk because they have sex with other women (Brotman, Ryan, and Cormier 2003). The sexual health realities among transgender people is equally challenging and may include sexual practices that health care providers are unaware of (such as receptive genital sex by male-to-female transgender people) and unsure of how to care for in screening and education (Bauer et al. 2012). There is a distinct lack of education regarding sexuality—let alone comprehensive or culturally safe LGBTQ health education—in medical and other health professional training in Canada, and North America more generally (Shindel and Parish 2013). The third case study demonstrates the downstream negative care implications of health care providers'

> ### Case 3
>
> "I didn't come out to my first family doctor because I'm from a small town up North. At that point, in my late teens, I hadn't come out to my family or friends, and I didn't want anyone to find out I was gay. I actually didn't know anyone who was gay, and it wasn't even mentioned in my sex ed classes in high school. I wasn't sure how my doctor would take it if I did tell him that I was attracted to men. He'd been my doctor since I was born, and he'd never asked me any questions about sex or offered any test. When I did move down to the city, I started having sex with some new guys. I went to a walk-in when I needed to get checked for STIs. They put a swab into my penis which was so painful that I never went back to get tested again, scared of the pain. I met a friend who introduced me to a new family doctor, who asked me right up front who I like to have sex with. I know this doctor has a lot of gay guys in this practice, so I finally felt comfortable asking questions and learning to protect my own health. I don't feel judged if I've had an encounter that wasn't safe, and I need to deal with that after the fact. He's never done a urethral swab, and I know now that it's not the right way to check for STIs. I feel safer knowing that all the right tests have been done and get done regularly with this new doctor. I feel so grateful that I've become a part of a community that can support me, that directed me towards a health professional that understands and helps. Really, I just wish I had found someone earlier that would have helped educate me about my sexual health, because getting care made me feel more comfortable coming out. It's taken me until my late thirties to get to this place."

poor education and ignorance, and the restorative opportunities and optimal wellness that culturally competent care can provide. This chapter should only serve as the beginning of a lifelong journey to appreciate the full diversity of human sexuality, with additional resources and continuing education opportunities available.

LGBTQ communities have promoted change in health policy and practices that have benefited our broader society. In the face of the AIDS epidemic, LGBTQ activists persistently demanded change to drug approval and access pathways that have resulted in enduring differences (Edgar and Rothman 1990). LGBTQ individuals have also forwarded rights and discrimination discourses, including activism to achieve marriage equality for same-sex couples (Taylor et al. 2009), repealing discriminatory practices in the military and other institutions (Yerke and Mitchell 2013), and problematizing the human rights framework (Mertus 2007).

MOVING FORWARD

Within a health promotion approach, an approach that focuses on enabling populations to remain healthy across the life course, the question of what contributes to LGBTQ health and well-being is often absent from our evidence base (Rootman et al. 2012, 21). A shift to a more upstream, primary prevention perspective is warranted to more deeply understand and learn from these health outcomes among LGBTQ populations across the life course. The complex interplay of social and structural factors on the health outcomes among these diverse communities of sexual and gender minorities requires a rethinking of how we approach health across the life course. These intersecting determinants of health interact in complex ways with other aspects of these individuals' identities and social locations to produce particular vulnerabilities to, but also often resiliencies against, low rates of health service access and negative health outcomes (Colpitts and Gahagan 2016b). An example of this is provided in the fourth case study, where a lesbian woman living in Ontario recounts her cervical cancer diagnosis back in the 1980s when she was 21.

For clinicians and other health care providers, we support the Institute of Medicine and the Joint Commission, which have recommended asking about SOGI in clinical settings (Cahill and Makadon 2014). Research with primary health care patients in the United States who were mainly heterosexual and racially diverse demonstrated high levels of acceptability to these questions. Health policy and institutions in Canada should move to support the inclusion of such data within patient health records. In this regard, it is critical that health care providers, health researchers, and policy-makers understand and integrate SOGI into their work and, perhaps more importantly, utilize these concepts correctly. These approaches cannot stereotype or be reductionist, but instead must allow for and embrace diversity in expressions of SOGI.

Case 4

"The doctor had said to me, 'how many partners have you been with?' And I said 'One.' And he refused to believe me. He said 'You're lying.' ... And, he kept saying to me 'I won't treat you if you won't come clean.' ... I said, 'I've had relationships with other women,' because I didn't want to say lesbian. And I remember at the time thinking I was very terrified to say that. And he had said, 'With other men?' And I said, 'No, no, not at all.' And, he was just very adamant that I could not have had this disease unless I had had multiple [male] partners." Later she describes a turning point in her relationships with her health care provider: "I wanted to find a doctor who was gay friendly, who wasn't going to look down over eyeglasses at me because I was gay. And it was at that point that I decided, 'from this point on in my life, I am not going to be in the closet. I have to be out medically, professionally, socially. I have to be out.'"

Excerpt from and more information about the Cancer's Margins study is available from Taylor and Bryson (2016).

CRITICAL THINKING QUESTIONS

1. What assumptions do you have about LGBTQ people and why?
2. How does Canadian society recognize and normalize heterosexuality and being cis-gender? How do we assume someone is heterosexual or cis-gender in our conversations or on medical and social service forms? What are the sexual orientations and gender identities, at least assumed, of people who hold more power in our society (e.g., political, business, religious, and cultural leaders)?
3. What forms of interpersonal and structural violence can you identify that are faced by LGTBQ populations?
4. How could we reconcile and improve the experiences of LGBTQ people within our health and social care systems?

ADDITIONAL RESOURCES

1. The Rainbow Health Ontario (RHO)'s glossary of terms, which was created by the 519 Church Street Community Centre: http://www.rainbowhealthontario.ca/glossary/.
   This is a helpful resource to understand the diversity of terminology employed in LGBTQ communities and the particular nuance and meaning of each word.

2. The Institute of Medicine's 2011 report, *The Health of Lesbian, Gay, Bisexual, and Transgender People: Building a Foundation for Better Understanding*: http://www.nationalacademies.org/hmd/Reports/2011/The-Health-of-Lesbian-Gay-Bisexual-and-Transgender-People.aspx.
   This resource provides a comprehensive review of the state of health of LGBTQ populations as well as recommendations for a way forward to improving health.

REFERENCES

Abramovich, Ilona Alex. 2012. "No Safe Place to Go—LGBTQ Youth Homelessness in Canada: Reviewing the Literature." *Canadian Journal of Family and Youth* 4: 29–51.

Bauer, Greta R., Robb Travers, Kyle Scanlon, and Todd A. Coleman. 2012. "High Heterogeneity of HIV-Related Sexual Risk among Transgender People in Ontario, Canada: A Province-Wide Respondent-Driven Sampling Survey." *BMC Public Health* 12: 292.

Brennan, David J., Lori E. Ross, Cheryl Dobinson, Scott Veldhuizen, and Leah S. Steele. 2010. "Men's Sexual Orientation and Health in Canada." *Canadian Journal of Public Health* 101: 255–8.

Brotman, Shari, Bill Ryan, and Robert Cormier. 2003. "The Health and Social Service Needs of Gay and Lesbian Elders and Their Families in Canada." *Gerontologist* 43: 192–202.

Cahill, Sean, and Harvey J. Makadon. 2014. "Sexual Orientation and Gender Identity Collection Update: U.S. Government Takes Steps to Promote Sexual Orientation and Gender Identity Collection through Meaningful Use Guidelines." *LGBT Health* 1: 157–60.

Colpitts, Emily, and Jacqueline Gahagan. 2016a. "'I Feel Like I Am Surviving the Health Care System': Understanding LGBTQ Health in Nova Scotia, Canada." *BMC Public Health* 16: 1005. https://doi.org/10.1186/s12889-016-3675-8.

Colpitts, Emily, and Jacqueline Gahagan. 2016b. "The Utility of Resilience as a Conceptual Framework for Understanding and Measuring LGBTQ Health." *International Journal for Equity in Health* 15: 60. https://doi.org/10.1186/s12939-016-0349-1.

Crenshaw, Kimberle. 1991. "Mapping the Margins: Intersectionality, Identity Politics, and Violence against Women of Color." *Stanford Law Review* 43 (6): 1241–99.

Dean, Laura, Ilan H. Meyer, Kevin Robinson, Randall L. Sell, Robert Sember, Vincent M. B. Silenzio, Deborah J. Bowen, et al. 2000. "Lesbian, Gay, Bisexual, and Transgender Health: Findings and Concerns." *Journal of the Gay and Lesbian Medical Association* 4: 102–51.

Edgar, Harold, and David J. Rothman. 1990. "New Rules for New Drugs: The Challenge of AIDS to the Regulatory Process." *Milbank Quarterly* 68 (s1): 111–42.

Fenway Institute. 2014. *The Case for Designating LGBT People as a Medically Underserved Population and as a Health Professional Shortage Area Population Group*. Boston: Fenway Institute. http://www.fenwayhealth.org/documents/the-fenway-institute/policy-briefs/MUP_HPSA-Brief_v11-FINAL-081914.pdf.

Gahagan, Jacqueline, and Emily Colpitts. 2017. "Understanding and Measuring LGBTQ Pathways to Health: A Scoping Review of Strengths-Based Health Promotion Approaches in LGBTQ Health Research." *Journal of Homosexuality* 64 (1): 95–121. http://dx.doi.org/10.1080/00918369.2016.1172893.

Greensmith, Cameron, and Sulaimon Giwa. 2013. "Challenging Settler Colonialism in Contemporary Queer Politics: Settler Homonationalism, Pride Toronto, and Two-Spirit Subjectivities." *American Indian Culture and Research Journal* 37: 129–48.

Hankivsky, Olena. 2014. *Intersectionality 101*. Vancouver: Institute for Intersectionality Research and Policy.

King, Michael, Joanna Semlyen, Sharon S. Tai, Helen Killaspy, David Osborn, Dmitri Popelyuk, and Irwin Nazareth. 2008. "A Systematic Review of Mental Disorder, Suicide, and Deliberate Self Harm in Lesbian, Gay and Bisexual People." *BMC Psychiatry* 8: 70.

Lee, Edward Ou Jin, and Shari Brotman. 2011. "Identity, Refugeeness, Belonging: Experiences of Sexual Minority Refugees in Canada." *Canadian Review of Sociology* 48: 241–74.

Mertus, Julie. 2007. "The Rejection of Human Rights Framings: The Case of LGBT Advocacy in the US." *Human Rights Quarterly* 29 (4): 1036–64.

Mink, Michael D., and Ali A. Weinstein. 2014. "Stress, Stigma, and Sexual Minority Status: The Intersectional Ecology Model of LGBTQ Health." *Journal of Gay & Lesbian Social Services* 26: 502–21.

Mulé, Nick J., and Miriam Smith. 2014. "Invisible Populations: LGBTQ People and Federal Health Policy in Canada." *Canadian Public Administration* 57 (2014): 234–55.

O'Neill, Brian. 2013. "Toward Inclusion of Lesbian, Gay, and Bisexual People." In *Canadian Social Policy: Issues and Perspectives*, edited by Anne Westhues and Brian Wharf, 315–32. Waterloo, ON: Wilfrid Laurier University Press.

Public Health Agency of Canada (PHAC). 1999. *Toward a Healthy Future: Second Report on The Health of Canadians*. Ottawa: PHAC. http://www.nccdh.ca/resources/entry/toward-a-healthy-future.

Public Health Agency of Canada (PHAC). 2013. *Population-Specific HIV/AIDS Status Report: Gay, Bisexual, Two-Spirit, and Other Men Who Have Sex with Men*. Ottawa: PHAC. http://www.phac-aspc.gc.ca/aids-sida/publication/ps-pd/men-hommes/assets/pdf/pshasrm-revspdhb-eng.pdf.

Public Health Agency of Canada (PHAC). 2014. "Chapter 1: National HIV Prevalence and Incidence Estimates for 2011." In *HIV/AIDS Epi Update*. Ottawa: PHAC. http://www.phac-aspc.gc.ca/aids-sida/publication/epi/2010/1-eng.php.

Quinn, Gwendolyn P., Matthew B. Schabath, Julian A. Sanchez, Steven K. Sutton, and B. Lee Green. 2015. "The Importance of Disclosure: Lesbian, Gay, Bisexual, Transgender/Transsexual, Queer/Questioning, and Intersex Individuals and the Cancer Continuum." *Cancer* 121: 1160–3.

Rootman, Irving, Sophie Dupéré, Ann Pederson, and Michel O'Neill, eds. 2012. *Health Promotion in Canada: Critical Perspectives on Practice*. Toronto: Canadian Scholars' Press.

Shindel, Alan W., and Sharon J. Parish. 2013. "Sexuality Education in North American Medical Schools: Current Status and Future Directions (CME)." *Journal of Sexual Medicine* 10: 3–18. https://doi.org/10.1111/j.1743-6109.2012.02987.x.

Statistics Canada. 2015. "Sexual Orientation." In "Same-Sex Couples and Sexual Orientation … by the Numbers." Last updated June 25. http://www.statcan.gc.ca/eng/dai/smr08/2015/smr08_203_2015#a3.

Taylor, Evan T., and Mary K. Bryson. 2016. "*Cancer's Margins*: Trans* and Gender Nonconforming People's Access to Knowledge, Experiences of Cancer Health, and Decision-Making." *LGBT Health* 3 (1): 79–89. https://doi.org/10.1089/lgbt.2015.0096.

Taylor, Verta, Katrina Kimport, Nella Van Dyke, and Ellen Ann Andersen. 2009. "Culture and Mobilization: Tactical Repertoires, Same-Sex Weddings, and the Impact on Gay Activism." *American Sociological Review* 74 (6): 865–90.

Trussler, Terry, and David Ham. 2016. *Gay Generations: Life Course and Gay Men's Health—Findings from the National Sex Now Survey*. Vancouver: Community Based Research Centre for Gay Men's Health.

Yerke, Adam F., and Valory Mitchell. 2013. "Transgender People in the Military: Don't Ask? Don't Tell? Don't Enlist!" *Journal of Homosexuality* 60 (2–3): 436–57.

CHAPTER 14

"Prescribing Income": A Multi-level Approach to Treating Social Determinants for Health Providers

Ritika Goel and Gary Bloch

LEARNING OBJECTIVES

After reading this chapter, you should be able to:

1. Illustrate, with examples, health provider advocacy on social determinants of health.
2. Using income as an example, appreciate how health providers can act at various levels to mitigate the negative impacts of the social determinants of health:
   - Micro: using a clinical tool to identify poverty and improve patient finances;
   - Meso: through the development of health team partnerships and innovative programs targeted at addressing the social determinants of health (SDH); and
   - Macro: through policy advocacy, including the engagement and mobilization of other health providers.

Health providers on the front lines have long been aware of a disconnect between the services they offer and the needs of their patients who experience social marginalization. These patients' stories, and the health evidence, point to the powerful impact of social context on health, but health providers have not traditionally been trained to address that context directly.

In this chapter, we will outline the evolution of a series of health provider actions, over the last decade, that demonstrate our ability to act on a social determinant of health. We use a framework of social accountability to demonstrate tangible action on income at multiple levels (Buchman et al. 2016). At the micro level, the development of a clinical tool has allowed providers to screen for and intervene into poverty with individual patients. At the meso level, we explore the journey of one clinic in downtown Toronto to optimize its team to address income and other social determinants. At the macro level, we discuss the engagement and mobilization of health providers to advocate for a reduction in poverty at the policy level, calling for upstream solutions to the health impacts of living with low income.

TAKING DIRECTION FROM THE COMMUNITY

In 2005, a group of health providers in Toronto were contacted by the Ontario Coalition against Poverty (OCAP), a grassroots advocacy organization that engages and mobilizes people living in poverty in the Toronto area to push for policy change, to participate in a campaign to raise social assistance rates. OCAP identified a little-known income benefit, known as the Special Diet Allowance, which allowed those living on social assistance to access up to 250 dollars of extra funds if a health provider deemed they qualified. OCAP suggested setting up community clinics to assess individuals for this benefit. Given the impact that poverty has on one's health, the involved health providers determined that it was justifiable to prescribe the full 250-dollar supplement to each person who came to the clinics based on an evidence-based diagnosis of poverty. Health providers effectively prescribed income to treat poverty. After a few months, the Ontario government changed the program regulations to drastically reduce the ability to prescribe the full allowance. But by this point, thousands of individuals had received a significant boost in their social assistance income, and a unique partnership had been forged between health providers, social activists, and people living in poverty.

Following the lead of this community organization resulted in a direct increase in incomes of low-income individuals and made a bold statement to government that the incomes provided to social assistance recipients were grossly inadequate. This campaign demonstrates that allowing communities that are directly affected by social challenges to direct our advocacy is not only ethical but often leads to more successful, sustainable outcomes.

ADVOCACY AT THE MICRO LEVEL: THE CLINICAL TOOL ON POVERTY

After the special diet clinics, it became clear that there was an appetite among health providers to address poverty as a social determinant of health, but that they lacked the skills to carry out this intervention in their regular work. One of the authors developed a clinical tool on poverty for family physicians—the Poverty Tool (Bloch 2015)—to meet this need. The Poverty Tool, replicated in figure 14.1, offers a simple three-step approach to addressing poverty in a typical 15-minute family medicine appointment. It proposes universal screening for income, an incorporation of the evidence linking poverty and health into clinical assessments, and a series of questions to help link patients with high-yield income benefit programs. It is similar to clinical tools on complex chronic illnesses like diabetes and cardiovascular disease. The goal is to reframe a social issue like poverty as a clinical issue that can be identified and addressed in the course of usual medical care.

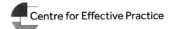 **Centre for Effective Practice**

Poverty: A Clinical Tool for Primary Care Providers (ON)

Poverty is not always apparent: In Ontario 20% of families live in poverty.

① Screen Everyone

"Do you ever have difficulty making ends meet at the end of the month?"
(Sensitivity 98%, specificity 40% for living below the poverty line)

② Poverty is a Risk Factor

Consider:
New immigrants, women, Indigenous peoples, and LGBTQ+ are among the highest risk groups.

Example 1:
If an otherwise healthy 35-year-old comes to your office, without risk factors for diabetes other than living in poverty, you consider ordering a screening test for diabetes.

Example 2:
If an otherwise low-risk patient who lives in poverty presents with chest pain, this elevates the pre-test probability of a cardiac source and helps determine how aggressive you are in ordering investigations.

③ Intervene

Ask Everyone: **"Have you filled out and sent in your tax forms?"**

- Ask questions to find out more about your patient—their employment, living situation, social supports, and the benefits they receive. Tax returns are required to access many income security benefits: e.g., GST / HST credits, child benefits, working income tax benefits, and property tax credits. Connect your patients to Free Community Tax Clinics.
- Even people without official residency status can file returns.
- Drug Coverage: up-to-date tax filing is required to access Trillium plan for those without Ontario Drug Benefits. Visit drugcoverage.ca for more options.

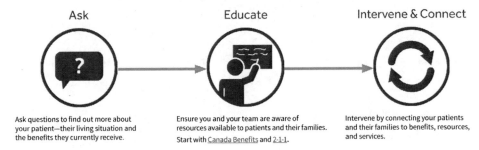

Figure 14.1: Steps to Addressing Poverty for Primary Care Providers

Source: Bloch (2015), https://thewellhealth.ca/poverty/.

The Poverty Tool has been presented at dozens of national and international conferences, accredited continuing medical education sessions, and a TEDx talk (Ontario College of Family Physicians n.d.b). Workshops on the Poverty Tool and concepts of caring for marginalized patients are now routinely conducted in undergraduate and postgraduate medical training sessions across Ontario, and have been embedded in the core curriculum of the University of Toronto's undergraduate medical program (Undergraduate Medical Education, University of Toronto n.d.). Provincial and national medical associations are promoting the tool (College of Family Physicians of Canada 2016) and have published reports on how they can act on the social determinants of health (Canadian Medical Association 2013).

The Poverty Tool has served as a catalyst for a new type of discussion about primary care providers addressing the social determinants of health on the front lines of care—one that has shifted from lamenting the impact of the SDH to opening up the possibility that providers can decrease that impact on their patients' health.

INTERVENTIONS AT THE MESO LEVEL: BUILDING A COORDINATED PROGRAM OF SDH INTERVENTIONS IN THE ST. MICHAEL'S HOSPITAL ACADEMIC FAMILY HEALTH TEAM

One health team in Toronto has taken the lead in developing and piloting a series of team-based initiatives aimed at reducing the impact of the social determinants of health. The St. Michael's Hospital Academic Family Health Team (SMHAFHT) serves over 45,000 patients through six clinical sites in downtown Toronto, with more than 75 family physicians, 40 resident physicians, and over 100 other health staff. There are five core initiatives in this program of social action (Porter 2015).

First, SMHAFHT members were part of the development and piloting of an initiative to collect sociodemographic information on all patients coming in contact with the health system in central Toronto (Mount Sinai Hospital 2015). This information allows the health team to better understand who it serves and to evaluate and target differential outcomes for vulnerable patients.

Second, in 2013, the team developed a new position—the Income Security Health Promoter—focused solely on improving patients' income. This is achieved through 1) direct individual case management, 2) patient and health team education, and 3) systemic advocacy. The two health promoters now see approximately five hundred unique patients per year. Internal evaluation data show a median increase of over 1,700 dollars per year for patients who access the program (personal communication with Alyssa Swartz, Income Security Health Promoter, October 2017).

Third, the team engaged in a novel partnership with another service sector to create a medicolegal partnership, known as the Health Justice Initiative, based on models popular in the United States. The SMHAFHT, in partnership with Legal Aid Ontario, now has an on-site lawyer and support staff, who focus on addressing the legal needs of the team's most vulnerable and lowest income patients. They provide this service through 1) direct legal support for individual clients, 2) legal education for patients and health team members, and 3) systemic law reform on issues identified through this practice.

Fourth, the SMHAFHT has hired a community engagement specialist, who focuses on bringing the community's perspective into program planning and evaluation, as well as bringing the health team's voice to the community, to promote initiatives that will improve community health, with a specific equity perspective. While this approach has been taken for years by community health centres in Ontario, it is rare in mainstream primary health care delivery models (Collins, Resendes, and Dunn 2014).

Fifth, the team initiated Reach Out and Read (2014), an approach to improving literacy popular in the United States. This program provides free books and literacy counselling at well-child visits and has been shown to improve literacy rates and cognitive outcomes, especially among low-income children (Zuckerman and Khandekar 2010). The SMHAFHT has partnered with the Toronto Public Library and First Book Canada while drawing on multiple sources of private and public funding to enable providers to give children six free books through their first five years of life.

In order to coordinate between and guide these initiatives, an interdisciplinary Social Determinants of Health Committee, with broad representation from different health specialties, management, trainees, and community members, was created in 2013. The committee is now moving beyond the development of specialized programs and focusing on building the capacity of the entire SMHAFHT to adopt an equity lens on its work and on its health outcomes (Pinto and Bloch 2017).

Many of these initiatives are being evaluated through a rigorous program of research. These include a randomized controlled trial of the income security health promotion program, as well as studies of the Health Justice Initiative and ongoing evaluation and development of the sociodemographic data collection. Other centres in Canada have started to replicate these programs, including new medicolegal partnerships in two sites in Ontario and a social prescribing program through the Basics for Health Society in Vancouver.

ADVOCACY AT THE MACRO LEVEL: MOBILIZING HEALTH PROVIDERS TO SYSTEMIC ADVOCACY

While the interventions above may directly improve the health of patients by addressing upstream social determinants, a true reduction in health inequities will require a change in the social policies and structures that allow those inequities to continue.

Health Providers against Poverty emerged from the Special Diet Campaign as an advocacy group of health providers specifically targeting the health impacts of living with low income. It has been a prominent advocacy force since 2005.

The Decent Work and Health Network was created to address the health risks posed by the increase in precarious employment and inadequate legal protections for many workers. It was formed after health providers became involved in advocacy efforts to increase the minimum wage. Health providers collaborated with a grassroots advocacy and workers' support organization, the Workers' Action Centre.

Health providers have pushed for a basic income in Ontario, which has in part led to the initiation of a basic income pilot by the Ontario government. Additionally, one of the authors was asked to take part in an intensive working group tasked with the development of the Roadmap for Change, a 10-year path to income security reform in Ontario (Ontario Ministry of Community and Social Services 2017). Health providers have written op-eds, held press conferences, signed open letters, lobbied elected representatives, performed deputations, made policy submissions, joined rallies, engaged in creative actions, and more.

Health provider organizations have also been engaged in systemic advocacy. The Ontario College of Family Physicians' Committee on Poverty and Health focuses on educating primary care providers and medical trainees, as well as establishing partnerships with health and social service organizations (Ontario College of Family Physicians n.d.a). The College of Family Physicians of Canada's Social Accountability Working Group (Meili and Buchman 2013) seeks to bring social accountability to the core of family medicine, and, similarly, the Association of Faculties of Medicine of Canada and the Canadian Medical Association have incorporated a strong focus on social determinants of health (Canadian Medical Association 2013).

The last decade has seen a significant shift in the approach to advocacy in the health community. The creation of local, provincial, and national committees focused on addressing social determinants, along with the development of advocacy bodies, points to the potential for health providers to truly become involved in efforts to address these issues from a systemic perspective. Bringing an evidence-based health equity lens can offer a crucial new element to ongoing efforts to bring about policy change towards improving the social determinants of health.

CRITICAL THINKING QUESTIONS

1. When advocating on an issue, it is important to try to engage with those directly affected. Think about different ways in which health provider advocates may take their cues from communities who are affected.
2. As a health provider, how would you explore potential avenues for advocacy on a particular social determinant of health using partnerships and programs?
3. Develop a policy advocacy plan for addressing a particular social determinant of health in a local setting known to you. Consider your goal, audience, target, allies, and tactics.

RECOMMENDED READINGS

1. Ontario Medical Review—Series on Poverty and Health
    a. Part 1: "Why Poverty Is a Medical Problem" (Dorman et al. 2013)
    b. Part 2: "Office Interventions for Poverty" (Raza, Bloch, and ter Kuile 2013)
    c. Part 3: "Office Interventions for Poverty: Child Health" (Morinis and Feller 2013)
    d. Part 4: "Office Interventions for Poverty: Racialized Groups" (Green, Labelle, and Vien 2013)
    e. Part 5: "Policy and Population Approaches to Poverty" (Rachlis et al. 2013)
2. Canadian Family Physician—Series on Social Accountability
    a. "Practising Social Accountability: From Theory to Action" (Buchman et al. 2016)
    b. "Social Accountability at the Micro Level: One Patient at a Time" (Goel et al. 2016)
    c. "Social Accountability at the Meso Level: Into the Community" (Woollard et al. 2016)
    d. "Social Accountability at the Macro Level: Framing the Big Picture" (Meili et al. 2016)

REFERENCES

Bloch, G. 2015. *Poverty: A Clinical Tool for Primary Care Providers.* Toronto: Centre for Effective Practice. https://thewellhealth.ca/wp-content/uploads/2016/12/Poverty_flow-Tool-Final-2016v4.pdf.

Buchman, S., R. Woollard, R. Meili, and R. Goel. 2016. "Practising Social Accountability: From Theory to Action." *Canadian Family Physician* 62 (1): 15–18.

Canadian Medical Association. 2013. *What Makes Us Sick?* Ottawa: Canadian Medical Association. https://www.cma.ca/Assets/assets-library/document/fr/advocacy/What-makes-us-sick_en.pdf.

College of Family Physicians of Canada. 2016. "Poverty: A Clinical Tool for Primary Care Providers." http://www.cfpc.ca/Poverty_Tools/.

Collins, Patricia, Sarah Resendes, and James Dunn. 2014. "The Untold Story: Examining Ontario's Community Health Centres' Initiatives to Address Upstream Determinants of Health." *Health Care Policy* 10 (1): 14–29.

Dorman, K., R. Pellizzari, M. Rachlis, and S. Green. 2013. "Why Poverty Is a Medical Problem." *Ontario Medical Review* 80 (9): 15–19.

Goel, R., S. Buchman, R. Meili, and R. Woollard. 2016. "Social Accountability at the Micro Level: One Patient at a Time." *Canadian Family Physician* 62: 287–90.

Green, S., M. Labelle, and V. Vien. 2013. "Office Interventions for Poverty: Racialized Groups." *Ontario Medical Review* (November): 25–29.

Meili, R., and S. Buchman. 2013. "Social Accountability: At the Heart of Family Medicine." *Canadian Family Physician* 59 (4): 335–6.

Meili R., S. Buchman, R. Goel, and R. Woollard. 2016. "Social Accountability at the Macro Level: Framing the Big Picture." *Canadian Family Physician* 62 (10) 785–8.

Morinis, J., and A. Feller. 2013. "Office Interventions for Poverty: Child Health." *Ontario Medical Review* (November): 20–23.

Mount Sinai Hospital. 2015. *Measuring Health Equity: Demographic Data Collection in Health Care*. Toronto: Human Rights & Health Equity Office, Sinai Health System. http://toronto-healthequity.ca.

Ontario College of Family Physicians. n.d.a. "Poverty and Health Committee." Accessed August 28, 2017. http://ocfp.on.ca/who-we-are/2014-15-board-members-and-committees/poverty-and-health-committee.

Ontario College of Family Physicians. n.d.b. "Primary Care Interventions in Poverty." Accessed August 28, 2017. http://ocfp.on.ca/cpd/povertytool.

Ontario Ministry of Community and Social Services. 2017. *Income Security: A Roadmap for Change*. Toronto: Ministry of Community and Social Services. http://www.ontario.ca/incomesecurity.

Pinto, Andrew, and Gary Bloch. 2017. "Framework for Building Primary Care Capacity to Address the Social Determinants of Health." *Canadian Family Physician* 63 (11): e476–82.

Porter, Catherine. 2015. "St. Michael's Hospital Health Team Offers Prescription for Poverty." *Toronto Star*, May 23. http://www.thestar.com/news/insight/2015/05/23/st-michaels-hospital-health-team-offers-prescription-for-poverty.html.

Rachlis, M., R. Goel, C. Mackie, R. Pellizzari, and L. Simon. 2013. "Policy and Population Approaches to Poverty" *Ontario Medical Review* (November): 30–34.

Raza, D., G. Bloch, and S. ter Kuile. 2013. "Office Interventions for Poverty." *Ontario Medical Review* (October): 21–24.

Reach Out and Read. 2014. *Reach Out and Read*. http://www.reachoutandread.org.

Undergraduate Medical Education, University of Toronto. n.d. "Transition to Clerkship (TTC 301Y)." Accessed August 28, 2017. http://www.md.utoronto.ca/courses-0.

Woollard, R., S. Buchman, R. Meili, R. Strasser, I. Alexander, and R. Goel. 2016. "Social Accountability at the Meso Level: Into the Community." *Canadian Family Physician* 62: 538–40.

Zuckerman, B., and Aasma Khandekar. 2010. "Reach Out and Read: Evidence Based Approach to Promoting Early Child Development." *Current Opinion in Pediatrics* 22 (4): 539–44. https://doi.org/10.1097/MOP.0b013e32833a4673.

CHAPTER 15

Models of Primary Care Delivery for Under-Served Populations in Inner-City Settings

Dale Guenter, Abe Oudshoorn, and Joe Mancini

LEARNING OBJECTIVES

After reading this chapter, you should be able to:

1. Identify the main principles of primary health care.
2. Explain how specific social determinants of health can lead to compromise in a person's ability to access and engage with primary health care.
3. Identify programs and services that can make primary health care more comprehensive and more accessible, especially for people experiencing homelessness.
4. Identify alternative approaches to developing services for under-served inner-city populations.

PRINCIPLES OF PRIMARY HEALTH CARE

Preceding chapters have made apparent how social conditions are linked to health status and how housing status has an impact as a critical determinant of health. Those who deliver health services are also aware of a limitation of the effectiveness of health care for people with particularly precarious biopsychosocial situations. In this chapter, we will consider how the philosophy of primary health care (PHC) makes it well-suited to address the social determinants of health, as well as several examples of how PHC has been designed for under-served populations. We will focus primarily on models that extend the reach of PHC to people who are precariously housed.

The Declaration of Alma-Ata, led by the World Health Organization in the former USSR in 1978, is an important historical event for PHC and therefore a good place to begin the discussion. During the week of September 6–12, 1978, countries of the world gathered to call for "urgent action by all governments, all health and development workers, and the world community to protect and promote the health of all the people of the world" (WHO 1978, 1). The conference on primary health care led to a consolidation and global affirmation of the foundational principles of PHC and positioned it as a human right:

> The Conference strongly reaffirms that health, which is a state of complete physical, mental and social wellbeing, and not merely the absence of disease or infirmity, is a fundamental human right and that the attainment of the highest possible level of health is a most important world-wide social goal whose realization requires the action of many other social and economic sectors in addition to the health sector. (WHO 1978, 1)

While the declaration's aspiring goal of "Primary Care for All by the Year 2000" was not met, it remains an important approach to improving health through the provision of PHC. The declaration states that primary health care includes the following:

- Being relevant to the economic and sociocultural conditions of the community being served, and distributed equitably
- Using promotive, preventative, curative, and rehabilitative approaches to the main health needs of the community
- Using appropriate technology that is affordable, feasible, and relevant to the needs of community
- Using a multi-sectoral approach with integration of services from varied sectors relevant to the community and its health issues
- Being established through community participation in priorities and planning
- Ensuring an appropriately trained and supported workforce to deliver services

PHC is the arm of health services that is closest, most accessible, and most responsive to all people. It may be a package of approaches that would take into account the biopsychosocial nature of illness. Since Alma-Ata, numerous care models have evolved, in different jurisdictions and contexts, with the aim of fulfilling the principles of PHC to ensure effective care for all in a given population.

It is generally understood that PHC will be most accessible when services are universally funded. In Canada, government legislation and funding of health services evolved over several decades, with federal legislation taking its current form in 1965. Although this has ensured equitable access to many health services, it has become clear over time that a generic approach to primary health care delivery does not serve all populations effectively. Weinreb and Bassuk (1990) highlighted some specific barriers to accessing health care for people precariously housed, such as lack of appropriate transportation, fragmentation of health care services, difficulty maintaining therapeutic relationships, and lack of child care. Thus, a variety of unique approaches has evolved, often adapted and particularized in order to increase effectiveness for groups with unique circumstances.

We will now explore the development and key elements of several models of health service that have attempted to express PHC principles for under-served populations. These models have evolved to meet the needs of a large variety of people with precarious circumstances including the elderly, cultural or ethnic minorities such as newcomers and Indigenous groups, students, and people experiencing poverty.

COMMUNITY HEALTH CENTRES

The community health centre (CHC) movement in Canada can be traced to the 1920s when CHCs were the first sign of the publicly funded health care system. The important feature of the CHC movement in Canada is its holistic approach: to have medical care, health promotion, and community development all wrapped into the same organization. In principle, these activities are delivered through an integrated team of clinicians and other professionals with skills deemed valuable to the unique needs of the specific community being served. These roles are then able to "enfold" an individual in interdisciplinary relationships that can address many facets of that person's issue at the same time. At its best, a team's mandate arises organically from within the community to be served—though at times, the process of creating and sustaining a CHC operates from the top down. They are governed by directors drawn from, and passionate about, the elevation of the social and health situation of the citizens of the community.

CHCs have evolved to meet the needs of many different populations, including people who experience homelessness. Their funding structure and organization in Canada have increased in formality, accountability, and sense of mandate. Different provinces have taken on the funding and development of CHCs to varying degrees. Quebec stands out as the jurisdiction with the greatest commitment to a unique CHC sector. It established the Centres locaux de services communautaires (CLSC), beginning in the 1970s, as health services were taken over by the province from numerous religious providers (Bozzini 1988). Currently, about 150 of these centres are distributed throughout all regions of the province, each providing a spectrum of free services that address the biopsychosocial needs of the unique community that they serve.

Community-oriented primary care (COPC) might be considered a conceptual outgrowth of the principles of PHC, with a particular emphasis on assessing and intervening on a population level (Longlett, Kruse, and Wesley 2001). COPC articulates the approaches and tools that enable a comprehensive understanding of a community's needs (rather than only the individuals who present to a clinic for care), intervening to improve on this situation at both the population and individual levels, and mobilization of that community to participate in both assessment and intervention. Members of a community might be defined by geography, ethnicity, age, shared values, or any other features that identify a group's shared interests as they relate to health (Institute of Medicine 1996).

In Ontario, CHCs became organized as an entity separate from the rest of the health sector in the 1970s. They espoused a holistic style of PHC, and have grown to over 70 centres distributed throughout the province with an explicit mandate to provide comprehensive, community-based primary care to populations who face barriers to care (e.g., rural, impoverished, new Canadians). Within this model, provincial funding is available for comprehensive care teams, including family physicians, nurses, nurse practitioners, social workers, community developers, psychologists, psychiatrists, diabetes educators, and other allied health providers.

CHCs in Canada have used many unique strategies and partnerships to increase their accessibility and effectiveness to people experiencing homelessness. Just a sample of these approaches include providing services embedded in homeless shelters or addiction treatment agencies; needle exchange programs for injection drug use; public health staff to enhance health promotion activities; financial and legal services; job-finding and skill-building programs; community garden programs; and language programs. In addition, many of these centres have developed creative strategies to decrease barriers to access of services, such as funding for public transit, child care services for mothers, and translation services. The goal of these encompassing programs is to locate health as one component of the broad reality of the person being served, and as one outcome of improvement in a spectrum of other social and psychological circumstances. Muldoon and colleagues (2010) have demonstrated that CHCs don't just address the health and social needs of individuals; rather, they positively

Homeless Veterans in the United States

An American project, presented and evaluated by O'Toole and colleagues (2015) focuses on engaging people experiencing homelessness into primary care, in this case with a focus on homeless veterans. Their concern was the extent to which people experiencing homelessness access acute care facilities in communities where primary care is available. Hospital care is both costly and disjointed, leading to less than ideal outcomes for both the system and the individual. PHC approaches are promising ways to improve engagement with community-based and more effective services. In O'Toole et al.'s (2015) study, the authors found that interventions that included introducing homeless veterans to primary care clinics and the primary care team increased likelihood of long-term engagement into primary care, from under 40 percent to as high as 88.7 percent. The primary care settings included homeless-focused teams working in partnership with generalized primary care, allowing individuals to access care permanently within the same site, although potentially changing teams as housing status changed.

This model of outreach is an example of an approach to "softening the barriers" between the person's daily lived reality and the culture and structure of services being offered in medical primary care.

Adding what may often be a more approachable service provider between the health care providers and the individuals needing care shortens what may feel like an insurmountable psychological leap. In doing this, access to and engagement with care are improved.

alter the community context in which de-housing and re-housing occurs. In achieving this, CHCs are well positioned as bridges for people to transition to effective engagement with the rest of the health care system and what are often its less approachable services.

HEALTH CARE ON THE MARGINS IN CANADA

Across Canada, it is possible to identify a wide variety of health service delivery models that are built on the principles of Alma-Ata and PHC, but have not grown out of the formal CHC sector. These are often organically evolving, loosely organized, community-focused, community-led, person-centred, partnership-dependent entities. They have frequently been an outgrowth of a perceived gap in comprehensiveness or accessibility for a fairly specific group of people. Like CHCs, they aim to reduce the barriers to receiving PHC, bringing service as close as possible to those being served. And they aim to be comprehensive, by strengthening the social and psychological dimensions of the person's situation before, or in parallel with, their biomedical situation. Here, we will explore the evolution of two of these programs in two different Ontario communities.

CHARACTERISTICS OF PRIMARY CARE AND OTHER MODELS OF CARE FOR THE UNDER-SERVED

Although somewhat focused on an American context of payment for access, and still considering homeless-focused primary care clinics, Weinreb and Bassuk (1990) present some preliminary considerations that can be advanced to build a model of maintaining primary care in spite of a change in housing status: 1) transience associated with homelessness leading to geographic separation; 2) complexities of behaviours and conditions associated with homelessness leading to termination of the relationship by either the physician, the individual experiencing homelessness, or both; and 3) access to alternative sites of care that are simply more convenient, timely, or likely to yield the outcomes desired by the individual. The considerations the authors offer begin to address these particular factors, including primary care provision that goes beyond health and engages patients in interventions to address income and housing challenges.

Additionally, Weinreb and Bassuk (1990) look at confronting barriers to health care access, such as addressing transportation needs, coordinating fragmented health care services, maintaining therapeutic relationships, and supporting child care for homeless families. Practically, primary care providers can consider some of the following questions: 1) How can they address behaviours associated with addiction in a manner that does not remove patients from access to care? 2) How can they ensure "warm transfers" to appropriate services for those patients who travel as a result of homelessness? 3) How can they provide support around the determinants of health that take primacy over medical health needs? 4) How can they keep current with treatment that patients are receiving across multiple sites of care? Answering these questions begins to uncover opportunities for primary care providers to better support individuals as they transition through various housing statuses. This chapter will now explore two case studies of community-driven health care for the under-served to illustrate these principles.

Hamilton Shelter Health Network—Dale Guenter

It all started with a simple lunch date in 2005 with two family doctors and a nurse, all who had worked in different settings within Hamilton's inner city. Was there a way to improve on what we had experienced in many years of working in the inner city? We brought our passions and our visions to the table. We left with ideas about what our aspiration was and a plan for whom else to invite into dialogue.

People whose lives are disjointed, chaotic, and painful often land in the inner city, where services and shelters are more accessible, shadows for hiding are abundant, friends are near, and the drug trade is active. Because of this, housing insecurity concentrates in the inner city as well. As in many cities, Hamilton's central neighbourhoods are known through anecdote and systematic data to have health outcomes much lower, and health service utilization much higher, than other neighbourhoods. In fact, some measures are well within developing country norms.

We were interested in the people whose material and psychological insecurities were the most extreme, which also means that most of the rest of society simply does not fit for them. Often, this includes experiences of trauma, cognitive and behavioural challenges, poor education, and scarcity of resources. Our health and social systems tend to consider these people *non-compliant*, a term that places blame on the people most in need and suggests that they are making some conscious attempt to ignore those of us who want to help. Appointments are missed, laboratory tests left undone, prescriptions unfilled, rents unpaid, apartments unkempt. Robust science now tells us that post-traumatic stress, poor physical and mental health, and homelessness are all constantly feeding each other. None is likely to improve unless all three do so in concert.

And so, from this, we wondered whether the clinical care we were involved in was still missing the mark, failing to provide service in a manner that could really work. We wondered whether by taking good clinicians into many of the buildings and spaces where people lived (shelters and transitional housing), and where they spent much of their time (addiction, mental health, and social services), we might begin to align ourselves better with their lives, rather than them with ours.

Eventually, about 20 people representing the following key organizations were meeting regularly to discuss: Hamilton Public Health Services, Hamilton Health Sciences, St. Joseph's Health Care, Wesley Urban Ministries, Mission Services, Salvation Army, Good

Shepherd Centres, Canadian Mental Health Association, Wayside House, Community Care Access Centre, and McMaster University's Department of Family Medicine and School of Nursing. By 2009, this advisory group transformed into a board of directors, and the new organization was named Shelter Health Network (SHN). Soon after, a specific pocket of funding was awarded to pay for family physicians and several specialty services. In spite of a variety of attempts, acquiring funding for nursing and allied health was not successful. But the collaborators were insistent that service for this clientele be comprehensive and relevant to their complex social and psychological needs, and so partner social service organizations created a variety of approaches to funding a more comprehensive team that the physicians could work along with.

Clinical services were launched quickly. Women and men, immigrant families, and people addicted to substances, all of whom shared the unifying feature of experiencing precarious housing, began to receive primary health care, where previously they had had none. They were not required to make appointments or go to a separate medical clinic, but could access service when and where they were seeking housing or social services. Visits did not need to be rushed, so a more thorough and narrative assessment was possible—trusting relationships were pivotal. Bureaucratic processes for housing, food, and transportation were minimized. Clients were warmly accompanied as they made their transitions into the mainstream system.

Many clients presented to multiple agencies where our health services were located. We had chosen an Internet-based electronic medical record that could be read and written on from any location. This meant that providers across the SHN would always have the same and most current information about assessments, management plans, test results, and prescriptions.

As of 2017, the SHN continues to function with a variety of funding sources, no bank account of its own, and staff contributed by all of the partner agencies. Clinical care is now provided by nurses who are staff of the individual agencies, in collaboration with about 20 physicians working up to 3.5 full-time equivalents, including family physicians, psychiatrists, internists, and paediatricians. Services for mental health, addiction, opioid substitution, prenatal care, pain management, housing, language, and employment are all readily available. The physicians also support two residential addiction treatment facilities, one of which provides "managed alcohol" as a harm reduction strategy to its residents who are deemed to be resistant to all other forms of treatment. A hepatitis C outreach team has received separate funding to provide social and counselling support to people with hepatitis C and precarious lives, in order to increase their willingness to receive curative treatment. Thousands of individuals have been served in the time since the SHN first began, and many of those have made the step to mainstream primary care clinics as their lives have stabilized and their capacity has increased.

Developing Psychiatric Outreach and Primary Care at St. John's Kitchen—Joe Mancini

The Working Centre was established in Kitchener-Waterloo, Ontario, during the recession of 1982. While the recession soon ended, this was the beginning of a new phase of capitalism that had fewer qualms about leaving larger numbers of workers unemployed and less attached to the labour market. Over the next 30 years, wave after wave of plant closings throughout the Waterloo region reshaped the labour force. The factory worker with a Grade-12 education or less found fewer job opportunities.

When the Working Centre established St. John's Kitchen in 1985, we recognized that we were providing a place of refuge for individuals caught in the cycle of being excluded from the labour market. Our goal was to redistribute surplus food by involving patrons in the work of cooking, serving, and cleaning up the daily meal. This engenders solidarity through cooperative work. By the 1990s, a regular day consisted of 250 visitors that included people who were dealing with addictions and mental health issues, as well as physical limitations and injuries. There were street kids and refugee families, and ages ranged from youth to middle-aged adults seeking employment. In St. John's Kitchen, the majority found a way to lessen isolation: a common gathering place to escape the rooming houses they lived in.

St. John's Kitchen recognizes that unemployment and homelessness are socially induced outcomes that flow from a societal bias against those who do not compete effectively in the labour market. By creating a daily meal service where those left out can serve each other creates a new kind of spirit that opens the possibilities for engagement.

DEVELOPMENT OF OUTREACH SERVICES

Our starting point to counter alienation was to build relationships and to integrate hospitality in our model. In 2003, we established Kitchener's first "downtown street outreach worker" with funding from the City of Kitchener. These workers are available in downtown Kitchener and Waterloo to support people who are homeless and at risk of becoming homeless. They problem-solve together around issues related to finances, housing, health, and legal matters.

Soon, "streets to housing workers" were added with the goal of assisting about 40 individuals who are chronically homeless. The workers first build relationships as they work together to find housing and, if such housing is lost, to assist in finding new housing.

In 2006, after 22 years at St. John's Anglican Church, where our original focus was simply hospitality and a meals service, St. John's Kitchen moved to a new location. We had recently worked with a volunteer retired psychiatrist who did street work one day a week. In our new location, we recognized the importance of expanding our mental health and outreach services. We built a medical clinic, laundry, showers, and an open kitchen fully visible to the large dining area. By this time, as our outreach services were starting to develop, we could identify a large group of individuals, living on the outskirts of society, with minimal connections to families, institutions of care, and housing, and who were daily patrons at St. John's Kitchen. We were committed to maintaining our open supportive culture as we developed new ways of helping.

Downtown Outreach has evolved as a series of services that constitute an indispensable network of support that aims to increase our sense of belonging to each other. It is the goal of outreach to walk with many individuals abandoned by family and society, people who have been deprived and have deprived themselves from nourishing social relationships. Dislocated individuals have few places to turn. It is our role to gently encourage connectedness. Is the answer a doctor with mental health experience, a friend who can walk with one through the pain, an outreach worker that re-establishes an income source, a judge in the mental health court who offers compassion, or a local retailer who takes an individual under her wings? Every attempt is another undertaking to create further community, a way for a wounded individual to bounce their character off another in the search for healing.

Our first ideas centred around recognizing how individuals who use St. John's Kitchen were alienated from the health care system. The health system, to us, was a bureaucratic machine without care. It reflected the competitive and efficient values of dominant society. To engage in the health system, an individual needed a stable address; they had to deal with nurses and receptionists; they had to show up to appointments and then follow up and ask the right questions. They had to trust the same doctors who projected distrust back at them.

We recognized that the health system was another form of ostracization that added stresses and further marginalized the people it aimed to help, while generating resentment and anger from its so-called clients. For the homeless, the medical system, like the labour market and the education system, are walls with small doors that refuse to open.

BUILDING SOCIAL SOLIDARITY

St. John's Kitchen has been a place of refuge for 30 years. It is a place of work, where the main job each day is the preparation and serving of a nutritious meal. It is a place of social solidarity, as it fully involves the community who come each day for a meal with the work of preparing, serving, and cleaning up the daily meal.

The disaffection of workers from the labour market is the main social problem that generates long-term unemployment, teaching and reinforcing a kind of disillusionment with society. The work of St. John's Kitchen, relying on the dedication of hundreds of people, is a commitment to create a place that lessens the harsh realities that poverty inflicts. In the face of growing dislocation, it now includes health professionals, outreach workers, volunteers, and peers who participate in creating an integrated community that builds meaning and connection through hospitality.

continued

PSYCHIATRIC OUTREACH

In downtown Kitchener at the turn of the millennium, there was a distinct rise in the number of homeless people dealing with the combination of mental health and addiction issues. The downtown BIA (Business Improvement Area) started a community process to bring together social services, neighbourhood groups, and institutional organizations to address this growing issue. The Kitchener Downtown Community Collaborative created a process that yielded new energy aimed at supporting people. The downtown street outreach worker role expanded to three positions, as did the more focused streets to housing worker role. This work was complimented by the Psychiatric Outreach Project (POP).

The early experiment with a street-based psychiatrist proved that the development of a community-based health service would advance our relationship-building work. When St. John's Kitchen opened its new location at 97 Victoria, we had the opportunity to redesign 7,500 square feet on the second floor. We allocated about 800 square feet to the medical clinic that occupies a prime area at the top of the stairs and beside the elevator lift. POP starts with outreach workers who build relationships and then complements this work with psychiatric nurses and a doctor offering direct medical support. POP turns the medical model upside down by bringing the resources to where the people are, leaving behind professional status and rigid appointment schedules; whether at the clinic or on the street, a flexible, welcoming approach is essential. By locating the clinic as an integrated part of St. John's Kitchen, access to the clinic is seen as natural and non-threatening. We insist that the same non-judgmental approach that is the hallmark of St. John's Kitchen is the same approach at the medical clinic.

The model has expanded to include dealing with physical illness, which is an important form of engagement. People find trust and support through interacting with the nurses and doctors who provide help with wound care, illnesses that require penicillin, or a quick check on an ailment that is causing anxiety. The medical clinic provides practical services that lead to discussion and connections. This is a model of integrated supports.

Dr. George Berrigan (2012) summarized the POP approach in this way:

As a family practitioner, I am used to being my own boss. At POP, I work in a different way, here we work in a circle. We are reaching out to individuals who have major illnesses, addictions and mental health issues. These are truly the walking wounded and who is there to listen to their pleas? This is why the model of care is that of a circle. We who do this work are outliers as the model of professional service is usually based on top-down approaches. The model we are using helps us avoid the tunnel vision we all have. Rather than only hearing the story of an individual from one perspective our team usually hears the perspective of the doctor, the nurse, the social worker and the outreach worker. Each hears in a different way and we put together a more accurate story. (6)

The front desk of the medical clinic is just 15 feet from the busy open stairs, which three to four hundred people use each day on their way to the dining area. It is important that when the door is open, the medical clinic welcomes everyone in a way that emphasizes that all people matter and that professionalism is not a barrier to relationships. People are encouraged to talk about the stuff that is important to them. This is what builds relationships.

The POP clinic is complemented by the village of supports that have evolved at St. John's Kitchen, including the innumerable free services that we have cobbled together, like the showers, laundry, public phones, the daily meal, food pantry distribution, the daily community interactions, the grieving process through hosting memorial funeral services, and opportunities for work and volunteering. Each of these efforts are crucial access points of relationship building that add to our downtown outreach and POP and medical clinic work. These support circles are working with in excess of one thousand individuals each six-month period. This integrated model with other complementary services creates circles of support that help people find their way through the fog of dislocation.

ADDITION OF A NURSE PRACTITIONER

For 10 years the St. John's Kitchen medical clinic has operated through cross-stitching together four different kinds of resources. When we built the clinic we secured the services of a number of doctors who could provide a combination of primary care with the addition of mental health and addiction supports. The Psychiatric Outreach Project was privately developed but eventually found funding through the Waterloo Wellington LHIN in a program called Specialized Outreach Supports that brought three psychiatric outreach nurses to the clinic. The LHIN, Waterloo Region, and Kitchener and Waterloo all contributed to the downtown street outreach workers, who are on the ground building relationships and helping people get access to legal, housing, and income services and assistance to get to medical appointments. These resources have been held together through fundraising by the Working Centre.

When the Grand River Hospital Board visited St. John's Kitchen to learn about the model, it started a two year conversation between the LHIN, the hospital, and the Working Centre. Eventually it was agreed that the Grand River Hospital would transfer one nurse practitioner role to the St. John's Kitchen medical clinic. When this position started in early 2018 there was no slack. Immediately, the nurse practitioner was busy providing primary care at the clinic and on the street. Whether providing wound care or addressing the effects of increased drug use, the addition of this role has substantially added to the support the medical clinic can provide.

CRITICAL THINKING QUESTIONS

1. Consider using a web-based electronic health record in which all PHC providers from different locations document and view clinical information. How might this improve care and health outcomes for people who are precariously housed?
2. List three characteristics of a person that might make it difficult for them to engage in, or stay with, health care from a traditional primary care clinic. For each of these, list two strategies that might make these barriers smaller.
3. If you were a teenage mother of three children living on social assistance and precariously housed, what services would you value most that would make attending primary health care appealing?

REFERENCES

Berrigan, George. 2012. "Healthy Community, Healthy Minds." *Good Work News* 111: 6. http://www.theworkingcentre.org/sites/default/files/Dec2012gwn.pdf.

Bozzini, Luciano. 1988. "Local Community Services Centers (CLSCs) In Québec: Description, Evaluation, Perspectives." *Journal of Public Health Policy* 9 (3): 346–75. https://doi.org/10.2307/3342640.

Institute of Medicine. 1996. *Primary Care: America's Health in a New Era*. Washington, DC: National Academy Press.

Longlett, Shirley K., Jerry E. Kruse, and Robert M. Wesley. 2001. "Community-Oriented Primary Care: Historical Perspective." *Journal of the American Board of Family Practice* 14 (1): 54–63. http://www.jabfm.org/content/14/1/54.long.

Muldoon, Laura, Simone Dahrouge, William Hogg, Robert Geneau, Grant Russell, and Michael Shortt. 2010. "Community Orientation in Primary Care Practices Results from the Comparison of Models of Primary Health Care in Ontario Study." *Canadian Family Physician* 56 (7): 676–83.

O'Toole, Thomas P., Erin E. Johnson, Matthew L. Borgia, and Jennifer Rose. 2015. "Tailoring Outreach Efforts to Increase Primary Care Use among Homeless Veterans: Results of a Randomized Controlled Trial." *Journal of General Internal Medicine* 30 (7): 886–98. https://doi.org/10.1007/s11606-015-3193-x.

Weinreb, Linda F., and Ellen L. Bassuk. 1990. "Health Care of Homeless Families. A Growing Challenge for Family Medicine." *Journal of Family Practice* 31 (1): 74–80.

World Health Organization (WHO). 1978. "Declaration of Alma-Ata." Adopted at the International Conference on Primary Health Care, Alma-Ata, USSR, September 6–12.

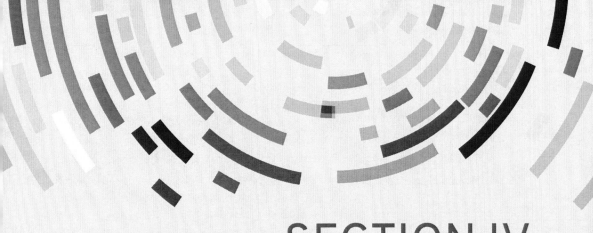

SECTION IV

REFUGEE AND MIGRANT POPULATIONS

SECTION INTRODUCTION BY SHPRESA ALIU-BERISHA

I was born in a small village in Kosovo, which at that time belonged to Yugoslavia. I was the only girl of four children. When I was quite young, my parents decided to move to the big city with the hope of better schooling and a more prosperous future for us all. In retrospect, I look back on a seemingly ideal childhood, safe and surrounded by family and friends. In my community, there was no difference between rich and poor; we were all the same.

My passion for healing began in the beautiful country fields where my grandmother lived. There she would show me plants that we used, traditionally, for healing. At the age of seven, I told my parents that one day I, too, would become a healer. I soon began working toward my goals.

Before entering medical school in Pristina, Kosovo's capital and largest city, I already had my future mapped out. I envisioned myself in my early 30s, working as a doctor with a family and a home. Indeed, by age 34, my vision was reality: I had my profession, my dream home with my husband, and a daughter, Shega. I was also expecting a second child. Suddenly, my dream turned to nightmare as the political situation in Yugoslavia worsened. Instead of preparing a new bedroom for the baby, we were preparing to flee the war.

If you have never experienced war, you probably don't know what it's like to be always planning for a worst-case scenario. I made my husband promise that if something happened to me, he should leave me behind to save our daughter, Shega, even though I was pregnant. Inside Pristina, the city I loved, I lived in the fear of bullets. I did not fear one hitting my head or chest, but my belly, where my unborn daughter, Vesa, was growing. We did all we could to shelter Shega from the war; we played loud music and we danced. We pretended that everything was okay and that it would continue that way indefinitely. Of course, children often pick up on much more than they let on. As it turns out, she, too, was protecting us, also trying to let us know that everything would be okay.

I was three months pregnant when the war in Kosovo escalated; I no longer had access to prenatal care. However, with the burden of pregnancy, it was also difficult to decide to leave. In April of 1999, the decision was made for us: we were forced to leave, each pushed in separate directions, at gunpoint. For about 30 minutes, we lost Shega. When we found her crying in a crowd of people, I cannot forget her face and words: "Thank you, mommy and daddy, for finding me." But I could find no good answer to her question, "Why did those masked people make us leave our home?" and only responded, "We need to leave."

Arriving in Macedonia, we claimed refugee status, a concept quite foreign to me. I was traumatized. I had to sleep on the floor and eat less than desirable food just to survive. All of this may have contributed to my hypertension. I felt lucky to be safe but couldn't shake the thought that so many other women, still trapped inside Kosovo, were not. Many were raped and murdered. Some would either deliver their babies in the mountains or risk becoming a casualty of war.

After six long weeks spent in Macedonia as war refugees, we arrived in Canada. This would be our final stop. I was fortunate enough to find a great obstetrician within the first week of my arrival. She immediately began treating my hypertension, and two weeks later I gave birth to a healthy baby girl, Vesa. It still frightens me to this day, particularly with what I know as a doctor, when I consider what may have happened had I been unable to access treatment for my hypertension: seizures, kidney failure, or, even worse, harm to Vesa or myself.

I had my two healthy daughters and husband by my side in my new country, and we were safe. This stirred an unbelievable mix of emotions. I was grateful, yet I feared for my family and had no idea if my parents were still alive. In Canada, we moved forward with our lives. We met new friends, who have had a huge impact on our lives. They helped to show us around and helped us spiritually, as well, as we adjusted to our new home.

The Interim Federal Health Program (IFHP) provided for our urgent health needs, but what strikes me, in retrospect, is the fact we had no access to counselling services to help us recover from the impact of the trauma we experienced. Having escaped during pregnancy, I could never forget the other pregnant women who could not flee that warzone. I could not shake off the realization that many women would become pregnant due to rape. The tragedies of war have always extended beyond the front lines.

To this day, I am still not sure how my family managed to move forward. I had to collect myself and provide love for my two daughters. I had to shelter them from the horrible and continuous effects of fleeing from a warzone. Luckily, much of the rest of my family, including my brothers and their families, also arrived in Canada with us. We were able to provide each other with support. We gradually started adapting to the new country and culture, making many great friends in the process. Once again, I went about envisioning my future, but this time here in Canada. I had to decide if I would allow the war to continue to influence me negatively, or whether I could turn this around and do something positive. I decided I would try out the latter.

For many months after the war, I spent sleepless nights thinking about the logic of war and people I knew who had died. At one point, I justified war as a force that moves societies forward. Of course, this is no justification. It just seemed that no place in the world was safe from war, and at no time has the world ever been free of war. In the end, I came to the conclusion that war is the most horrific thing that can happen to a person. But it does happen nonetheless, and the experience will change you forever. It was not my choice to become a war refugee. It was, however, my choice to stay in my new country, Canada, and to start life all over again. I could never forget my past; all I could hope was that my family and I were finally safe. And if we are lucky, we will never have to relocate.

I had my third daughter, Zana, in Canada. This was around the time my husband, Gazmend, went back to school. After he finished his education, I started my own journey, fully aware of all the challenges I would face to get to the end of the road. I wanted to become a practising physician in Canada. It took me two and a half years to finish all my exams. I finally obtained a position in McMaster's Family Medicine Residency Program. This process was very long and difficult. I had to finish three major exams prior to even being considered for an interview. After the year 2000, only a tiny fraction of applicants, 60 international medical graduates (IMGs), have been accepted to residency programs annually in Ontario. All this time, I felt that as a parent and partner, my first obligation was to feed my family.

As I set about working as a family doctor in Canada, I wanted to give back to the same group of people that I arrived with: immigrants and refugees. I was privileged to hear many other stories from war-torn countries such as Somalia, Bosnia, Iraq, and Afghanistan: stories of struggle, sacrifice, hardship, and loss—stories similar to my own. We all had something in common: we were all fleeing out of necessity, and it was never a choice. All anyone wanted was a safe place for the ones they loved. Everyone was motivated by survival, not just for themselves but also for their family members. A mother's love for her child is the same all over the world.

Now, as a family doctor, I have 1,700 patients under my care. Each day is a new story that deepens my book of life. However, not a single day goes by that I fail to recall the first chapter—my first 34 years spent in Kosovo, the country of my birth. I also cannot forget the respect I feel for Canada, the country that opened its doors to my family and me. As refugees, we have all struggled through our own unique transitions, but we have a home within this country. In our family, all are working, most of us in our chosen fields. Immigrants, and specifically refugees, then, do not only bring stories of trauma and loss but also a powerful look at life through different eyes. They bring experience, skills, and training to this country.

In this section, Michaela Hynie introduces the social determinants of health for refugee populations with unique challenges prior to and after their arrival in Canada. Meb Rashid, Vanessa Redditt, Andrea Hunter, and Kevin Pottie present an approach to and the guidelines for the care of refugee populations presenting to primary care. Hanna Gros identifies issues facing detained migrant populations, which may be even more horrific than the situations from which they flee, producing, unmasking, or magnifying mental health challenges and preventing adequate treatment. Finally, Janet McLaughlin and Michelle Tew describe unique strategies needed for the care of farm workers, a temporary migrant population to Canada, that is meant to fill an increasing need. As you read through this section, remember the powerful, often untold stories of patients. As a health care provider, I often work with the voiceless, whose severe trauma fails to get the attention it needs. I share my story here on behalf of those victims of war and violence. Remember what you can do to help those who unwillingly fled from their roots in order to survive.

Timeline: A Brief History of Migration and Marginalization

Neil Arya

Canada's recorded history of forced migration is long and complex. The history begins with the internal displacement of Indigenous peoples by European settlers—a displacement that continues today but is often invisible in discussions of forced migration (see Chapter 3 by Freeman in this volume). In the seventeenth and eighteenth centuries, what became Canada also participated in forced migration of slaves, primarily from the African continent, abolishing slavery only in 1834, with the British Parliament's Slavery Abolition Act. However, Upper and Lower Canada and the colony of Nova Scotia also served as refuge for those fleeing slavery. With the creation of the United States, many loyal to the British Crown migrated to Upper and Lower Canada, including 3,000 Black Loyalists who received asylum and resettlement in Nova Scotia, while later, the Underground Railroad brought 30,000 freed or escaped slaves. In the 1800s, famines brought Irish immigrants and others seeking economic opportunities.

Race has consistently played a role in Canadian migration patterns. In 1885, a "head tax" was placed on Chinese immigration; this was increased over the next 30 years and was only repealed in 1947. Other regulations included an Order-in-Council adopted by the Canadian government in 1908, imposing a "continuous passage rule," excluding people who could not make a direct journey to Canada from immigration, that while used for "undesirables" from the Indian subcontinent was not applied to Europeans. When a group of 376 Indian Sikhs from Punjab on board the *Komagatu Maru* attempted to dock in 1914, after two months in the harbour and an unsuccessful court challenge, they were forced to leave. Another Order-in-Council in 1911 (PC 1324) prohibited "any immigrants belonging to the Negro race, which race is deemed unsuitable to the climate and requirements of Canada" (quoted in Yarhi 2016).

Immigration from Eastern Europe increased from the beginning of the last century to the 1960s, as many fled unfavourable conditions: economic, environmental, and political. Despite occasional suspicions related to concerns about socialist sympathizers, this immigration was largely welcomed. But under Section 38 of the Immigration Act, which, by an Order-in-Council, allowed Cabinet to prohibit any race, nationality, or class of immigrants, Doukhobors, Mennonites, and Hutterites were excluded in 1919, due to their "peculiar habits, modes of life and methods of holding property" (quoted in Canadian Council for Refugees 2000, 3). This order was revoked three years later for Mennonites and Hutterites when it became apparent that many were simply escaping the Russian Revolution. Jews fleeing Nazi Germany were less welcome, sometimes because of political suspicions but often purely because of race. In 1939, the *St. Louis*, which had sailed from Germany with over nine hundred passengers, returned to Europe, failing to find refuge in North America, including when trying to dock in Halifax. A quarter to a third of its passengers later died in death camps. From 1933 to 1939, only five thousand Jews from Europe were accepted; even in the immediate post-war period, between 1945–1948, only another eight thousand Holocaust survivors were allowed. Anti-Semitism, led by the director of the immigration branch, Frederick Blair, with the support of the Mackenzie King Liberal government, was rife throughout the Canadian establishment. Said an unnamed immigration officer in 1939, when questioned about how many Jews should be accepted, "None is too many"; this would become the title of a book by Irving Abella and Harold Troper. Jews also had a capital requirement of 5,000 to 20,000 dollars to enter Canada. In 1942, a policy expelling Japanese Canadians from within a hundred miles of the Pacific was enacted, resulting in the internment of 22,000 Japanese Canadians until the end of the war.

In the post-war period, perhaps in response to labour needs, an Order-in-Council in 1946 opened up options to family sponsorship options. Meanwhile, internationally, a recognition of refugees as rights bearers and states as duty bearers began with the UN Declaration of Human Rights in 1948. The United Nations Relief and Works Agency (UNRWA) was established for Palestine in 1949 and the United Nations High Commissioner for Refugees (UNHCR) in 1950. In 1951, the UN Convention Relating to the Status of Refugees finally defined *refugees*, differentiating between those who might be political as opposed to environmental and economic migrants, and created a policy of "non-refoulement," making it illegal to send people back to their troubled countries. (Initially, these were only meant to apply to refugees from Europe.) Canada's delay to sign on until 1969 related to the security concerns of bringing in potential Communists. A policy giving temporary health coverage to refugees from post–Second World War Europe was established in 1957, well before universal health care was established in Canada.

Policies became more welcoming in the 1960s and 1970s—for example, in 1962 with the elimination of ethnicity requirements for immigration, and in 1971 with adoption of an official multicultural policy by the federal government. When 50,000 South Asians were kicked out of Uganda by Idi Amin, 7,000 were welcomed to Canada in 1972–1973. With the 1976 Immigration Act, Canada finally developed a formal system that defined refugees and distinguished between irregular immigrants at borders, allowing claims within and at borders, and established private and government sponsorship categories. Chileans, Lebanese, and US war resisters all came to Canada during the 1970s. In 1979, a private sponsorship of refugees program was developed, just in time for Canada to accept 60,000 "Vietnamese boat people" from Vietnam, Laos, and Cambodia. The government initially matched the first 21,000 privately sponsored, but interest proved much greater than anticipated. Now, in 2018, after the Syrian influx, we have almost 300,000 refugees from all countries in total that have been accepted through this unique program since 1979.

The 1980s brought Central Americans fleeing civil wars in several countries, foremost from El Salvador. The 1985 Supreme Court Singh decision—that the right to life, liberty, and security also applied to claimants—allowed them an oral hearing. However, fears of Sikh and Tamil boats in 1987 led to the more restrictive Bill C-84, the Refugee Deterrents and Detention Act, leading to new mechanisms for detaining and rejecting claimants, especially those who might be involved with criminal activity, including the establishment of the Immigration and Refugee Board in 1989 to review claims. Waves of new refugees, among them Bosnians and Kosovars from the former Yugoslavia, Somalis, and Afghans, came in the 1990s.

In 2002, as Europeans developed policies regarding the first port of entry in the aftermath of 9/11, Canada signed a Safe Third Country Agreement with the United States (enacted in 2004) that, with few exceptions, required refugees to make an application for asylum in the first of the two countries entered. Advocates have expressed concern regarding lack of proper process and safety in the US, especially with the Trump administration. The Immigration and Refugee Protection Act 2001–2002 replaced that of 1985. While section 38(1) included an exclusion of migrants who might reasonably be expected to cause excessive demand on health or social services mirroring section 19(1) of the 1985 Act, which had proved a barrier to those with HIV and with many disabilities, exception 2c gave protected persons an exemption from this provision, meaning that they could no longer be considered inadmissible on health grounds.

Major groups of refugees coming to Canada in this century include those from Iraq, Iran, and Afghanistan, the Burmese Thai border, Bhutan, Congo, the Horn of Africa, and Colombia. In 2012, concerned about a swarm of "queue-jumpers"—the tide of those seeking our gold-plated health care—the Harper Conservative government proposed Bill C-31, Protecting Canada's Immigration System Act. While giving the government minister the right to determine which countries were "safe" with reduction in oversight and appeal before deportation, it also cut IFHP benefits to such individuals. Together with a barbaric practices snitch line and Canadian values test, this seemed designed to exploit a general fear of foreigners, and Muslims in particular. After foot-dragging by the Harper government responding to the Syrian crisis, a new Liberal government was elected, explicitly welcoming 25,000 refugees at the end of 2015 and beginning of 2016, and more than 40,000 Syrian refugees in total, including a mixture government and privately sponsored.

More information on many aspects of migration history can be found through simple Internet searches. Additionally, more information can be found in the Additional Resources and Source Material section.

REFERENCES

Canadian Council for Refugees. 2000. *Report on Systemic Racism and Discrimination in Canadian Refugee and Immigration Policies.* Montreal: Canadian Council for Refugees. http://ccrweb.ca/files/arreport.pdf.

Yarhi, Eli. 2016. "Order-in-Council P.C. 1911-1324—the Proposed Ban on Black Immigration to Canada." September 30. http://www.thecanadianencyclopedia.ca/en/article/order-in-council-pc-1911-1324-the-proposed-ban-on-black-immigration-to-canada/.

ADDITIONAL RESOURCES AND SOURCE MATERIAL

Dench, Janet. 2000. "A Hundred Years of Immigration to Canada 1900–1999." Canadian Council for Refugees, May. http://ccrweb.ca/en/hundred-years-immigration-canada-1900-1999.

Epp, Marlene, ed. 2017. *Refugees in Canada: A Brief History.* Ottawa: Canadian Historical Association. http://www.cha-shc.ca/download.php?id=2488.

Government of Canada. 2017. "Canada: A History of Refuge." Last modified May 26. http://www.cic.gc.ca/english/refugees/timeline.asp.

CHAPTER 16

Social Determinants of Refugee Health

Michaela Hynie

LEARNING OBJECTIVES

After reading this chapter, you should be able to:

1. Have a general understanding of the nature of refugee migration.
2. Understand how the physical and social conditions of pre-migration and the migratory process itself may have an impact on short-term and long-term health outcomes of refugees.
3. Reflect on the living conditions in refugee camps from a social determinants of health perspective.
4. Gain insight into how post-migration factors at several levels have an impact on the health and well-being of resettled refugees in Canada.

INTRODUCTION

In 1951, the United Nations approved the Convention Related to the Status of Refugees (United Nations General Assembly 1951). Over 140 countries are signatories to this convention, including Canada (United Nations 2010). The Convention definition of a *refugee* is someone who,

> owing to a well-founded fear of being persecuted for reasons of race, religion, nationality, membership of a particular social group or political opinion, is outside the country of his nationality, and is unable to, or owing to such fear, is unwilling to avail himself of the protection of that country. (United Nations General Assembly 1951)

This chapter considers the social determinants of health for those migrants who are deemed to meet the Convention definition, or for individuals who are seeking asylum on these grounds. The social and material hardship and trauma that is often endured by refugees and asylum seekers creates unique vulnerabilities and challenges. Moreover, because of their political status, they also have unique pathways of migration, settlement, and integration. Individuals who meet this definition of forced migration and fear of persecution are afforded certain rights and protections under international conventions that are not available to those who migrate for other reasons, such as extreme poverty, natural disaster, or environmental degradation (Docherty and Giannini 2009). The latter individuals are considered voluntary migrants, even though, for some, their migration may be more forced than voluntary (Bates 2002). While international policies toward newcomers are based on distinct migration categories, the reality is that there are multiple drivers of migration, and the boundaries between forced and voluntary migration is often not clear, especially among the most marginalized and vulnerable people (Van Hear 2011). The social determinants described here may therefore apply to a broader range of migrants who may be forced from their homes by intolerable conditions; however, those who arrive in a country without formal refugee designation may have access to even fewer resources and formal protections than Convention refugees.

WHO IS A REFUGEE?

Refugee

A *refugee* is a person who has been forced to leave their country 1) because of a "well-founded" fear of persecution on the basis of their race, religion, sexual orientation, political opinions, or membership in a social group; and 2) whose state cannot or will not protect them from this persecution. Refugees are those individuals whose claims of persecution have been recognized by the state in which they have sought sanctuary or the United Nations High Commissioner for Refugees (UNHCR). Signatories of the UN Convention Related to the Status of Refugees agree to provide temporary sanctuary to refugees and not to return them to the country that they are fleeing (the principle of *non-refoulement*). Some can become permanent residents in some hosting countries, but the vast majority are only allowed temporary residence.

Asylum Seeker

An *asylum seeker* is a person who has crossed an international border seeking sanctuary and is seeking recognition as a refugee but whose case has not yet been decided. Asylum seekers must demonstrate that they are fleeing persecution in order to be awarded refugee status and be recognized as a refugee. In some countries, this can take years. If their claims are not accepted, they are normally required to leave the country in which they are seeking sanctuary and can be deported back to the country they are fleeing if they do not leave voluntarily.

Resettled Refugee

A *resettled refugee* is a person who is officially recognized as a refugee and who has been offered permanent residency in another third country.

Internally Displaced Person (IDP)

An *internally displaced person* is a person who is forcibly displaced from their home for the same reasons as refugees but does not cross international borders. The majority of those who are forcibly displaced by violence and persecution are in fact displaced within their own countries.

Migrant

A *migrant* is a person who crosses international borders but does not meet the Convention definition of a refugee. Their migration may or may not be voluntary—for example, those fleeing starvation, extreme poverty, or climate change are often forced to move in order to survive but are not eligible for recognition as refugees and thus are not afforded the same right to sanctuary (UNHCR 1977, 2014).

PATTERNS OF REFUGEE MIGRATION

In 1951, when it first started keeping statistics on those displaced by conflict or persecution, UNHCR recorded 2.12 million persons of concern. These numbers vary dramatically from year to year depending on regions of conflict. Despite the variability, it is clear that the number of refugees has grown, increasing in the mid-1970s and growing exponentially in recent years (see figure 16.1). As of December 2015, there were 65.3 million forced migrants around the world (UNHCR 2016). Of these, 21.3 million were forced to flee across international borders, making them refugees, either under the protection of UNHCR (16.1 million) or Palestinians registered by the United Nations Relief and Works Agency (UNRWA) for Palestine Refugees. An additional 3.2 million were asylum seekers—people who have claimed refugee status but whose claims have not yet been decided. The remaining 40 million are internally displaced within their own countries.

Most refugees flee to neighbouring low-income countries, often in great numbers, and seek asylum there, placing a strain on populations that may already be struggling with difficult material conditions and limited resources (UNHCR 2013). The absolute numbers of refugees residing in these countries can be staggering. At the time of writing, the countries hosting the largest number of individuals with accepted refugee claims are Turkey (2.5 million), Pakistan (1.6 million), Lebanon (1.1 million), the Islamic Republic of Iran (979,400), Ethiopia (736,100), and Jordan (664,100). For small countries like Lebanon and

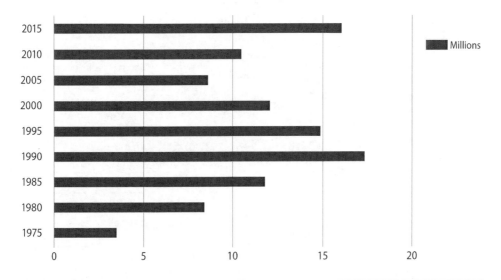

Figure 16.1: Number of Refugees by Year (in Millions)

Source: UNHCR (2017).

Jordan, this means that they are currently providing temporary shelter to refugee populations that are, respectively, 26 percent and 10 percent of the entire size of the country's population. By comparison, in 2015, the industrialized countries with the highest numbers of individuals with recognized refugee claims all had much smaller numbers of refugees and host populations of several million people. For example, while the United States was hosting 273,148 refugees, its population in 2015 was 321.4 million. Refugees thus made up less than one tenth of a percent of the United States' population (see table 16.1).

It should be noted, however, that 2015 saw the largest number of asylum claims in history—those who are requesting refugee status but whose claims are not yet decided (UNHCR 2016). The engagement of industrialized countries is much larger if asylum seekers are considered, particularly for Germany, which already had the largest number of recognized refugees in the world. In 2015, Germany was also hosting the largest number of asylum seekers in the world (see table 16.2). The number of new claims declined by over 70% in 2016 and are continuing to decline (Amnesty International 2018). It should be noted that Canada, which is among the top countries for hosting refugees, has very few asylum claims because of its relatively isolated geographic location. The number of asylum claims has increased recently, however, from 23,930 in 2016 to 50,445 in 2017 (CIC 2018).

In the 1990s, approximately 70 percent of refugees were residing in low- to middle-income countries, with the largest refugee camps existing in Africa, mostly in Kenya and Tanzania. By 2014, the proportion of refugees hosted in low- and middle-income countries rose to 86 percent, in large part because of the conflict in Syria. The importance of relative proximity of sending and receiving countries in determining where refugees are hosted is clear if one looks at the top three hosting countries and the top three sending countries for refugees from 1975 to 2015 (see table 16.3).

Table 16.1. Refugees Hosted in 2014 as a Percentage of Total Population in Top-Six Receiving Countries

Country	Refugees Hosted, 2014[a]	Total Population, 2010[b]	Refugees as a Percentage of Population (%)
Turkey[c]	1,500,000	72,140,000	2.2
Pakistan	1,500,000	173,150,000	0.9
Lebanon	1,500,000	4,340,000	26.5
Islamic Republic of Iran	982,000	74,460,000	1.3
Ethiopia	659,500	87,100,000	0.8
Jordan	654,000	6,460,000	10.1

a UNHRC (2015a).
b United Nations (2015).
c Turkey is both the highest in hosting refugees and the third-highest industrialized country in which refugees sought asylum in 2014.

Table 16.2. Numbers of Refugees and Asylum Seekers in Select Industrialized Countries

	Refugees (Accepted Claims)	Asylum Seekers (Claims Pending)
Germany	316,058	420,569
United States	273,148	286,146
Sweden	168,461	156,991
Canada	135,865	19,542
United Kingdom	122,996	45,773
Italy	117,986	60,105

Source: UNHCR (2017).

Table 16.3. Top Three Sending and Receiving Countries for Refugees, 1975 to 2015

	Top Sending Countries			Top Receiving Countries		
	First	Second	Third	First	Second	Third
2015	Syria	Afghanistan	Somalia	Turkey	Pakistan	Lebanon
2010	Afghanistan	Iraq	Somalia	Pakistan	Iran	Syria
2005	Afghanistan	Sudan	Burundi	Pakistan	Iran	Tanzania
2000	Afghanistan	Burundi	Iraq	Pakistan	Iran	Germany
1995	Afghanistan	Rwanda	Liberia	Germany	Iran	United States
1990	Afghanistan	Ethiopia	Mozambique	Pakistan	Iran	Malawi
1985	Afghanistan	Ethiopia	Iraq	Pakistan	Iran	Somalia
1980	Ethiopia	Afghanistan	Angola	Somalia	Pakistan	DR Congo
1975	Angola	Guinea	Rwanda	United States	DR Congo	Côte d'Ivoire

Source: UNHCR (2017).

FROM TEMPORARY REFUGE TO PERMANENT RESIDENCY: THE CANADIAN CONTEXT

Refugee status was originally conceived of as a temporary solution to forced displacement, although it can last a lifetime. The UNHCR notes that there are currently over 23 protracted refugee situations that have lasted longer than 20 years, with many of those displaced living in temporary asylum for decades (UNHCR 2016). Hosting refugees involves providing temporary asylum. In contrast, resettling refugees is one of three durable solutions for refugees that is promoted by the UNHCR. *Resettlement* refers to permanent residency in a third country. The other two durable solutions are voluntary repatriation to the country of origin or integration into the hosting country (UNHCR 2011). Only a minority of refugees are permanently resettled in a third country; in 2015, resettlement only occurred for 107,100 of 23.1 million refugees.

There are two main routes to permanent settlement for refugees in Canada. Refugees can make a claim for asylum and permanent residency on arrival in the country, or they can be sponsored, have their claim accepted, and be resettled from abroad. Historically, approximately half of all refugees resettling in Canada were accepted through overseas resettlement programs. With the Syrian resettlement initiative of 2015–2017, the number of resettled refugees doubled, but the target for 2017 is returning to pre-2015 levels (25,000). Among resettled refugees who arrive in Canada with permanent residency status, about half arrive as government-assisted refugees (GARs). These are individuals whose first year of financial and settlement support is provided by federal funding and government-funded agencies—similar to what Canadians on social assistance receive from their respective provincial governments—and they receive settlement support through local settlement agencies. The other half are privately sponsored refugees (PSRs), who are sponsored by non-governmental organizations, community groups, faith groups, or groups of private citizens. For PSRs, financial obligations and settlement and social supports are borne by the sponsoring group for up to a year. A smaller minority of refugees with special needs may receive support through the Joint Assistance Sponsorship program, with joint government and private sponsorship extending for two years. Finally, as of 2013, a smaller proportion are resettled through a blended program—the Blended Visa Office-Referred (BVOR) program—where the financial support is shared by private groups and the government, but the resettlement services are provided by government-funded agencies (Blended Visa Office-Referred refugees) (CIC 2015b).

Those who apply for refugee status upon arrival in Canada are deemed refugee claimants. Refugee claimants must present their claim for refugee status before the Immigrant Review Board. Once they are determined to be eligible to make a claim, but before they have had their claim heard, they may be eligible for social assistance (IRCC 2017). They can also apply to Immigration, Refugees and Citizenship Canada for work permits once they have passed their medical examination—although in practice, this can take time. However, those who have come from one of the 42 "Designated Countries of Origin" (DCOs) are ineligible for work permits until their claim is accepted, or until they have been in the country for 180 days, whichever comes first (IRCC 2013). DCOs have been deemed "safe countries" by the Canadian government but include some of the top source countries, such as Hungary and Mexico, which had acceptance rates of 35 percent and 29 percent, respectively, in 2014, challenging their status as "safe" (Keung 2015). Determination of an individual's refugee status may rest in the hands of a single judge, adding a layer of subjectivity. Refugee claimants that are denied refugee status—"failed refugee claimants"—may nevertheless be fleeing tremendous hardship despite not being recognized as individuals fleeing persecution.

Debate exists regarding the effectiveness of Canada's unique private sponsorship program in supporting successful resettlement and integration. Some argue that PSRs receive more attentive care, form stronger relationships with other Canadians outside of their co-ethnic group, and integrate more successfully. But research also suggests that early gains in income, a marker of successful integration, are not sustained, despite the fact that PSRs may be arriving in Canada with higher levels of education and better English/French language skills than those arriving as GARs (Hynie and Hyndman 2016). As attention has turned to the Syrian resettlement initiative and Canada's intention to export the private sponsorship model, more research is being conducted on these models, which may shed more light on their relative merits.

Social Determinants of Health

It is now widely accepted that the health of individuals and populations is influenced by the social conditions of their lives (Commission on Social Determinants of Health 2008). As discussed elsewhere in this book (see Chapter 2 by Raphael), it has consistently been shown that those with greater status and access to resources have better health outcomes along multiple measures of health and well-being. These differences are the result of political and social structures that create inequalities within and between populations and in this way generate and sustain unequal conditions in people's lives (Irwin and Scali 2010).

It is argued that there are three paths through which these structural systems influence health and well-being (Brunner and Marmot 2005). Structural factors determine access to material resources, such as housing and safe environments, and access to social and health services. Material conditions and access then have a direct impact on health by creating unhealthy living conditions. A second pathway through which structural variables operate is through social relationships. Social structures affect social and community relationships, including situations of exclusion and discrimination, employment opportunities, and access to supportive relationships (cf. Dahlgren and Whitehead 1991). These social variables affect health indirectly through psychological states such as stress or feelings of support and perceptions of control over one's life and living conditions (Bambra et al. 2009). These psychological variables in turn result in physiological changes, such as increased cortisol levels, which are then associated with health outcomes, such as increased risk of coronary heart disease (Miller, Chen, and Cole 2009). A third pathway through which social structures affect health outcomes is by shaping and supporting different health-related behaviours, such as drinking, smoking, or eating patterns.

PRE-MIGRATION CONDITIONS AND CONSEQUENCES FOR HEALTH AND MENTAL HEALTH

Material Conditions

The severity of the social, political, and material conditions from which refugees are fleeing have often focused researchers' attention on pre-migration social determinants of health, including exposure to trauma, poor living conditions, and inadequate or non-existent health care (Cronkright and Ramalya 2014; Pryce and Madhar 2014). Refugees are often forced to leave their homes with minimal preparation and few resources, and their migratory path to safety is typically treacherous (Gerard and Pickering 2014).

Many refugees are required to settle into refugee camps, where material deprivation can be severe. Refugee camps were intended as short-term solutions, but most camps have resulted from protracted situations and can exist for decades. Refugee camps often house many more individuals than they were intended for, resulting in overcrowding, inadequate housing, poor sanitation, and limited access to clean water and food (Loewenberg 2011). In one review of water sanitation in UNHCR camps, it was found that over 40 percent of camps were below UNHCR standards for water availability, and more than 25 percent failed to meet the standards for number of latrines (Cronin et al. 2008).

Consequently, refugee camps are often characterized by elevated rates of infectious diseases, such as tuberculosis, and of diseases associated with poor sanitation (Murshidi et al. 2013; Pryce and Madhar 2014). In household surveys in two African refugee camps (in Ghana and Kenya), Cronin and colleagues (2008) found that those respondents reporting a case of diarrhea in the last 24 hours collected 26 percent less water. Moreover, their analysis of UNHCR data found a significant relationship between the incidence of diarrhea, malaria, and rates of Global Acute Malnutrition, reinforcing the interconnected nature of living conditions and a range of measures of morbidity.

Increasingly, however, refugees are settling into urban areas rather than refugee camps, but there too they face inadequate food and shelter, as well as hazardous environmental conditions that expose them to additional health risks (UNHCR 2012). In Jordan, for example, 84 percent of Syrian refugees live outside of camps in both urban and rural regions. A household survey of those living outside of camps documented that about 68 percent lived below the poverty line, 47 percent were living in situations assessed as bad or urgent, and 40 percent lived with poor sanitary conditions. As the Syrian situation continues, these refugees are slipping further into vulnerability and poverty (UNHCR 2015b).

Health Care Access

Refugee camps typically provide some medical facilities but not enough for the number of individuals living in them (Murshidi et al. 2013). Those refugees living in urban settings in low-income countries often have no, or very limited, access to any health care (UNHCR 2012). An outlier is the Jordanian government's commitment to providing free services to Syrian refugees, with over three quarters accessing health care and over half of their children enrolled in formal education—an indication of the critical role that policy plays in refugee health and well-being (UNHCR 2015a). This situation is an exception, however, and because of the limited health care, many refugees arrive in Canada with untreated or undiagnosed medical conditions (Hynie, Canic, and Korn 2014), as well as elevated risk of future illnesses (Dookeran et al. 2010).

Social and Community Relationships

By definition, Convention refugees are fleeing experiences of persecution and discrimination, often accompanied by extreme violence. The social conditions are of extreme community disruption. Families are often scattered and separated for extended periods of time, disrupting normal sources of emotional support and stability (Boyden et al. 2002). Moreover, there are high rates of intimate partner violence reported in displaced families (Rothkegel et al. 2008). Within refugee camps, social conditions can be dangerous, particularly for girls and women, with sexual and gender-based violence officially recognized as one of the most prevalent protection issues (Crisp 2000). In some countries, refugees face challenges registering and acquiring personal identification, leaving them stateless, vulnerable to exploitation, and without the protection of basic rights (de Bruijn 2009). Refugees living outside of camps also face high levels of exclusion, discrimination, and, often, violence. In urban settings, access to food and shelter can only be achieved through employment, which is typically only available through the informal sector, which also further exposes refugees to exploitation and violence (UNHCR 2012).

The short-term impact of forced migration on health is well documented. Refugees arrive with higher rates of infectious diseases, as well as diseases associated with poor sanitation, including parasites and hepatitis; families experiencing forced migration also have elevated rates of child mortality and morbidity (Avogo and Agadjanian 2010; Hargreaves et al. 2004; Dookeran et al. 2010; Lifson et al. 2002). A substantial body of research on post-migration mental health has documented elevated rates of mental health challenges among refugees (Fazel, Wheeler, and Danesh 2005; Porter and Haslam 2005). In many cases, the emphasis on post-migration mental health assumes, either implicitly or explicitly, that these mental health issues are a result of pre-migration trauma, and as noted above, refugees experience high levels of stress and distress in the pre-migration context (Miller and Rasmussen 2010). However, refugees also face a number of challenges to integration and resettlement in their new countries of residence that place them at continued risk of poor mental health following permanent settlement (Hynie, Canic, and Korn 2014; Hynie 2017; Li, Liddell, and Nickerson 2016; Mawani 2014).

POST-MIGRATION CONDITIONS AND CONSEQUENCES FOR HEALTH AND MENTAL HEALTH

Material Conditions

As noted above, sponsored refugees arrive in Canada under a range of programs that provide both material and integration support. Those arriving as GARs normally receive one year of financial support and access to a variety of formal settlement services for education, housing, and health care needs (CIC 2015a). Those arriving under private sponsorship (PSRs) receive equivalent levels of financial support for up to one year, plus informal settlement support. Those who arrive through the blended program (BVOR) receive six months of financial support from the government and six months from private sponsors, plus formal settlement support. Some of those in the blended program may receive ongoing financial support from their combined sponsorship for up to 24 months. In contrast, refugee claimants do not receive settlement support but are eligible to apply for social assistance or for a work permit after their application has been accepted and while they await their hearing, unless they are from one of the Designated Countries of Origin, in which case they must wait 180 days or until they receive a positive decision, whichever comes first (IRCC 2013).

Poverty is a common concern among refugees to Canada. Financial support is at minimum equivalent to that provided by government social assistance (CIC 2015c) and varies from province to province, with supplements possible for housing under special circumstances (CIC 2015b). For example, a single adult living in Ontario would receive approximately 700 dollars per month. Two adults with two children under the age of 18 would receive approximately 840 dollars, plus the Ontario child benefit of up to 230 dollars per month per child. During the time that they are receiving this financial support, refugees are allowed to earn up to 50 percent of their Resettlement Assistance Program (RAP) benefits through employment, after which point their RAP benefits are reduced by the amount equal to their excess earnings (CIC 2015b). However, both settlement workers and refugees themselves note that the levels of financial support are often barely sufficient to meet the costs of basic needs, particularly for singles and large families (Hynie, Canic, and Korn 2014). Moreover, sponsored refugees to Canada must pay for the cost of their airfare, documents, and medical exams, which they typically do through a loan from the Canadian government, which can amount to a large sum for large families and is a source of stress and anxiety for many refugees (Hynie, Canic, and Korn 2014; Shakya et al. 2014). Syrians arriving between November 4, 2015, and February 29, 2016, were not required to repay the cost of transportation. Monthly payments must start 12 months after arrival, but, as of 2018, they are interest free (Government of Canada 2018). Rates of poverty are influenced by local economic situations, shelter costs, employment opportunities, and ease of accessing financial support, such that conditions may be more difficult for refugees in some cities relative to others (Hiebert 2013; Hynie, Canic, and Korn 2014).

A major source of concern for refugees is access to employment, for reasons of income but also because of their desire to feel like contributing members of the community (Beiser and Hou 2001; Hynie, Canic, and Korn 2014). Recently arrived refugees in Canada showed steadily decreasing rates of employment from the 1980s to the early 1990s (Social Research and Demonstration Corporation 2001), with 55 percent or less of those arriving in the early to mid-1990s achieving any employment income (full- or part-time) after five years of residence, reflecting what appears to be a pattern of increasing social exclusion. Recent refugees report struggling to find employment that is commensurate with their previous education and skills, often citing the elusive "Canadian experience" as a barrier to finding employment, in addition to challenges associated with language skills (Hynie, Canic, and Korn 2014). Refugee claimants can face unique employment challenge because of the DCO policies described above.

Upon arrival, refugees often struggle to find safe and affordable housing, frequently finding themselves segregated into low-income neighbourhoods (Ley and Smith 2000; Murdie 2008). Refugees are destined to particular locations in Canada and may find themselves in settings with particularly challenging housing conditions. Poor quality housing has been associated with negative mental and physical health outcomes, including elevated rates of infectious diseases like tuberculosis, chronic diseases such as chronic respiratory illnesses, and injuries including lead poisoning. Housing may be particularly important to children's health, as a family's struggle to afford adequate housing has been associated with poorer nutrition for their children (Krieger and Higgins 2002).

Finding adequate housing is particularly difficult for those with large families, as affordable large homes are typically not available, and for those with disabilities, who can spend many years waiting for assisted housing (Hynie, Canic, and Korn 2014). A study of newcomers in Montreal, Toronto, and Vancouver found that a surprisingly high proportion of refugees relative to other newcomers had spent time in temporary housing, some staying in shelters or with friends, and other measures indicative of precariousness and the danger of homelessness in this population (Hiebert 2013). The precariousness of housing was even greater for refugee claimants, who had less access to settlement support and lower incomes than refugees.

Although education is seen as a priority by many refugees, particularly youths, they face numerous barriers to completing education that could provide locally recognized accreditation, improved language skills, and access to higher income employment. Beyond linguistic limitations, there may be system barriers such as the loss or non-recognition of previous educational documents or "aging out" of the high school system prior to being prepared for university. Refugee youths' educational pathways are frequently disrupted and delayed by forced migration and so they may take longer to complete their secondary education than their non-refugee peers, but free secondary education is typically only offered to youth under the age of 18 or 19 (depending on the region or province). The aforementioned economic challenges are also a barrier for youth's educational aspirations. A short-term need to provide immediate income can conflict with long-term goals of education, as youth refugees report withdrawing temporarily from university studies in order to contribute more to the family's income (Shakya et al. 2010).

Health Care Access

The challenge of meeting basic resettlement needs such as housing, food, and financial support for one's family is a source of stress and can take priority over seeking health care, resulting in a second pathway through which difficult material conditions can influence health for this population (Asgary and Segar 2011). However, refugees who seek to access health care report numerous barriers. Like many newcomers, refugees are unfamiliar with the Canadian health care system, and they may face additional challenges in gaining an understanding of the system because of the complexity of refugee health insurance, language barriers, and the large systemic differences between the health care available to them in their previous country of asylum and Canada (Hynie, Canic, and Korn 2014).

Canada's universal health care coverage is normally managed through provincial insurance, and the procedures working with the Interim Federal Health Program (IFHP) can seem difficult to health care practitioners, who may therefore opt not to see patients with IFHP coverage unless they pay for their own care. Newbold, Cho, and McKeary (2013) found that in Hamilton, few health care providers were willing to accept IFHP insurance coverage and thus were unwilling to treat refugees. When the federal government temporarily changed IFHP coverage, between June 2012 and April 2016, to a more complex system, whereby privately sponsored refugees were no longer covered for supplemental benefits and refugee claimants from some countries were no longer covered for supplemental or primary care, the system became so complex that many additional health care providers began withdrawing services because they lacked the resources to navigate such a complex system (Hynie, Korn, and Canic 2014; see also Berger et al., Chapter 27 in this volume). Qualitative research with migrants with varying migration statuses in Toronto, Ontario, found that migrants perceived a two-tier health care system: one for those with OHIP and one for everyone else, including those with IFHP insurance (Campbell et al. 2014). This suggests that these barriers to accessing care are also being experienced by at least some migrants as a form of discrimination.

Research has consistently found language and a lack of appropriate interpretation services is a major barrier to accessing care, especially for more recently arrived refugees (Asgary and Segar 2011; Newbold, Cho, and McKeary 2013). A lack of adequate interpretation services is a common challenge that affects both immigrants and refugees (McKeary and Newbold 2010) but may be felt more acutely by refugees. First, refugees arrive in Canada much less likely to speak either official language than do immigrants. Data on recent GAR arrivals in Ontario found that around 75 to 85 percent spoke little to no English or French (Korn 2014). Second, their relatively low incomes make it difficult for them to pay for interpretation services themselves when interpreters or family members are not available (Newbold, Cho, and McKeary 2013), creating very real barriers to accessing care. Cultural appropriateness of available care adds another layer of challenge, and may be particularly acute in the context of mental health care (Hynie, Canic, and Korn 2014).

Social Conditions

Social exclusion of refugees in Canada occurs in both direct and indirect ways. Racism and discrimination may underlie many of the barriers that refugees face in accessing housing, employment, or health care (Edge and Newbold 2013). For example, Hiebert (2013) found that refugees reported discrimination in accessing appropriate housing. Accommodation in health care access, especially around interpretation, was associated with negative staff attitudes (Hynie, Canic, and Korn 2014). A study with refugee youth in Ontario found that they struggled against assumptions that they would be unable to succeed in school by virtue of their refugee status. As a result, they were being streamed into non-academic programs in high school rather than academic streams preparing them for university (Hynie, Canic, and Korn 2014; Shakya et al. 2010).

Perhaps the most extreme form of social exclusion is detention. Refugee claimants (as well as failed claimants and other non-citizens) may be held in detention for extended periods of time, sometimes in penal institutions (see Gros, Chapter 18 in this volume). Over the last five years, between 6,500 and 9,000 non-citizens (including refugee claimants) were detained annually (Canada Border Services Agency 2017). The passage of Bill C-4 in 2011 created a new category of "designated foreign nationals": individuals who arrived as part of a group of "irregular arrivals." Designated foreign nationals are only allowed a first review of their detention 12 months following their detention (Béchard 2011). Bill C-4 is framed as a federal initiative to deter smuggling of refugee claimants through marine arrivals. The detrimental mental health impact of detention has been documented in both adults and children after relatively short periods of detention, raising concerns about the long-term consequences of this new policy (Kronick, Rousseau, and Cleveland 2011).

However, other, less intentional, forms of exclusion also arise and affect a broader range of newcomers. Linguistic barriers make it difficult for refugees to participate in the employment sector, access services, and navigate social systems. Moreover, structural barriers arise when institutions do not accommodate refugee-specific challenges, such as lost or unfamiliar qualifications for education, missing information about exact birth dates, and presenting with IFHP insurance coverage. These effectively exclude refugees from accessing needed services and opportunities (Hynie, Canic, and Korn 2014; Shakya et al. 2010).

Accessing adequate social support can mitigate the impact of these social determinants. Co-ethnic communities can be a tremendous source of social support for refugees, providing information, emotional support, and material support that help them navigate their new environment and buffer the negative impacts of migration. However, social isolation and difficulties in building connections to other communities is a persistent challenge (Stewart 2014). Social support needs may not be fully met for those who migrate without family members, and achieving adequate support may be particularly difficult for refugee claimants and those with precarious migration status (Hynie, Crooks, and Barragan 2011).

The detrimental impacts of discrimination and social exclusion on immigrant health have been documented in the "healthy immigrant effect," whereby immigrants arrive in Canada healthier than the average Canadian and then show decreases in perceived and observed measures of health over time (de Maio and Kemp 2010). This effect is particularly marked for visible minorities, and those who have experienced discrimination. Similar effects are observed in mental health (McKenzie 2003). For example, in a cross-sectional and longitudinal survey with over 5,600 new refugees in the UK, Campbell (2012) found that poorer mental health outcomes were associated with unemployment, poor English language skills, infrequent contact with social support networks, jobs that did not meet their skills and qualifications, difficulties managing money, dissatisfaction with housing, and experiences of physical or verbal attacks. Two years later, worsening mental health was associated with decreasing satisfaction with housing, experiences of attacks, and employment at jobs for which they were overqualified, while mental health improvements were associated with employment, better money management, and the alleviation of physical or verbal attacks.

SUMMARY

Refugees and refugee claimants confront severe social and material conditions both prior to migration and following arrival in their country of settlement. Although early experiences place them at risk for health problems, the challenges they confront in the process of integrating into a new country further threaten their health and well-being. Some of these challenges will improve with time, as refugees learn to navigate their new environment, but many of these challenges arise from systemic factors that create extended situations of poverty and exclusion. The health of refugees is therefore a political, material, social, and medical issue, and one that must be considered from all of these perspectives if it is to be adequately addressed.

CRITICAL THINKING QUESTIONS

1. How might health and well-being change over time post-settlement for resettled refugees? What are the implications of these health pathways for providing appropriate health care?
2. Are refugee experiences similar to those of immigrants, only more extreme, or are they qualitatively different? If yes, in what way? If not, why not?
3. How might variables like gender, age, and education shape the likelihood of exposure to various social determinants of health for refugees, both prior to and following

migration? As a health care provider, how might you take these differences into account, if at all?
4. What are the boundaries of care for health care workers when working with refugees? How can and should health care providers address the broader determinants of health?

ADDITIONAL RESOURCES

1. *Canadian Medical Association Journal*: http://www.cmaj.ca
   The journal has a searchable database with several articles on various aspects of refugee health, including treatment guidelines for physical and mental health, and studies on the epidemiology of various health issues among refugee populations. Use the term *refugee* in the search window to find relevant articles.

2. The International Organization for Migration (IOM): https://health.iom.int
   The IOM has created frameworks for thinking about migrant health that incorporate a clear social determinants of health perspective. These are described on their home page under IOM Approach to Migrant Health and their description of the Public Health Approach to Migrant Health. The site is also useful for its Thematic Reports and Policy Papers, which can be found under the site's "Policy" menu.

3. Unite for Sight: http://www.uniteforsight.org/refugee-health/module1
   Unite for Sight has a training module for refugee health care in refugee camps. It includes an extensive reading list and case studies addressing both the physical and social determinants of health for refugees in camps, including information about economic conditions, relationships with host communities, and mental health.

4. United Nations High Commissioner for Refugees (UNHCR): http://www.unhcr.org/about-us.html
   This website is a portal to an enormous amount of information about the work of the UNHCR in the area of forced migration, including:
   - definitions of different categories of migrants
   - the history of international policy regarding forced migration (including extensive historical archives)
   - detailed statistics on migration patterns of those under the UNHCR mandate, including source countries, receiving countries, and age and gender breakdowns of forced migrants
   - annual global reports summarizing migration trends for each year
   - evaluations of a range of programs and situations, from conditions in refugee camps, to resettlement programs in particular countries, to evaluations of their own implementation of UNHCR policies

5. The World Health Organization (WHO): http://www.who.int/migrants/en/
   The WHO website provides excellent resources for refugee and migrant health. The website includes annual world health statistics, international treatment guidelines, and a range of reports on health care systems.

REFERENCES

Amnesty International. 2018. *Amnesty International Report 2017/18: The State of the World's Human Rights.* London: Amnesty International Ltd. https://www.amnesty.org/en/documents/pol10/6700/2018/en/.

Asgary, Ramin, and Nora Segar. 2011. "Barriers to Health Care Access among Refugee Seekers." *Journal of Health Care for the Poor and Underserved* 22 (2): 506–22.

Avogo, Winfred Aweyire, and Victor Agadjanian. 2010. "Forced Migration and Child Health and Mortality in Angola." *Social Science & Medicine* 70 (1): 53–60.

Bambra, Clare, M. Gibson, A. Sowden, K. Wright, M. Whitehead, and M. Petticrew. 2009. "Tackling the Wider Social Determinants of Health and Health Inequalities: Evidence from Systematic Reviews." *Journal of Epidemiology and Community Health* 64: 284–91.

Bates, Diane C. 2002. "Environmental Refugees? Classifying Human Migrations Caused by Environmental Change." *Population and Environment* 23 (5): 465–77.

Béchard, Julie. 2011. "Legislative Summary of Bill C-4: An Act to Amend the Immigration and Refugee Protection Act, the Balanced Reform Act and the Marine Transportation Security Act." *Library of Parliament Research Publications*, August 30. Publication no. 41-1-C2E. http://www.parl.gc.ca/About/Parliament/LegislativeSummaries/bills_ls.asp?Language=E&ls=c4&Parl=41&Ses=1&source=library_prb.

Beiser, Morton, and Feng Hou. 2001. "Language Acquisition, Unemployment and Depressive Disorder among Southeast Asian Refugees: A 10-Year Study." *Social Science & Medicine* 53 (10): 1321–34.

Boyden, Jo, Jo de Berry, Thomas Feeny, and Jason Hart. 2002. "Children Affected by Armed Conflict in South Asia: A Review of Trends and Issues Identified through Secondary Research." Refugee Studies Centre Working Paper, Oxford, February.

Brunner, Eric, and Michael Marmot. 2005. "Social Organization, Stress and Health." In *Social Determinants of Health*, edited by Michael Marmot and Richard G. Wilkinson, 17–43. Oxford: Oxford University Press.

Campbell, Mark. 2012. "Social Determinants of Mental Health in New Refugees in the UK: Cross-Sectional and Longitudinal Analyses." *Lancet* 380 (suppl 3): S27.

Campbell, Ruth, A. Klei, Brian Hodges, David Fisman, and Simon Kitto. 2014. "A Comparison of Health Access between Permanent Residents, Undocumented Immigrants and Refugee Claimants in Toronto, Canada." *Journal of Immigrant Minority Health* 16 (1): 165–76.

Canada Border Services Agency. 2017. "Arrests, Detentions and Removals." Last modified November 6. http://www.cbsa-asfc.gc.ca/security-securite/arr-det-eng.html.

Citizenship and Immigration Canada (CIC). 2015a. *Government-Assisted Refugee Resettlement in Canada*. Ottawa: CIC. http://www.cic.gc.ca/english/pdf/pub/GAR_eng.pdf.

Citizenship and Immigration Canada (CIC). 2015b. *In Canada Processing of Convention Refugees Abroad and Members of the Humanitarian Protected Persons Abroad Classes—Part 2 [Resettlement Assistance Program (RAP)]*. Ottawa: Citizenship and Immigration Canada. http://www.cic.gc.ca/english/resources/manuals/ip/ip03-part2-eng.pdf.

Citizenship and Immigration Canada (CIC). 2015c. *Privately Sponsored Refugee Resettlement in Canada*. Ottawa: Citizenship and Immigration Canada. http://www.cic.gc.ca/english/pdf/pub/PSR_eng.pdf.

Citizenship and Immigration Canada (CIC). 2018. *Asylum Claims Processed by Canada Border Services Agency (CBSA) and Immigration, Refugees, and Citizenship Canada (IRCC) Offices, January 2011–May 2018*. Ottawa: Citizenship and Immigration Canada. https://www.canada.ca/en/immigration-refugees-citizenship/services/refugees/asylum-claims/processed-claims.html.

Commission on Social Determinants of Health. 2008. *Closing the Gap in a Generation: Health Equity through Action on the Social Determinants of Health*. Geneva: World Health Organization.

Crisp, Jeff. 2000. "A State of Insecurity: The Political Economy of Violence in Kenya's Refugee Camps." *African Affairs* 99 (39): 601–32.

Cronin, A. A., D. Shrestha, N. Cornier, F. Abdalla, N. Ezard, and C. Aramburu. 2008. "A Review of Water and Sanitation Provision in Refugee Camps in Association with Selected Health and Nutrition Indicators—The Need for Integrated Service Provision." *Journal of Water and Health* 6 (1): 1–13.

Cronkright, Peter, and Astha K. Ramalya. 2014. "Chronic Disease Management." In *Refugee Health Care: An Essential Medical Guide*, edited by Aniyizhai Annamalai, 115–47. New York: Springer.

Dahlgren, Göran, and Margaret Whitehead. 1991. "Policies and Strategies to Promote Social Equity in Health." Stockholm: Institute for Future Studies.

de Bruijn, Bart. 2009. "The Living Conditions and Well-Being of Refugees." United Nations Development Programme Human Development Reports Research Paper, 2009/25, New York, July.

de Maio, Fernando G., and Eagan Kemp. 2010. "The Deterioration of Health Status among Immigrants to Canada." *Global Public Health* 5 (5): 462–78. https://doi.org/10.1080/17441690902942480.

Docherty, Bonnie, and Tyler Giannini. 2009. "Confronting a Rising Tide: A Proposal for a Convention on Climate Change Refugees." *Harvard Environmental Law Review* 33 (2): 349–403.

Dookeran, Nameeta, M., Tracy Battaglia, Jennifer Cochran, and Paul L. Geltman. 2010. "Chronic Diseases and its Risk Factors among Refugees and Asylees in Massachusetts, 2001–2005." *Preventing Chronic Diseases* 7 (3): A51.

Edge, Sara, and Bruce Newbold. 2013. "Discrimination and the Health of Immigrants and Refugees: Exploring Canada's Evidence Base and Directions for Future Research in Newcomer Receiving Countries." *Journal of Immigrant and Minority Health* 15 (1): 141–8.

Fazel, Mina, Jeremy Wheeler, and John Danesh. 2005. "Prevalence of Serious Mental Disorder in 7000 Refugees Resettled in Western Countries: A Systematic Review." *Lancet* 365: 1309–14. https://doi.org/10.1016/S0140-6736(05)61027-6.

Gerard, Alison, and Sharon Pickering. 2014. "Gender, Securitization and Transit: Refugee Women and the Journey to the EU." *Journal of Refugee Studies* 27 (3): 338–59.

Government of Canada. 2018. "Regulations Amending the Immigration and Refugee Protection Regulations." *Canada Gazette, Part II*, 152 (4). http://www.gazette.gc.ca/rp-pr/p2/2018/2018-02-21/html/sor-dors22-eng.html.

Hargreaves, James R., Mark A. Collinson, Kathleen Kahn, Samuel J. Clark, and Stephen M. Tollman. 2004. "Childhood Mortality among Former Mozambican Refugees and Their Host in Rural South Africa." *International Journal of Epidemiology* 33 (6): 1271–8.

Hiebert, Daniel. 2013. "Precarious Housing and Hidden Homelessness among Refugees, Asylum Seekers, and Immigrants in Montreal, Toronto, and Vancouver: Introduction and Synthetic Executive Summary." Government of Canada. Last modified December 12. https://www.canada.ca/en/employment-social-development/programs/communities/homelessness/immigrants-precarious.html.

Hynie, Michaela. 2017. "The Social Determinants of Refugee Mental Health in the Post-migration Context: A Critical Review." *Canadian Journal of Psychiatry*, December 4. https://doi.org/10.1177/0706743717746666.

Hynie, Michaela, Katarina Canic, and Ashley Korn. 2014. *An Impact Evaluation of Client Support Services for Government Assisted Refugees*. Final report for YMCA and Citizenship and Immigration Canada. https://www.slideserve.com/malina/an-impact-evaluation-of-client-support-services-for-government-assisted-refugees.

Hynie, Michaela, Valerie A. Crooks, and Jackeline Barragan. 2011. "Immigrant and Refugee Social Networks: Determinants and Consequences of Social Support among Women Newcomers to Canada." *Canadian Journal of Nursing Research* 43 (4): 26–46.

Hynie, Michaela, and Jennifer Hyndman. 2016. "From Newcomer to Canadian: Making Integration for Refugees Work." *Policy Options*, May 17. http://policyoptions.irpp.org/fr/magazines/mai-2016/from-newcomer-to-canadian-making-refugee-integration-work/.

Hynie, Michaela, Ashley Korn, and Katarina Canic. 2014. "Refugee Integration in Ontario: A Tale of Six Cities. Institutional Adaptation to Health Policy Changes for Government Assisted Refugees." Paper presented at the meeting of the International Association of Studies in Forced Migration, Bogota, Colombia, July 15–18.

Immigration, Refugees and Citizenship Canada (IRCC). 2013. "Backgrounder—Designated Countries of Origin." Last modified February 1. http://www.cic.gc.ca/english/department/media/backgrounders/2012/2012-11-30.asp.

Immigration, Refugees and Citizenship Canada (IRCC). 2017. *How Canada's Refugee System Works*. Last modified April 3. https://www.canada.ca/en/immigration-refugees-citizenship/services/refugees/canada-role.html.

Irwin, Alec, and Elena Scali. 2010. "Action on the Social Determinants of Health: Learning from Previous Experiences." Social Determinants of Health Discussion Paper 1 (Debates). Geneva: World Health Organization.

Keung, Nicholas. 2015. "Canada's Refugee Acceptance Rate Up Despite Asylum Restrictions." *TheStar.com*, March 1. http://www.thestar.com/news/immigration/2015/03/01/canadas-refugee-acceptance-rate-up-despite-asylum-restrictions.html.

Korn, Ashley. 2014. "Client Support Services: The Regional and Local Overview." Unpublished Report. Toronto: YMCA.

Krieger, James, and Donna L. Higgins. 2002. "Housing and Health: Time Again for Public Health Action." *American Journal of Public Health* 92 (5): 758–68.

Kronick, Rachel, Cecile Rousseau, and Janet Cleveland. 2011. "Mandatory Detention of Refugee Children: A Public Health Issue?" *Paediatrics & Child Health* 16 (8): e65-7.

Ley, David, and Heather Smith. 2000. "Relations between Deprivation and Immigrant Groups in Large Canadian Cities." *Urban Studies* 37 (1): 37–62. https://doi.org/10.1080/0042098002285.

Li, Susan S. Y., Belinda J. Liddell, and Angela Nickerson. 2016. "The Relationship between Post-migration Stress and Psychological Disorders in Refugees and Asylum Seekers." *Current Psychiatry Reports* 18: 82. https://doi.org/10.1007/s11920-016-0723-0.

Lifson, Alan R., Dzung Thai, Ann O'Fallon, Wendy A. Mills, and Kaying Hang. 2002. "Prevalence of Tuberculosis, Hepatitis B Virus, and Intestinal Parasitic Infections among Refugees to Minnesota." *Public Health Reports* 117 (1): 69–77.

Loewenberg, Samuel. 2011. "Humanitarian Response Inadequate in Horn of Africa Crisis." *Lancet* 378 (9791): 555–8. https://doi.org/10.1016/S0140-6736(11)61276-2.

Mawani, Farah N. 2014. "Social Determinants of Refugee Mental Health." In *Refuge and Resilience: Promoting Resilience and Mental Health among Resettled Refugees and Forced Migrants*, edited by Laura Simich and Lisa Anderman, 27–50. New York: Springer.

McKeary, Marie, and Bruce Newbold. 2010. "Barriers to Care: The Challenges for Canadian Refugees and Their Health Care Providers." *Journal of Refugee Studies* 23 (4): 523–45.

McKenzie, Kwame. 2003. "Racism and Health." *British Medical Journal* 326: 65–66.

Miller, Gregory, Edith Chen, and Steve W. Cole. 2009. "Health Psychology: Developing Biologically Plausible Models Linking the Social World and Physical Health." *Annual Review of Psychology* 60: 501–24.

Miller, Kenneth E., and Andrew Rasmussen. 2010. "War Exposure, Daily Stressors, and Mental Health in Conflict and Post-conflict Settings: Bridging the Divide Between Trauma-Focused and Psychosocial Frameworks." *Social Science & Medicine* 70 (1): 7–16.

Murdie, Robert A. 2008. "Pathways to Housing: The Experiences of Sponsored Refugees and Refugee Claimants in Accessing Permanent Housing in Toronto." *Journal of International Migration and Integration* 9 (1): 81–101.

Murshidi, Mujalli Mhailan, Mohamed Qasem Bassam Hijjawi, Sahar Jeriesat, and Akram Eltom. 2013. "Syrian Refugees and Jordan's Health Sector." *Lancet* 382 (9888): 206.

Newbold, K. Bruce, Jenny Cho, and Marie McKeary. 2013. "Access to Health Care: The Experience of Refugee and Refugee Claimant Women in Hamilton, Ontario." *Journal of Immigrant and Refugee Studies* 11 (4): 431–49.

Porter, Matthew, and Nick Haslam. 2005. "Predisplacement and Postdisplacement Factors Associated with Mental Health of Refugees and Internally Displaced Persons: A Meta-analysis." *JAMA* 294 (5): 602–12.

Pryce, Douglas J., and Asha M. J. Madhar. 2014. "Viral Hepatitis." In *Refugee Health Care: An Essential Medical Guide*, edited by Aniyizhai Annamalai, 79–93. New York: Springer.

Rothkegel, Sibylle, Julian Poluda, Charlotte Wonani, Juliette Papy, Eva Engelhardt-Wendt, Barbara Weyermann, and Reinhard Henning. 2008. *Evaluation of UNHCR's Efforts to Prevent and Respond to Sexual and Gender-Based Violence in Situations of Forced Displacement*. Geneva, Switzerland: UNHCR. http://www.unhcr.org/48ea31062.pdf.

Shakya, Yogendra B., Sepali Guruge, Michaela Hynie, Arzo Akbari, Mohamed Malik, Sheila Htoo, Azza Khogali, Stella Abiyo Mona, Rabea Murtaza, and Sarah Alley. 2010. "Aspirations for Higher Education among Newcomer Refugee Youth in Toronto: Expectations, Challenges, and Strategies." *Refuge* 27 (2): 65–78.

Shakya, Yogendra B., Sepali Guruge, Michaela Hynie, Sheila Htoo, Arzo Akbari, Barinder (Binny) Jandu, Megan Spasevksi, Nahom Berhane, and Jessica Forster. 2014. "Newcomer Refugee Youth as 'Resettlement Champions' for Their Families: Vulnerability, Resilience and Empowerment." In *Refuge and Resilience: Promoting Resilience and Mental Health among Resettled Refugees and Forced Migrants*, edited by Laura Simich and Lisa Andermann, 131–54. New York: Springer.

Social Research and Demonstration Corporation. 2001. *A Statistical Profile of Government-Assisted Refugees*. Report submitted to Citizenship and Immigration Canada, May 1. http://www.srdc.org/uploads/statistical_profile.pdf.

Stewart, Miriam J. 2014. "Social Support in Refugee Resettlement." In *Refuge and Resilience: Promoting Resilience and Mental Health among Resettled Refugees and Forced Migrants*, edited by Laura Simich and Lisa Andermann, 91–107. New York: Springer.

United Nations. 2010. *Convention and Protocol Relating to the Status of Refugees*. Geneva: United Nations High Commissioner for Refugees. http://www.unhcr.org/3b66c2aa10.

United Nations. 2015. "World Population Prospects: The 2012 Revision." United Nations, Department of Economic and Social Affairs, Working Paper No. ESA/P/WP.228. Program Division, Population Estimates and Projections Section. http://esa.un.org/unpd/wpp/publications/Files/WPP2012_HIGHLIGHTS.pdf.

United Nations General Assembly. 1951. "Convention Relating to the Status of Refugees." United Nations Treaty Series. Geneva: United Nations. http://www.ohchr.org/EN/ProfessionalInterest/Pages/StatusOfRefugees.aspx.

United Nations High Commissioner for Refugees (UNHCR). 1977. "Note on Non-refoulement, EC/SCP/2." UNHCR, August 23. http://www.unhcr.org/afr/excom/scip/3ae68ccd10/note-non-refoulement-submitted-high-commissioner.html.

United Nations High Commissioner for Refugees (UNHCR). 2011. *Refugee Protection and Mixed Migration: The 10-Point Plan in Action*. Geneva: UNHCR. http://www.unhcr.org/protection/migration/4d52864b9/refugee-protection-mixed-migration-10-point-plan-action.html.

United Nations High Commissioner for Refugees (UNHCR). 2012. *The State of the World's Refugees: In Search of Solidarity*. Oxford: Oxford University Press.

United Nations High Commissioner for Refugees (UNHCR). 2013. *Hosting the World's Refugees: Global Report, 2013*. Geneva: UNHCR. http://www.unhcr.org/539809daa.html.

United Nations High Commissioner for Refugees (UNHCR). 2014. *Protecting Refugees & the Role of UNHCR*. Geneva: UNHCR. http://www.unhcr.org/509a836e9.html.

United Nations High Commissioner for Refugees (UNHCR). 2015a. *UNHCR Asylum Trends 2014: Levels and Trends in Industrialized Countries*. Geneva: UNHCR. http://www.unhcr.org/551128679.html.

United Nations High Commissioner for Refugees (UNHCR). 2015b. *Living in the Shadows: Jordan Home Visits Report, 2014*. Geneva: UNHCR. http://unhcr.org/jordan2014urbanreport/home-visit-report.pdf.

United Nations High Commissioner for Refugees (UNHCR). 2016. *UNHCR Global Trends: Forced Displacement in 2015*. Geneva: UNHCR. http://www.unhcr.org/556725e69.html.

United Nations High Commissioner for Refugees (UNHCR). 2017. "Population Statistics." http://popstats.unhcr.org/en/overview#_ga=1.195124712.535301527.1428525829.

Van Hear, Nicholas. 2011. *Mixed Migration: Policy Challenges*. Oxford: The Migration Observatory at the University of Oxford. http://www.migrationobservatory.ox.ac.uk/wp-content/uploads/2016/04/PolicyPrimer-Mixed_Migration.pdf.

CHAPTER 17

Health Issues in Refugee Populations

Meb Rashid, Vanessa Redditt, Andrea Hunter, and Kevin Pottie

LEARNING OBJECTIVES

After reading this chapter, you should be able to:

1. Appreciate the unique health needs of refugee populations.
2. Understand the key components of a comprehensive health assessment for newly arrived refugees, including special considerations for children and youth, and the evidence base for these guidelines.
3. Identify components of sensitive and respectful practice in providing health care for refugees.

Case Study

A 32-year-old woman presents to your clinic 10 days after arriving in Canada. She speaks Korean and you access a phone interpreter to speak to her. She is quiet, almost withdrawn, but willingly answers all of your questions. You determine that she is a refugee claimant, originally from a small town in North Korea. She has arrived alone in Canada, and, although the details are vague, she suggests that she has children and a husband who passed away. She is currently staying at a shelter for newly arrived refugees but has no other contacts in the city.

UNIQUE HEALTH CONSIDERATIONS FOR REFUGEE PATIENTS

Approximately 250,000 newcomers resettle in Canada each year, about 10 percent of whom are refugees (Minister for Immigration, Refugees, and Citizenship Canada 2016). Unlike other immigrant groups, most refugees have endured significant trauma, such as war and torture, prior to migrating to Canada. Furthermore, many refugees originate from countries with a high burden of infectious diseases. Refugees may have also experienced limited access to health care and poor living conditions. Furthermore, this population typically has less access to health care and experiences higher levels of poverty (Guendelman, Schauffler, and Pearl 2001; Ornstein 2000; Crockett 2005; Sanmartin and Ross 2006; Schulpen 1996). As a result of such factors, refugees often have unique health issues that require careful consideration by clinicians (Pottie et al. 2011; McKeary and Newbold 2010). The preceding chapter (Hynie, Chapter 16) provides an important overview of refugee migration patterns and domestic policies and pre-migratory, migratory, and post-migratory factors shaping refugee health.

HEALTH CARE COVERAGE FOR REFUGEES IN CANADA

Those who are recognized as refugees prior to migration—government-assisted and privately sponsored refugees (GARs and PSRs, respectively)—are granted provincial health insurance upon arrival to Canada and are on a trajectory towards becoming Canadian citizens. They are also provided health insurance by the Interim Federal Health Program (IFHP) to cover the costs of medications and other supplemental services during the first year of their resettlement. These benefits are similar to those covered by provincial social assistance programs (IRCC 2018). Refugee claimants are provided health insurance through the IFHP for both basic medical services (similar to provincial health insurance) and supplemental coverage. Once accepted as refugees, they can apply for provincial health insurance.

REFUGEE CARE GUIDELINES

Over the past decade, researchers and practitioners began to recognize the need for guidance to address the unique needs of migrant populations (IOM 2008; Gushulak et al. 2011). Health equity is an evidence-based science that aims to address unfair and unjust health inequality outcomes (O'Neill et al. 2014). These culturally and linguistically diverse populations often suffer poorer health outcomes related to previous exposures, refugee status, language proficiency, gender, and socioeconomic status (Pottie et al. 2011; Ng, Pottie, and Spitzer 2011). Beach et al. (2006) led a systematic review on ethnic and visible minorities that clearly showed health inequities but also interventions that could improve health care. Numerous bodies have developed guidelines for health care providers caring for refugee patients (Centers for Disease Control and Prevention 2014; Murray et al. 2009). However, among industrialized countries, source countries of refugee migrants may differ significantly. As such, recommendations from the United States, Australia, or other nations may not be universally applicable to the Canadian context.

The 2011 Canadian Collaboration for Immigrant and Refugee Health (CCIRH)'s "Evidence-Based Clinical Guidelines for Immigrants and Refugees" provide an evidence-based, practical approach to the care of newcomers (Pottie et al. 2011). These guidelines were driven by primary care providers across Canada, who collaborated in developing a consensus on the priority preventable and treatable health conditions for newly arriving migrants (Swinkels et al. 2011). A user-friendly online checklist for migrants from specific regions has also been adapted from the Canadian guidelines and can be found at http://www.ccirhken.ca. Furthermore, the collaboration created a series of short podcasts that pragmatically explore guideline implementation with patients (Cochrane Podcasts: Immigrant Health: https://www.cochrane.org/evidence/podcasts?title=&body_value=Immigrant+health). Recommendations have also been adapted to address the specific needs of Syrian refugees, responding to the large numbers of Syrian refugees resettling in Canada (Pottie et al. 2015).

Additionally, the Canadian Pediatric Society has developed an extensive set of evidence-based guidelines, clinical and advocacy tools, and training materials for health providers focused on newcomer children through Caring for Kids New to Canada (http://www.kidsnewtocanada.ca).

APPLYING REFUGEE GUIDELINES IN PRACTICE

There is tremendous variability in the needs of different refugee populations (Gushulak et al. 2011; McKeary and Newbold 2010). The politician urgently fleeing violence may have a very different health risk profile than the individual who has languished in a refugee camp for decades. Different refugee groups and individuals may present with dramatically diverse histories of exposure to violence, the duration of such threats, and the perils of their migration journeys (UNHCR 2015). Similarly, the sociodemographic profile, language competencies, and education levels of refugee groups and individuals—even from the same country—can vary immensely. Individuals differ substantially in their coping mechanisms, such that similar trauma can result in profoundly different impacts. Factors such as individual coping mechanisms, personality traits, the ability and desire to articulate symptoms, expectations and beliefs about illness, and culture can also affect illness presentations (Kirmayer et al. 2011; McKeary and Newbold 2010). The Canadian guidelines for refugee care demonstrate that care must be informed by the person's age, region or country of origin, migration history, refugee status, income, and language, among other factors (Pottie et al. 2011).

Despite such heterogeneity, some common challenges confront refugee populations, including a higher burden of infectious diseases, exposure to trauma, and limited previous primary care (Pottie et al. 2011). Consideration of these common themes, as well as a patient's unique pre-migration history and migratory pathway, is essential in effectively providing care for these individuals.

THE IMMIGRATION MEDICAL EXAM

All refugees receive an immigration medical exam (IME) (IRCC 2013), which is intended to screen for burden of illness and certain transmissible infections for public health considerations; it is not designed to provide comprehensive clinical care for individual refugees (Gushulak et al. 2011). The exam consists of a basic history and physical exam, HIV and syphilis testing for those 15 years of age and older, a chest X-ray for those 11 years and older, and urinalysis for those 5 years and older. For GARs and PSRs, the IME is performed before their arrival in Canada and is generally valid for up to one year. Thus, when refugees connect to health care in Canada, testing may be dated, and clinicians may consider repeating exams, when indicated. For refugee claimants, the exam is conducted in Canada soon after a refugee claim is initiated. Of note, however, health needs do not constitute grounds for inadmissibility for refugees.

DISCUSSING MEDICAL HISTORY WITH REFUGEE PATIENTS

Fostering a bond of trust with refugee patients is critical for exploring a comprehensive history and promoting follow-up. Eliciting a complete history may require numerous visits, and different aspects of a patient's health status may only be revealed with time. In addition to addressing immediate patient concerns during an initial visit, clinicians should focus on ensuring that the patient feels comfortable and safe during the assessment. An explanation of patient confidentiality is important and can help to allay fears that medical information will be shared with authorities and somehow affect their refugee status.

For patients with limited English proficiency, use of a trained interpreter is recommended instead of relying on family members and colleagues. Using a family member for interpretation can diminish the reliability of information (due to translation errors, nondisclosure of sensitive information, or altered meanings to protect family members) and can place individuals in the stressful role of negotiation broker between a health professional and family members. This is a particularly heavy responsibility for children and youth (Hilliard 2018b). Furthermore, it can disrupt family roles and dynamics (Hilliard 2018b).

Alongside a regular medical history, obtaining a thorough migration history is critical, including the country of one's birth, all countries visited during migration, and the length of time spent in each country. Health risks may vary considerably depending on the duration of time in transit after an individual leaves his or her source country, in addition to the specific geography and exposures of a particular migratory journey.

Some refugee patients have had little to no access to any primary care pre-migration; the history of previous preventative interventions, such as immunizations and cervical cancer screening, should be noted.

A thorough family history can provide valuable information on existing social stressors and supports, as well as hereditary diseases and risk factors. For example, it may emerge that patients are estranged from children or other family members, or that there have been deaths in the family. Noting the composition of a patient's family in Canada may also provide a sense of available social supports.

A social history, where appropriate, may include the highest educational level and employment history in the patient's country of origin. Literacy skills in the patient's first language should also be noted. Exploring a patient's current living situation and economic means may also be informative. This information may be helpful in linking refugees to language, educational, employment, and social services in Canada, as well as potentially assisting in appropriately tailoring treatment plans and patient education.

Individuals may present with a variety of concerns related to reproductive health. There may be an increase in unwanted pregnancy during the period soon after migration due to unmet contraceptive needs (Pottie et al. 2011). This may result in abortion, difficulties adopting healthy pregnancy recommendations, or limitation of women's ability to achieve educational, employment, and economic goals. Sensitively exploring contraceptive needs with patients, including providing education regarding emergency contraception, early in the migration process and connecting them with desired interventions can help address these concerns. Consider also regional trends in family planning methods, such as higher rates of intrauterine device (IUD) use in Eastern Europe, the Middle East, and Asia and injectable contraceptive use in some refugee camp settings (Pottie et al. 2011; UNHCR 2011); however, individual preferences can vary widely. On the other hand, women may arrive at various stages of pregnancy and require prenatal care, or they may desire pregnancy, presenting important opportunities for optimizing preconception health.

A thorough review of systems is essential, with emphasis on any history of fever (particularly for patients from malaria endemic regions), cough, night sweats, and weight loss. Rates of mental health issues are particularly high in refugee populations and inquiring about sleep and appetite may be a non-intrusive approach to broach these sensitive issues (Kirmayer et al. 2011).

CONSIDERATIONS FOR PHYSICAL EXAMINATIONS IN THE CARE OF REFUGEES

A thorough physical exam, as early as possible after arrival in Canada, is recommended. Early identification and treatment of illness can help to prevent further health complications.

Rates of chronic illnesses in refugee patients can be high, and as a result, vital signs, including blood pressure and body mass index, should be noted for all patients on their first visit (Pottie et al. 2011; Dookeran et al. 2010). As with other immigrant groups, many refugees gain weight after arrival in Canada, due to changes in access to and type of food and levels of physical activity (McDonald and Kennedy 2005). This weight gain may be appropriate for some refugees who have been exposed to prolonged deprivation, but for many others, weight gain may increase their risk of negative health outcomes.

Clinicians should be alert for clues of previously undiagnosed disease during the physical exam. Given higher rates of iron deficiency and potentially higher rates of hemoglobinopathies, depending on ethnic background, a clinical evaluation for signs of anemia is important (Pottie et al. 2011). A screening eye exam is crucial, as unrecognized visual loss is not uncommon among refugees and may significantly hamper integration (Pottie et al. 2011). Examination of the head and neck should focus particular attention on oral health status—studies have shown higher rates of dental caries among refugees and the benefits of early intervention (Pottie et al. 2011). Tooth pain with or without localized swelling, and when dental therapy cannot be started immediately, should typically be treated with anti-inflammatory medications and not antibiotics. The CCIRH guidelines also highlight a twofold increase in newcomers obtaining appropriate dental care when a primary care practitioner actively refers patients with dental pathology to a dental specialist (Pottie et al. 2011). A cardiovascular exam may reveal signs of unrecognized congenital or rheumatic heart diseases. A careful respiratory exam is particularly helpful in the context of respiratory symptoms or any concern for diseases such as tuberculosis. Enlargement of the liver and/or spleen may be detected with a thorough abdominal exam. Comprehensive examination for enlarged or irregular lymph nodes is important and can point to hematologic, malignant, or infectious disease. Clubbing of the digits may be an indicator of congenital heart disease, chronic lung infections (including pulmonary tuberculosis [TB]), cirrhosis of the liver, or whipworm infection, among other causes (Rutherford 2013). Dermatologic issues are common in refugee populations and a thorough dermatological exam also provides an opportunity to document any physical signs of previous violence or torture.

Refugees may have been exposed to sexual violence, increasing their risk of sexually transmitted infections in addition to other physical and psychological complications. Furthermore, many female refugees may have never undergone screening for cervical cancer (Pottie et al. 2011). A gynecological examination in women and a urological exam in men are recommended. In many circumstances, these exams may not be appropriate on an initial visit; unless urgently indicated, clinicians may choose to defer such examinations until the patient feels comfortable undergoing such testing. Culturally sensitive and patient-centred approaches, including tailored patient education, professional interpreters, and the availability of female providers, may help to improve uptake of cervical cancer screening and gynecologic examinations (Pottie et al. 2011; Wiedmeyer, Lofters, and Rashid 2012).

HEALTH ASSESSMENTS FOR REFUGEE CHILDREN

As with adult patients, a complete medical history and physical examination are essential to identifying and providing support or early intervention for a multitude of health issues in newcomer children. Particular areas of focus that are of more relevance to refugee children and youth are outlined below. More information about specific considerations for children is available at the Canadian Pediatric Society's Caring for Kids New to Canada website (http://www.kidsnewtocanada.ca).

Medical History

- Age should be verified. Age may be calculated differently in some contexts, and some families may not know their child's precise birth date (Hilliard 2018a). A bone age is sometimes helpful if growth or development do not match stated chronological age (Benson and Williams 2008).
- Consanguinity should be considered as part of family history in children/youth with developmental delay, dysmorphism, or neurological symptoms (Hilliard 2018a). Consanguineous unions are traditional and respected in some communities (Hamamy et al. 2011; Tadmouri et al. 2009).
- Dietary history and nutritional status are important factors in assessing growth and development, with complex underpinnings including food security, cultural differences in early childhood nutrition practices, and interplay with chronic infections and disease. Higher rates of micronutrient deficiencies and undernutrition exist in refugee and internationally adopted children (Mason et al. 2012; Park et al. 2011).
- Psychosocial issues may play a significant role in refugee children and youth adjusting to life in Canada; it often requires multiple visits and rapport built over time with health providers to explore these in depth. Clinicians should be alert to mental health issues in refugee children and youth, particularly post-traumatic stress disorder, depression, attachment disorders, and altered behaviour patterns (Attanayakea et al. 2009; Bronstein and Montgomery 2011; Hilliard 2018a).
- Exploration of previous illnesses, along with the family's access to health care in their country(ies) of origin, and any traditional forms of treatment that they sought, including "natural" remedies and over-the-counter products, is an essential component of a thorough medical history (Hilliard 2018a).

Physical Examination

- A physical examination should include growth parameters; developmental assessment; signs of congenital infections; dental, hearing, and vision screening; and a careful head-to-toe assessment.
- Sensitivity in conducting a genitourinary examination is critical, with attention paid to signs of congenital abnormalities not yet addressed (hypospadias, cryptorchidism, inguinal hernias), sexually transmitted infections (STIs), sexual abuse, or female genital mutilation/cutting (FGM/C).
- Careful attention should be paid to signs of congenital issues that may not have been addressed, or fully addressed, prior to migration, such as hydrocephalus or other neurological abnormalities, clubfeet (*talipes equinovarus*), developmental dysplasia of the hip, structural congenital heart abnormalities, inborn errors of metabolism, or endocrine conditions.

Child Discipline and Maltreatment

Customs and beliefs about parenting and child behaviour differ among families, populations, and cultures. Sensitive orientation to Canadian norms and laws is an important component of orientation for newcomers. For example, some traditional healing practices used in some cultures may raise suspicions of maltreatment in the Canadian context, including moxibustion, cupping, and "coining" or rubbing (Galanti 2008; Waxler-Morrison et al. 2006). Clinicians should explore these issues sensitively and seek to understand the cultural context of such practices while also providing education about the risk of skin injuries (Ward, Azzopardi, and Morantz 2018).

Developmental Disabilities across Cultures

Developmental disabilities including intellectual disabilities, sensory impairments (i.e., hearing and vision), communication and language disabilities, and physical disabilities are common among Canadian-born and newcomer children, and are often a significant source of stress and focus for families. Different cultures often have different perspectives of disabilities, their causes, and the treatment of children with developmental disabilities (Baxter and Mahoney 2018). Clinicians may also encounter families with varying views of treatment and expectations for children with developmental or physical disabilities. Some families may be reluctant to disclose difficulties. Other families may arrive to Canada with expectations that their child's chronic or complex medical issues will be addressed fully or "cured" and may voice frustration in initially accepting more supportive modalities and services. Care providers can play a critical role in addressing these concerns and in navigating available supports.

RECOMMENDED INVESTIGATIONS IN REFUGEE HEALTH ASSESSMENTS

Age-appropriate screening for cervical, breast, and colon cancer is warranted among refugees. The CCIRH guidelines suggest screening low-risk immigrant and refugee patients for diabetes at 35 years of age, given evidence of higher prevalence of diabetes and earlier age of onset among certain ethnic groups (Pottie et al. 2011). Canadian Cardiovascular Society guidelines recommend lipid screening in men and women 40 years and over, but advise earlier screening among certain ethnic groups at higher risk, such as individuals of South Asian descent, and in the presence of other risk factors (Anderson et al. 2016).

Many refugees are exposed to an increased risk of other conditions and should undergo screening for the following tests (please refer to http://www.ccirhken.ca and CCIRH guidelines [Pottie et al. 2011] for further details):

- **Complete Blood Count (CBC)**—Testing will detect iron deficiency anemia (microcytic anemia), beta thalassemia trait, or other hemoglobinopathies (low

MCV), and eosinophilia (which is often due to a parasitic infection in this population). Note that some patients of African descent will have lower levels of neutrophil counts that are not pathological; an otherwise normal CBC and history and physical are reassuring (Haddy, Rana, and Castro 1999).

- **Hepatitis B**—Hepatitis B serology, including hepatitis B surface antigen (HBsAg), hepatitis B core antibody (HBcAb), and hepatitis B surface antibody (HBsAb), should be obtained for all refugees. A recent meta-analysis found a pooled seroprevalence of hepatitis B infection in approximately 9.6 percent among refugees, and 48.5 percent were found to be non-immune (Rossi et al. 2012). Identification of hepatitis B infection can lead to early treatment and monitoring, thereby preventing disease progression, and can also help to protect close contacts through targeted immunization. Patients who are found to be hepatitis B non-immune can be offered vaccination, although public coverage of hepatitis vaccines vary by region.

- **Hepatitis C**—Hepatitis C serology rates have been shown to be higher in the regions of North Africa/Middle East, Central and East Asia, and Eastern Europe (WHO 2014). Many refugees have been exposed to hepatitis C in the absence of traditional risk factors; thus, it is prudent to check serology even where there is no history of intravenous drug use, exposure to blood products, or known parental exposure. About 3 percent of immigrants are infected with chronic hepatitis C virus (HCV) (up to 18 percent in certain populations), most of whom will be asymptomatic but the majority of whom will be eligible for treatment (Pottie et al. 2011). Routine screening for HCV is now more important as effective treatments emerge. Treatment response rate is better in those who have not yet developed chronic liver disease.

- **Varicella**—Among immigrants from tropical countries, a large proportion of adolescents (up to 50 percent) and adults (up to 10 percent) are susceptible to varicella and are at increased risk of severe varicella (Pottie et al. 2011; Greenaway et al. 2014). Given the potential severity of varicella infection in adulthood, individuals over 13 years who are non-immune should be identified with screening serology and vaccinated appropriately. Universally immunizing children under 13 years of age may be more cost-effective than checking serology (Pottie et al. 2011).

- **Enteric Parasites**—Most intestinal parasites have a limited lifespan, are not a public health risk, and do not cause symptoms in adults. However, two of the more important exceptions are schistosomiasis and strongyloides, which can persist asymptomatically for years before causing serious health complications. In the context of immunosuppression, untreated strongyloides can result in life-threatening disseminated infection or hyperinfection syndrome. Chronic, untreated schistosomiasis can result in significant bladder or liver damage. Both parasites are difficult to detect in stool samples and thus serological testing is indicated instead. Treatment is straightforward with one to two days of antiparasitic medications (typically two days ivermectin for strongyloides and one day praziquantel for schistosomiasis), with relatively high treatment effectiveness and favourable side-effect profiles (Pottie at al. 2011). Strongyloides testing should be performed for all refugees from areas where poor sanitation is a risk, now mainly considered in Africa or East Asia. Schistosomiasis has a particular, though shifting, geographic distribution, and testing is only required for patients from endemic areas (including, at the time of writing, Africa, the Middle East, Brazil, Venezuela, the Caribbean, China, Indonesia, the Philippines, Cambodia, and Laos) (Pottie et al. 2011; Chitsulo et al. 2000). Focusing on these two specific parasites and forgoing traditional stool testing for asymptomatic patients marks a shift in practice.

- **HIV and Syphilis**—Although HIV and syphilis testing are performed in individuals 15 years and older through the immigration medical exam, it may be prudent to retest, particularly if previous screening is remote or if there is history of possible new exposures. Of note, the IME often involves a VDRL (Venereal Disease Reference Laboratory) or RPR (rapid plasma reagin) test for syphilis screening, though in Ontario a treponemal specific antibody test is generally used. Screening for other STIs, such as chlamydia and gonorrhea, may also be considered.

- **Latent Tuberculosis Infection (LTBI)**—All refugees up to the age of 50 from areas of high TB incidence should be screened for latent tuberculosis infection if they are capable of tolerating LTBI treatment (Pottie et al. 2011; Canadian Thoracic Society of the Canadian Lung Association and PHAC 2013). High rates of TB in regions such as sub-Saharan Africa and Asia (200 to 300 smear positive pulmonary TB cases per 100,000 population regionally, with much higher rates in some countries) confer increased risk of latent TB among newcomers from these areas (Pottie et al. 2011; WHO 2016). Risk factors for reactivation of TB include HIV, immunosuppressive therapy, hemodialysis, diabetes, and recent infection in the past two years, among others (Canadian Thoracic Society of the Canadian Lung Association and PHAC 2013). Children under five years of age are at greatest risk of TB, and exposed infants under one year are at much higher risk of developing disseminated (miliary) TB and TB meningitis (Canadian Thoracic Society of the Canadian Lung Association and PHAC 2013). Of note, risk of developing active tuberculosis is highest after the first year of arrival to a low-incidence region and is twofold higher among refugees compared to other immigrant populations (Pottie et al. 2011; Canadian Thoracic Society of the Canadian Lung Association and PHAC 2013).

    Screening for LTBI can be undertaken by tuberculin skin testing or by immunoglobulin release assay (IGRA), but note that neither should be used if there is suspicion of active tuberculosis disease in adults. Refugees older than 50 years of age may be screened for LTBI if they are at a higher risk of reactivation; however, consideration for benefits of treatment must be balanced with the higher risk of isoniazid-related hepatotoxicity in this older age group. The Online TST/IGRA Interpreter tool, Version 3.0 (http:// www.tstin3d.com), can be helpful in interpreting TB test results. Individuals with LTBI treatment with isoniazid (INH) or another approved regimen can be considered based on the risk of reactivation, after ruling out active TB by chest X-ray and clinical assessment. Active pulmonary tuberculosis constitutes a significant public health risk requiring urgent notification to public health authorities. Treatment of LTBI requires close follow-up, including regular monitoring for adherence, hepatotoxicity, and other side effects. Concomitant vitamin B6 (pyridoxine) supplementation is recommended for those at higher risk of pyridoxine deficiency or neuropathy.

APPROACHING MENTAL HEALTH CONCERNS AMONG REFUGEE PATIENTS

There is a considerable burden of mental health conditions in refugee populations, often as a consequence of individuals' exposure to significant trauma (Fazel, Wheeler, and Danesh 2015; Kirmayer et al. 2011). In particular, clinicians should be aware of relatively high rates of depression and post-traumatic stress disorder among refugee patients; often these present as co-morbid conditions (Kirmayer et al. 2011; Pottie et al. 2011). Nevertheless, despite the often immense trauma many refugees have endured, the majority do not suffer from severe mental health issues and can recover well with appropriate supports. Additionally, traversing the refugee determination process is, in itself, very stressful for many refugee claimants. In such cases, many symptoms resolve once the process is complete, even without treatment.

Early recognition and treatment of mental health symptoms may facilitate recovery and integration. However, detection of mental health issues may be complicated due to stigma, cultural variations in expression and manifestations of disease, and linguistic barriers (Kirmayer et al. 2011). Furthermore, mental health concerns may present in variable ways at different points in the migratory journey; for some, distress is most acute in the early stages of resettlement, while for others, it may not manifest for months or years. A strong therapeutic alliance between clinician and patient may help facilitate disclosure of mental health concerns. Clinicians should be attuned to the presence of somatic symptoms, such as changes in sleep, appetite, and energy. These symptoms may signal underlying mental health issues, particularly in children and youth. Clinicians should also be alert to the signs and symptoms of post-traumatic stress disorder in particular and provide support and referrals as needed.

Screening for depression is recommended only in the presence of integrated systems that can provide appropriate patient follow-up (Pottie et al. 2011). Specific screening for exposure to trauma is not advised, as it may cause more harm than benefit in well-functioning individuals (Pottie et al. 2011). Individuals with significant mental health concerns may benefit from referral to specialized psychiatric services, such as centres for victims of torture and trauma.

Intimate partner violence (IPV) is a significant issue worldwide, including in Canada. Current guidelines recommend against routine screening for IPV among immigrants and refugees, due to risk of harms that may outweigh benefits (Pottie et al. 2011). However, it is important for clinicians to be alert to signs and symptoms that may indicate IPV and to explore further based on concerns and/or patient disclosure (Pottie et al. 2011). Indications of abuse are highly variable among women, from symptoms of depression, to social withdrawal, to physical bruises and injuries. Language barriers, social isolation, precarious immigration status, financial dependency, lack of familiarity with local laws and supports, and fear of authorities can compound newcomer women's vulnerability to abuse and limit their comfort with disclosure. The clinician-patient relationship is thus paramount in detecting these signals, in helping women feel comfortable to disclose, and in connecting women to available supportive services.

IMMUNIZATION CONSIDERATIONS FOR REFUGEES

Most adult refugees do not have access to their immunization records and should therefore receive a full primary series of immunizations, guided by federal and provincial vaccination policies (PHAC 2018). Children and youth also require catch-up vaccinations according to their age, guided by the applicable vaccination policies. Hepatitis B and varicella serotesting may help guide immunizations for these two conditions, utilizing a more cost-effective approach (Pottie et al. 2011). Where immunization records are available and appear accurate, such records are considered acceptable, and duplicate vaccinations can be avoided.

DOCUMENTATION REQUESTS FOR REFUGEE HEARINGS

Some refugee claimants may request a letter of documentation of their medical health for their refugee hearing. Such letters can provide valuable support for a refugee claim. Letters can document any physical scars or mental health issues that may have resulted from refugees' pre-migration trauma. They also provide refugees an opportunity to comment on issues such as memory and concentration, which may affect a patient's ability to respond to questions at his or her refugee hearing. It is important that clinicians restrict such documentation to medical issues; the letter should refrain from commenting on the credibility of a refugee's story.

ADVOCACY FOR REFUGEE PATIENTS

Refugees face a multitude of ongoing stressors in the post-migratory resettlement process, including experiences of language barriers, financial strain, unemployment, loss of status, shifts in gender and family roles, and social isolation. Addressing these social concerns is crucial for advancing the health of newcomers, from access to safe housing to employment to family reunification. In the course of clinical care, clinicians can identify these needs and help connect refugees to appropriate social and community resources. Clinicians and providers have a recognized role as health advocates at the individual patient or family level, at a system or population level, and within wider policy decisions (MacDonald 2018).

Cultural Competence and Cultural Humility

To effectively provide care to the rich diversity of the communities we serve, health and service providers must be aware of and sensitive to differences between their own backgrounds and the backgrounds of their patients. Culturally competent care can help to improve health outcomes by navigating communication barriers and cultural differences (Britton and American Academy of Pediatrics 2004; Betancourt et al. 2005).

The LEARN model is one framework for approaching cultural competence (Berlin and Fowkes 1983):

- **L**isten with sympathy and understanding to the patient's perception of a problem
- **E**xplain your perceptions of a problem
- **A**cknowledge and discuss differences and similarities
- **R**ecommend treatment
- **N**egotiate agreement

Cultural humility goes beyond cultural competence, focusing on a lifelong reflective process of understanding one's own individual and systemic biases (both implicit and explicit) and managing power imbalances (Vo and Mayhew 2018). It involves humbly acknowledging our role as learners in seeking to understand the complexity of another's experience. Cultural humility requires ongoing honest self-awareness and critique to recognize our own culturally influenced beliefs, judgments, limitations, and gaps in knowledge. This concept emphasizes that health or service providers do not need to understand every cultural group's health beliefs or traditions, particularly given the vast heterogeneity *within* cultural and religious groups and the many other factors that may influence an individual or family's experience and interaction with the health care system (Vo and Mayhew 2018). Instead, we can respectfully seek to understand the unique perspectives, priorities, values, and experience of each individual and family.

Furthermore, it is important for providers working with refugee and other marginalized populations to embrace cultural safety in their practice, a crucial concept discussed elsewhere in this book (see Tomascik, Dignan, and Lavallée, Chapter 4, and Cooper et al., Chapter 28, in this volume). It was initially developed as a nursing practice in New Zealand in relation to health care for Maori people. It seeks to disrupt damaging power imbalances and emphasizes the importance of building respectful bicultural exchange, in which knowledge is *shared* (Brascoupé and Waters 2009).

At an individual patient or family level, clinicians may encounter many opportunities to assist individuals and families in navigating local health and social support systems, recognizing the many layers of social determinants of health. Awareness of local resources and networks is critical to effectively assist individuals in accessing community resources for education, employment, financial assistance, and recreation.

Addressing individual and family needs may lead to identification of broader issues within this population warranting systems-level advocacy. Some examples of systems advocacy might include working within a clinical practice or institution to implement cultural competency/humility training for staff members, facilitating access to trained interpreters and community resources, or compiling multilingual family health information.

Working at a policy level to effect change expands the reach of advocacy efforts. As an example, in response to government cuts to the IFHP (health coverage for refugees) in 2012, health care providers and allies led successful nationwide advocacy efforts leading to a reinstatement of the program (see, in this volume, Berger et al., Chapter 27, and Arya, Chapter 28).

Thoughtful advocacy efforts at individual or family, systemic, and policy levels are critical for optimizing the health of refugees, from improving access to quality health care to addressing upstream social determinants of health. Strategies often require long-term engagement, mobilization of broader networks of support, and creative adaptation to effect positive change.

Case Study Revisited

This 32-year-old woman originally from North Korea is introduced to the clinical practice, and urgent concerns, including headaches, are addressed during the initial visit using a trained interpreter. The clinician gently explores her medical and social history and performs a physical exam. Her gynecological exam is deferred to a subsequent appointment, but her contraceptive needs are attended to during the first visit. She is sent for screening blood tests, including CBC, hepatitis B and C serology, varicella serology, strongyloides serology, syphilis screening, and HIV testing. She is rebooked in two weeks to review results and to commence her immunization series, as well as to undergo latent TB testing.

After numerous months of visits, she shares that her husband and children were caught trying to escape North Korea and she has not heard from them since. She discloses symptoms of depression and begins counselling therapy. She also engages in English classes and starts to establish some social connections through her school. Her condition improves significantly after her claimant process is completed and she is accepted as a refugee in Canada.

CONCLUSION

Immigrants arriving in Canada through the refugee system often face different health risks than Canadian-born individuals. This chapter has highlighted some of the challenges and health care responses for providers working with refugees in Canada. Attending to these issues early in the migration trajectory facilitates refugees' integration into Canadian society and can prevent further health complications.

CRITICAL THINKING QUESTIONS

1. What barriers to accessing health care do refugees commonly encounter?
2. What challenges might refugees face during the short- and long-term resettlement process in Canada? How may post-migratory living conditions and social circumstances in Canada shape their health? In what ways might these challenges and circumstances be unique for children and youth?
3. Building on the examples outlined in the text and reflecting on the challenges outlined above, what are other opportunities for advocacy efforts at the individual, systems, and public policy levels to promote enhanced well-being among refugees?
4. How can care providers sensitively address patients' different explanatory models of disease and illness beliefs?

ADDITIONAL RESOURCES

The Canadian Collaboration for Immigrant and Refugee Care website has links to key clinical guidelines, clinical guideline checklists, e-learning modules, and other resources: http://www.ccirhken.ca.

The 2011 Canadian Collaboration for Immigrant and Refugee Health (CCIRH)'s "Evidence-Based Clinical Guidelines for Immigrants and Refugees," published in the *Canadian Medical Association Journal (CMAJ)*, provides an evidence-based, practical approach to the care of newcomers: http://www.cmaj.ca/content/183/12/E824.

For further information regarding caring for newcomer child and youth populations, visit Canadian Pediatric Society's Caring for Kids New to Canada website: http://www.kidsnewtocanada.ca.

The Refugee Mental Health Project, through the Centre for Addiction and Mental Health and Portico Network, offers online courses, webinars, communities of practice, and other resources related to refugee mental health, with a focus on intersectoral and interprofessional collaboration: http://www.porticonetwork.ca/web/rmhp.

ACKNOWLEDGEMENTS

We would like to acknowledge the 87 authors of the Canadian Immigrant Health Guidelines for their contributions to the "Evidence-Based Guidelines on Immigrant and Refugee Health" (Pottie et al. 2011), as well as the wide team of authors, editors, and reviewers of the Canadian Pediatric Society's Caring for Kids New to Canada website.

REFERENCES

Anderson, Todd J., Jean Grégoire, Glen J. Pearson, Arden R. Barry, Patrick Couture, Martin Dawes, Gordon A. Francis, et al. 2016. "2016 Canadian Cardiovascular Society Guidelines for the Management of Dyslipidemia for the Prevention of Cardiovascular Disease in the Adult." *Canadian Journal of Cardiology* 32 (11): 1263–82.

Attanayake, Vindya, Rachel McKay, Michel Joffres, Sonal Singh, Frederick Burkle Jr., and Edward Mills. 2009. "Prevalence of Mental Disorders among Children Exposed to War: A Systematic Review of 7,920 Children." *Medicine Conflict and Survival* 25 (1): 4–19.

Baxter, Cecilia, and William Mahoney. 2018. "Development Disability across Cultures." Caring for Kids New to Canada, Canadian Pediatric Society. Last updated March. http://www.kidsnewtocanada.ca/mental-health/developmental-disability.

Beach, Mary Catherine, Tiffany L. Gary, Eboni G. Price, Karen Robinson, Aysegul Gozu, Ana Palacio, Carole Smarth, et al. 2006. "Improving Health Care Quality for Racial/Ethnic Minorities: A Systematic Review of the Best Evidence Regarding Provider and Organization Interventions." *BMC Public Health* 6 (1): 104.

Benson, Jill, and Jan Williams. 2008. "Age Determination in Refugee Children." *Australian Family Physician* 37 (10): 821–5.

Berlin, Elois Ann, and William C. Fowkes. 1983. "A Teaching Framework for Cross-cultural Health Care—Application in Family Practice." *Western Journal of Medicine* 139 (6): 934–38.

Betancourt, Joseph R., Alexander R. Green, J. Emilio Carrillo, and Elyse R. Park. 2005. "Cultural Competence and Health Care Disparities: Key Perspectives and Trends." *Health Affairs* 24 (2): 499–505.

Brascoupé, Simon, and Catherine Waters. 2009. "Cultural Safety: Exploring the Applicability of the Concept of Cultural Safety to Aboriginal Health and Community Wellness." *Journal of Aboriginal Health* 5 (2): 6–41.

Britton, Carmelita V., and American Academy of Pediatrics, Committee on Pediatric Workforce. 2004. "Ensuring Culturally Effective Pediatric Care: Implications for Education and Health Policy." *Pediatrics* 114 (6): 1677–85.

Bronstein, Israel, and Paul Montgomery. 2011. "Psychological Distress in Refugee Children: A Systematic Review." *Clinical Child and Family Psychology Review* 14 (1): 44–56.

Canadian Thoracic Society of the Canadian Lung Association and Public Health Agency of Canada (PHAC). 2013. "Canadian Tuberculosis Standards, 7th Edition." *Canadian Journal of Respirology* 20 (suppl A): 23A–53A.

Centers for Disease Control and Prevention. 2014. "Guidelines for the U.S. Domestic Medical Examination for Newly Arriving Refugees." Last updated February 6. http://www.cdc.gov/immigrantrefugeehealth/guidelines/domestic/domestic-guidelines.html.

Chitsulo, Lester, Dirk Engels, Antonio Montresor, and Lorenzo Savioli. 2000. "The Global Status of Schistosomiasis and Its Control." *Acta Tropica* 77: 41–51.

Crockett, Maryanne. 2005. "New Faces from Faraway Places: Immigrant Child Health in Canada." *Pediatrics & Child Health* 10 (5): 277–81.

Dookeran, Nameeta M., Tracy Battaglia, Jennifer Cochran, and Paul L. Geltman. 2010. "Chronic Disease and Its Risk Factors among Refugees and Asylees in Massachusetts, 2001–2005." *Preventing Chronic Disease* 7 (3): 1–8.

Fazel, Mina, Jeremy Wheeler, and John Danesh. 2015. "Prevalence of Serious Mental Disorder in 7000 Refugees Resettled in Western Countries: A Systematic Review." *Lancet* 365 (9467): 1309–14. https://doi.org/10.1016/S0140-6736(05)61027-6.

Galanti, Geri-Ann. 2008. *Caring for Patients from Different Cultures*. 4th ed. Philadelphia: University of Pennsylvania Press.

Greenaway, Chris, Jean-François Boivin, Sonya Cnossen, Carmine Rossi, Bruce Tapiero, Kevin Schwartzman, Sherry Olson, and Mark Miller. 2014. "Risk Factors for Susceptibility to Varicella in Newly Arrived Adult Migrants in Canada." *Epidemiology and Infection* 142 (8): 1695–707. https://doi.org/10.1017/S0950268813002768.

Guendelman Sylvia, Helen Halpin Schauffler, and Michelle Pearl. 2001. "Unfriendly Shores: How Immigrant Children Fare in the U.S. Health System." *Health Affairs* 20: 257–66. https://doi.org/10.1377/hlthaff.20.1.257.

Gushulak, Brian D., Kevin Pottie, Janet Hatcher Roberts, Sara Torres, and Marie DesMeules. 2011. "Migration and Health in Canada: Health in the Global Village." *Canadian Medical Association Journal* 183 (12): E952–58. https://doi.org/10.1503/cmaj.090287.

Haddy, Theresa B., Sohail R. Rana, and Oswaldo Castro. 1999. "Benign Ethnic Neutropenia: What Is a Normal Absolute Neutrophil Count?" *Journal of Laboratory and Clinical Medicine* 133 (1): 15–22.

Hamamy, Hanan, Stylianos E. Antonarakis, Luigi Luca Cavalli-Sforza, Samia Temtamy, Giovanni Romeo, Leo P. Ten Kate, Robin L. Bennett, et al. 2011. "Consanguineous Marriages, Pearls and Perils: Geneva International Consanguinity Workshop Report." *Genetics in Medicine* 13 (9): 841–7.

Hilliard, Robert, ed. 2018a. "Medical Assessment of Immigrant and Refugee Children." Caring for Kids New to Canada. Last updated March. http://www.kidsnewtocanada.ca/care/assessment.

Hilliard, Robert, ed. 2018b. "Using Interpreters in the Health Care Setting." Caring for Kids New to Canada. Last updated March. http://www.kidsnewtocanada.ca/care/interpreters.

Immigration, Refugees, and Citizenship Canada (IRCC). 2013. "Chapter 4: Immigration Medical Examination, Panel Members' Handbook 2013." In *Panel Members' Handbook 2013*. Ottawa: IRCC. Last updated February 29, 2016. http://www.cic.gc.ca/english/resources/publications/dmp-handbook/index.asp#chap4.

Immigration, Refugees, and Citizenship Canada (IRCC). 2018. "Interim Federal Health Program: Summary of Benefits." Last updated March 23. http://www.cic.gc.ca/english/refugees/outside/summary-ifhp.asp.

International Organization for Migration (IOM). 2008. *The World Migration Report 2008: Managing Labour Mobility in the Evolving Global Economy.* Geneva: IOM. https://publications.iom.int/system/files/pdf/wmr_1.pdf.

Kirmayer, Laurence J., Lavanya Narasiah, Marie Munoz, Meb Rashid, Andrew G. Ryder, Jaswant Guzder, Ghayda Hassan, Cécile Rousseau, and Kevin Pottie. 2011. "Common Mental Health Problems in Immigrants and Refugees: General Approach in Primary Care." *Canadian Medical Association Journal* 183 (12): E959-67.

MacDonald, Noni, ed. 2018. "Advocacy for Immigrant and Refugee Health Needs." Caring for Kids New to Canada. Last updated March 2018. http://www.kidsnewtocanada.ca/beyond/advocacy.

Mason, John B., Jessica M. White, Linda Heron, Jennifer Carter, Caroline Wilkinson, and Paul Spiegel. 2012. "Child Acute Malnutrition and Mortality in Populations Affected by Displacement in the Horn of Africa, 1997-2009." *International Journal of Environmental Research and Public Health* 9 (3): 791-806.

McDonald, James Ted, and Steven Kennedy. 2005. "Is Migration to Canada Associated with Unhealthy Weight Gain? Overweight and Obesity among Canada's Immigrants." *Social Science and Medicine* 61 (12): 2469-81. https://doi.org/10.1016/j.socscimed.2005.05.004.

McKeary, Marie, and Bruce Newbold. 2010. "Barriers to Care: The Challenges for Canadian Refugees and Their Health Care Providers." *Journal of Refugee Studies* 23 (4): 523-45. https://doi.org/10.1093/jrs/feq038.

Minister for Immigration, Refugees, and Citizenship Canada. 2016. *Annual Report to Parliament on Immigration, 2016.* Ottawa: Government of Canada. Last updated October 31. https://www.canada.ca/en/immigration-refugees-citizenship/corporate/publications-manuals/annual-report-parliament-immigration-2016.html.

Murray, Ronan, David Burgner, Vicki Krause, Beverley-ann Biggs, and Jill Benson. 2009. *Diagnosis, Management and Prevention of Infections in Recently Arrived Refugees.* Surry Hills, Australia: Australasian Society for Infectious Disease. https://www.asid.net.au/documents/item/134.

Ng, Edward, Kevin Pottie, and Denise Spitzer. 2011. "Official Language Proficiency and Self-Reported Health among Immigrants to Canada" *Health Reports* 22 (4): 15-23.

O'Neill, Jennifer, Hilary Tabish, Vivian Welch, Mark Petticrew, Kevin Pottie, Mike Clarke, Tim Evans, et al. 2014. "Applying an Equity Lens to Interventions: Using PROGRESS Ensures Consideration of Socially Stratifying Factors to Illuminate Inequities in Health." *Journal of Clinical Epidemiology* 67 (1): 56-64.

Ornstein, Michael. 2000. *Ethnoracial Inequality in Toronto: Analysis of the 1996 Census. Metropolis Canada (CERIS).* Report prepared for the City of Toronto, Access and Equity Unit, Strategic and Corporate Policy Division, Chief Administrator's Office. https://povertyandhumanrights.org/docs/ornstein_fullreport.pdf.

Park, Hyun, Denise Bothe, Eva Holsinger, H. Lester Kirchner, Karen Olness, and Anna Mandalakas. 2011. "The Impact of Nutritional Status and Longitudinal Recovery of Motor and Cognitive Milestones in Internationally Adopted Children." *International Journal of Environmental Research and Public Health* 8 (1): 105–16.

Pottie, Kevin, Christina Greenaway, John Feigthner, Vivian Welch, Helena Swinkels, Meb Rashid, Lavanya Narasiah, et al. 2011. "Evidence-Based Clinical Guidelines for Immigrants and Refugees." *Canadian Medical Association Journal* 183 (12): E824–925. https://doi.org/10.1503/cmaj.090313.

Pottie, Kevin, Christina Greenaway, Ghayda Hassan, Charles Hui, and Laurence J. Kirmayer. 2015. "Caring for a Newly Arrived Syrian Refugee Family." *Canadian Medical Association Journal* 188 (3): 207–11.

Public Health Agency of Canada (PHAC). 2018. "Provincial and Territorial Immunization Information." Last updated January 19. http://www.phac-aspc.gc.ca/im/is-vc-eng.php.

Rossi, Carmine, Ian Shrier, Lee Marshall, Sonya Cnossen, Kevin Schwartzman, Marina B. Klein, Guido Schwarzer, and Chris Greenaway. 2012. "Seroprevalence of Chronic Hepatitis B Virus Infection and Prior Immunity in Immigrants and Refugees: A Systematic Review and Meta-analysis." *PLoS One* 7 (9): e44611. https://doi.org/10.1371/journal.pone.0044611.

Rutherford, John D. 2013. "Digital Clubbing." *Circulation* 127: 1997–99. https://doi.org/10.1161/CIRCULATIONAHA.112.000163.

Sanmartin, Claudia, and Nancy Ross. 2006. "Experiencing Difficulties Accessing First-Contact Health Services in Canada." *Health Policy* 1: 103–19.

Schulpen, Tom W. J. 1996. "Migration and Child Health: The Dutch Experience." *European Journal of Pediatrics* 155: 351–6.

Swinkels, Helena, Kevin Pottie, Peter Tugwell, Meb Rashid, and Lavanya Narasiah. 2011. "Development of Guidelines for Recently Arrived Immigrants and Refugees to Canada: Delphi Consensus on Selecting Preventable and Treatable Conditions." *Canadian Medical Association Journal* 183 (12): E928–32.

Tadmouri, Ghazi O., Pratibha Nair, Tasneem Obeid, Mahmoud T. Al Ali, Najib Al Khaja, and Hanan A. Hamamy. 2009. "Consanguinity and Reproductive Health among Arabs." *Reproductive Health* 6 (1): 17.

United Nations High Commissioner on Refugees (UNHCR). 2011. *Refocusing Family Planning in Refugee Settings: Findings and Recommendations from a Multi-country Baseline Study*. Geneva: UNHCR. http://www.unhcr.org/4ee6142a9.pdf.

United Nations High Commissioner for Refugees (UNHCR). 2015. *Global Report 2014*. Geneva: UNHCR. http://www.unhcr.org/gr14/index.xml.

Vo, Dzung, and Maureen Mayhew, eds. 2018. "Cultural Competence for Child and Youth Health Professionals." Caring for Kids New to Canada. Last updated March. http://www.kidsnewtocanada.ca/culture/competence.

Ward, Michelle, Corry Azzopardi, and Gillian Morantz, eds. 2018. "A Mindful Approach: Assessing Child Maltreatment in a Multicultural Setting." Caring for Kids New to Canada. Last updated April. http://www.kidsnewtocanada.ca/screening/maltreatment.

Waxler-Morrison, Nancy, Joan M. Anderson, Elizabeth Richardson, and Natalie A. Chambers, eds. 2006. *Cross-Cultural Caring: A Handbook for Health Professionals*. 2nd ed. Vancouver: UBC Press.

Wiedmeyer, Mei-ling, Aisha Lofters, and Meb Rashid. 2012. "Cervical Cancer Screening among Vulnerable Women." *Canadian Family Physician* 58: e521–6.

World Health Organization (WHO). 2014. *Guidelines for the Screening, Care and Treatment of Persons with Hepatitis C Infection*. Geneva: WHO. http://www.who.int/hiv/pub/hepatitis/hepatitis-c-guidelines/en/.

World Health Organization (WHO). 2016. *Global Tuberculosis Report 2016*. Geneva: WHO. http://www.who.int/tb/publications/global_report/en/.

CHAPTER 18

Mental Health Impact of Canadian Immigration Detention

Hanna Gros

LEARNING OBJECTIVES

After reading this chapter, you should be able to:

1. Explain some of the systemic challenges facing immigration detainees in Canada.
2. Consider what makes the immigration detention system particularly harmful to those who experience it.
3. Explore ways that health care professionals can help immigration detainees and impact advocacy in immigration detention.

BACKGROUND

Every year, thousands of migrants[1] are held in immigration detention in Canada (CBSA 2017). Between 2011 and 2016, nearly 40,000 migrants were detained in Canada (CBSA 2017). These individuals include some of the most vulnerable migrants: asylum seekers, individuals with mental health issues, torture survivors, pregnant women, and even children. When children are not placed under formal detention orders, they may be "housed" in detention in order to avoid separating them from their detained parents, or they may be separated from their parents and placed with child protective services. While immigration detainees are generally held in medium-security immigration holding centres, approximately a third are held in maximum-security wings of provincial jails (CBSA 2017). However, the majority of long-term detentions occur in maximum-security provincial jails—of the total number of days spent in detention across the country, two thirds are spent in jails (Kennedy 2017). As a result, although they are not serving criminal sentences, immigration detainees are often treated the same way as those detained under the criminal

> ### Personal Story: Uday
>
> By the time we met Uday,* he had been suffering from schizophrenia for over a decade. He had been managing his mental health long before he arrived in Canada in November 2011. Upon Uday's arrival at the Canadian border, Canada Border Services Agency (CBSA) officers detained him because they could not obtain proof of his identity or nationality and believed him to be a flight risk. Despite his persistent requests to access his medication from his suitcase after a long flight from Europe, CBSA officers insisted that he complete his interview.
>
> Shortly after, Uday had what he believed to be a seizure and was taken to hospital, and was then transferred directly to the Toronto Immigration Holding Centre. During a subsequent interview with CBSA, where Uday made his claim for asylum protection, he became agitated and caused some property damage. He was again taken to hospital and later transferred directly to a maximum-security jail. "I broke the phone and computer and then [they] put me in jail," he recalled. Although he had no criminal record and was not held on criminal charges, Uday continued to be detained in maximum-security jails for nearly three years until CBSA finally acknowledged that he was de facto stateless and allowed for his release.
>
> While in jail, Uday was provided with medication but received minimal individualized psychiatric attention. He told me that he would meet with a doctor for appointments that generally lasted only a few minutes. Uday's counsel confirmed that "his mental health condition played a large role in his inability to confirm his identity." Uday's counsel also noted that, despite the limited psychiatric care that Uday was receiving in jail, his mental health issues "posed a large barrier to securing his release due to concerns about his access to treatment [outside of detention]."
>
> As Uday recounted his experience in jail, he told us, "They treat[ed] us like garbage.... We had no rights at all."
>
> ---
>
> *Name has been changed in order to protect the individual's identity.

justice system. This not only has devastating effects on immigration detainees' mental health but also carries significant systemic disadvantages for those with pre-existing mental health issues.

Pursuant to Canada's Immigration and Refugee Protection Act, non-citizens may be detained for four main reasons: (1) if they are considered to be a flight risk, (2) if they are considered inadmissible and a danger to the public, (3) if their identity is not established, and/or (4) in order to complete an examination of their case (Immigration and Refugee Protection Act [IRPA] 2001). CBSA officers have the authority to detain non-citizens with the discretion to release them within 48 hours. Following the initial 48 hours, immigration detainees are subjected to a system of detention review hearings presided over by the Immigration Division of the Immigration and Refugee Board. Immigration Division adjudicators determine whether detention continues at the 48 hour mark, 7 days later, and subsequently every 30 days until release (IRPA 2001, s. 57).

Given that deprivation of liberty is among the most invasive acts that a state could impose on an individual, this deprivation must be justified within a robust justice system. Although the regularly scheduled detention review hearings are designed to ensure that detention continues to be justified, several flaws in this system may result in arbitrary and indefinite detention. First, Immigration Division adjudicators are not bound by any legal or technical rules of evidence and may rely on evidence that they consider credible or trustworthy in the circumstances (IRPA 2001, s. 173). This evidentiary standard pales in comparison to that required under the criminal justice system, although, as noted above, immigration detainees may experience the same deprivation of liberty as those on criminal hold. Second, despite the severe consequences that may result from detention review hearings, immigration detainees often do not have legal representation at these proceedings. Third, Immigration Division adjudicators may decide to continue detention if they are satisfied that it is warranted on a balance of probabilities (*Canada [Minister of Citizenship and Immigration] v. Thanabalasingham* 2004 [*Thanabalasingham*]). Again, this is in contrast to the criminal justice system, where deprivation of liberty requires proof of guilt beyond a reasonable doubt, which is a much higher standard. Fourth, before Immigration Division adjudicators may order release from detention, they must provide "clear and compelling reasons" to depart from previous decisions to continue detention (*Thanabalasingham* 2004). For this reason, in practice, the default decision is to continue detention, and immigration detainees are faced with the burden to prove that detention is no longer warranted. Finally, perhaps the most harmful aspect of the immigration detention system is that there is no legislatively prescribed limit to the length of time immigration detainees may be held, and detention may go on for months and even years with no end in sight.

The Canadian immigration detention system is in violation of international human rights law. In particular, the legal framework and policies that govern immigration detention may result in instances of arbitrary detention; cruel, inhuman, and degrading treatment; discrimination on the basis of disability; violations of the right to health; and violations of the right to an effective remedy. These human rights violations manifest in disturbing and profoundly detrimental consequences for immigration detainees' well-being and mental health. This is clearly reflected in the lived experiences of immigration detainees, who express overwhelming despair, anxiety, and helplessness because of their detention (Gros and van Groll 2015).

CONSEQUENCES FOR IMMIGRATION DETAINEES' MENTAL HEALTH

Immigration detention has a severe negative impact on mental health, whether or not detainees have pre-existing mental health issues. As one refugee lawyer has indicated, deterioration of mental health is "one of the most significant observable phenomena in immigration detention" (Gros and van Groll 2015, 26).

Mental health experts in Canada and around the world have consistently reported on the severely debilitating effects of immigration detention on mental health. In 2013, Janet Cleveland, a psychologist and legal scholar, conducted a study that demonstrated astounding differences in mental health between detainees who had been held for an average of 31 days and non-detainees (Cleveland and Rousseau 2013, 409). The study found the following: nearly a third of the detainees in the study had clinical post-traumatic stress disorder (PTSD) (twice as many as non-detainees); over three quarters of the detainees (and 52 percent of non-detainees) were clinically depressed; and nearly two thirds of the detainees were clinically anxious (compared to 47 percent of non-detainees) (414). Detainees in the same study reported several detention-related experiences that were highly correlated with anxiety, depression, and PTSD: powerlessness, concern about family back home, nothing to do except think about problems, uncertainty as to length of detention, loneliness, fear of being sent back home, boredom, and the sense that detention is unfair (414). Similar alarming patterns of mental health deterioration have been observed in the United Kingdom (Robjant, Robbins, and Senior 2009), the United States (Keller et al. 2003), and Australia (Joint Select Committee on Australia's Immigration Detention Network 2012, chap. 5).

Several international bodies have also highlighted the effects of immigration detention on mental health. The 2011 Global Roundtable on Alternatives to Detention of Asylum Seekers, Refugees, Migrants and Stateless Persons concluded that immigration detention causes "psychological illness, trauma, depression, anxiety, aggression, and other physical, emotional and psychological consequences" (UNHCR and OHCHR 2011, para. 10). In a 2012 report, the Special Rapporteur on the Human Rights of Migrants Francois Crépeau noted that immigration detention "systematically deteriorates the physical and mental condition of nearly everyone who experiences it" (United Nations General Assembly 2012, para. 48).

SYSTEMIC DISADVANTAGES FOR IMMIGRATION DETAINEES WITH PRE-EXISTING MENTAL HEALTH ISSUES

While immigration detention should be considered as a last resort, vulnerable persons with mental health issues are routinely and even presumptively held in maximum-security provincial jails (as opposed to medium-security immigration holding centres). CBSA (2017) justifies this practice on the basis that provincial correctional facilities provide "access to specialized care." Unfortunately, mental health care in provincial jails is alarmingly inadequate. Research indicates that while individuals suffering from schizophrenia or bipolar disorder are generally provided with medication, those with depression, PTSD, or anxiety disorders are often left untreated and unaddressed (Gros and van Groll 2015, 76). Psychiatric treatment beyond medication is lacking across the board.

Mental health issues may also pose a major impediment to securing release from detention. CBSA and the Immigration Division often requires immigration detainees to prove that they could access medication outside of jail in order to secure release from detention. However, this is particularly difficult for certain categories of non-citizens who may only receive health care coverage for conditions deemed to pose a danger to others (Gros and van Groll 2015, 76).

WHAT CAN HEALTH CARE PROVIDERS DO?

The immigration detention system clearly requires significant legislative and policy changes. However, health care providers are uniquely positioned to support immigration detainees, particularly by providing pro bono mental health assessments for immigration detainees held in provincial jails. Lawyers often rely on external psychiatrists to conduct mental health assessments of immigration detainees in order to establish the impact of detention on their clients' mental health, or to demonstrate that removal to the detainee's country of origin is inappropriate. Unfortunately, these assessments are incredibly costly and often require travel to distant jails.

Pro bono mental health treatments are also vital for individuals who are released from immigration detention. Health care providers may contribute to existing initiatives, such as the Canadian Centre for Refugee and Immigrant Health Care (http://www.ccrihc.ca), which provides medical treatment and assistance to uninsured newcomers to Canada.

Finally, health care providers may influence the situation of immigration detainees through advocacy. In particular, health care providers may draw on the extensive literature documenting the impact of social determinants on mental health to advocate for substituting incarceration with community-based care and programs. Equipped with scientific evidence and the stories of their patients, health care providers are uniquely situated to illustrate the negative repercussions of human rights violations, and to do so in a persuasive manner. This means that health care providers engaged in advocacy can help foster empathy and compassion towards those individuals who may otherwise be deemed simply as "foreign others."

CRITICAL THINKING QUESTIONS

1. Consider the severe mental health impact of immigration detention. Under what circumstances (if any) would the state be justified in depriving individuals' liberty and why?
2. Is the state justified in using certain measures against non-citizens that are illegal to apply against citizens? If yes, why? What are the limits to the state's power to use these measures?
3. What role can social science evidence play in policy debates about immigration detention? And why is social science evidence particularly compelling in these debates?

4. What role can immigration detainees' lived experiences play in policy debates about immigration detention? Why is this evidence particularly compelling in these debates?

ADDITIONAL RESOURCES

Gros, Hanna. 2017. *Invisible Citizens: Canadian Children in Immigration Detention*. Toronto: International Human Rights Program, University of Toronto Faculty of Law. http://ihrp.law.utoronto.ca/utfl_file/count/PUBLICATIONS/Report-InvisibleCitizens.pdf.

Gros, Hanna, and Yolanda Song. 2016. *"No Life for a Child": A Roadmap to End Immigration Detention of Children and Family Separation*. Toronto: International Human Rights Program, University of Toronto Faculty of Law. http://ihrp.law.utoronto.ca/utfl_file/count/PUBLICATIONS/Report-NoLifeForAChild.pdf.

Gros, Hanna, and Paloma van Groll. 2015. *"We Have No Rights": Arbitrary Imprisonment and Cruel Treatment of Migrants with Mental Health Issues in Canada*. Toronto: International Human Rights Program, University of Toronto Faculty of Law. http://ihrp.law.utoronto.ca/utfl_file/count/PUBLICATIONS/IHRP%20We%20Have%20No%20Rights%20Report%20web%20170615.pdf.

NOTE

1. The term *migrant* refers to non-citizens including foreign nationals, refugee claimants, failed refugee claimants, permanent residents who are in the process of being stripped of their permanent resident status, and former permanent residents.

REFERENCES

Canada Border Services Agency (CBSA). 2017. "Arrests, Detentions and Removals." Last modified November 6. https://www.cbsa-asfc.gc.ca/security-securite/arr-det-eng.html.

Canada (Minister of Citizenship and Immigration) v. Thanabalasingham, [2004] 3 FCR 572, 2004 FCA 4 (CanLII). http://canlii.ca/t/1g6nr.

Cleveland, Janet, and Cecil Rousseau. 2013. "Psychiatric Symptoms Associated with Brief Detention of Adult Asylum Seekers in Canada." *Canadian Journal of Psychiatry* 58 (7): 409–16. https://doi.org/10.1177/070674371305800706.

Gros, Hanna, and Paloma van Groll. 2015. *"We Have No Rights": Arbitrary Imprisonment and Cruel Treatment of Migrants with Mental Health Issues in Canada*. Toronto: International Human Rights Program, University of Toronto Faculty of Law. http://ihrp.law.utoronto.ca/utfl_file/count/PUBLICATIONS/IHRP%20We%20Have%20No%20Rights%20Report%20web%20170615.pdf.

Immigration and Refugee Protection Act, SC 2001, c. 27.

Joint Select Committee on Australia's Immigration Detention Network. 2012. *Final Report*. Canberra, Australia: Joint Select Committee on Australia's Immigration Detention Network. https://www.aph.gov.au/Parliamentary_Business/Committees/Joint/Former_Committees/immigrationdetention/report/index.

Keller, A., B. Rosenfeld, C. Trinh-Shervin, Chris Meserve, Emily Sachs, Jonathan A. Leviss, Elizabeth Singer, et al. 2003. "Mental Health of Detained Asylum Seekers." *Lancet* 362 (9397): 1721–3. https://doi.org/10.1016/S0140-6736(03)14846-5.

Kennedy, Brendan. 2017. "Canada's Immigration Detainees Being Locked Up Based on Dodgy Risk Assessments, Star Finds." *Toronto Star*, April 12. https://www.thestar.com/news/investigations/2017/04/12/canadas-immigration-detainees-being-locked-up-based-on-dodgy-risk-assessments-star-finds.html.

Robjant, K., I. Robbins, and V. Senior. 2009. "Psychological Distress amongst Immigration Detainees: A Cross-Sectional Questionnaire Study." *British Journal of Clinical Psychology* 48 (3): 275–86. https://doi.org/10.1348/014466508X397007.

United Nations General Assembly (UNGA). 2012. "Report of the Special Rapporteur on the Human Rights of Migrants, Francois Crépeau." UNGA, 20th Session, A/HRC/20/24.

United Nations High Commissioner for Refugees (UNHCR) and Office of the United Nations High Commissioner for Human Rights (OHCHR). 2011. "Global Roundtable on Alternatives to Detention of Asylum-Seekers, Refugees, Migrants and Stateless Persons: Summary Conclusions." Geneva, Switzerland, May 11–12. http://www.unhcr.org/refworld/docid/4e315b882.html.

CHAPTER 19

Migrant Farm Worker Health Care: Unique Strategies for a Unique Population

Janet McLaughlin and Michelle Tew

LEARNING OBJECTIVES

After reading this chapter, you should be able to:

1. Assess the key health issues facing migrant agricultural workers.
2. Explain the health care access barriers experienced by migrant workers.
3. Analyze ways that health practitioners can provide more accessible and effective care to migrant agricultural workers.
4. Consider why migrant agricultural workers may be particularly vulnerable to health concerns and what can be done to mitigate the root cause(s) of these issues.

Over the past decades, the presence of temporary foreign workers, or migrant workers, has expanded rapidly throughout the Canadian economy. In 2006, the number of temporary foreign workers exceeded the number of economic immigrants given permanent residence status for the first time (Faraday 2012). As of 2015, there were 154,859 work permit holders under the Temporary Foreign Worker Program (TFWP), with 46,827 of these in agriculture and 20,466 in caregiving (Government of Canada 2015). Migrant workers are employed in a wide range of sectors across the economy, ranging from fast food and domestic work to engineering. Provinces employing the highest number of these workers include (in order of numbers), Ontario, British Columbia, Alberta, and Quebec. Top source countries include the Philippines, Mexico, United States, India, Jamaica, and Guatemala (Curry 2014). Concerns have been raised over migrant workers' vulnerability to abuse, their sometimes high debts to recruiters, and poor monitoring and enforcement of their rights (Faraday 2012). Very little attention has been paid to their health needs.

This chapter discusses the health needs and care access issues of one of the longest-standing and most vulnerable groups of these migrant workers: those in agriculture. Despite these migrants having lived and worked in Canada for half a century with a variety of complex health risks, needs, and service access issues, only in the last few years have a few limited initiatives emerged that have focused on these workers' health and well-being. After describing the migrant agricultural worker population and their health risks and issues, this chapter will discuss some of the recent initiatives that have been piloted in Southern Ontario and make suggestions for how they can be replicated in other regions. Our findings, observations, and recommendations are based upon over a decade of work with this population, including quantitative and qualitative research studies and our roles in founding and participating in various migrant health educational and clinical initiatives.

Migrant agricultural workers have been coming to Canada since 1966 as part of the Seasonal Agricultural Worker Program (SAWP), a federal government initiative based on bilateral contracts with Mexico and Commonwealth Caribbean countries. Under the SAWP, workers enter Canada for seasonal contracts for up to eight months per year, often returning for successive years or even decades upon the invitation of employers. Since 2002, when the federal government expanded the TFWP across various sectors, agricultural workers have also been entering Canada through various newly introduced program streams, including a specific "agriculture stream" implemented in 2011. These streams

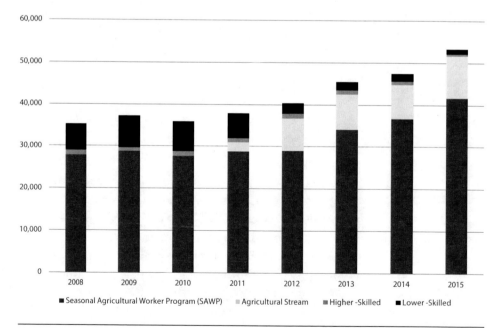

Figure 19.1: Temporary Foreign Worker Positions Approved across Various Program Streams, 2008–2015

Source: Employment and Social Development Canada (2016).

allow for the employment of workers from any country for up to 48 months at a time. As seen in figure 19.1, there were over 50,000 temporary agricultural worker positions approved in Canada as of 2015, with over 40,000 through the SAWP and the remainder through other TFWP streams (ESDC 2016).

While the majority of agricultural workers continue to come from Mexico and English-speaking Caribbean countries through SAWP, diverse states such as Thailand, the Philippines, and Guatemala are increasingly sending agricultural workers through the stream for low-wage positions (formerly known as the lower-skilled stream) and agricultural stream. Traditionally, SAWP workers were concentrated in Southern Ontario and Quebec; in recent years, their concentration has expanded from coast to coast, with employment in nearly every province. Employers determine both the gender and national origin of their labour force compositions. While preferences for nationalities have shifted over time, nearly all workers selected (97 percent) continue to be men, with women pegged for specific gendered tasks such as flower picking and peach packing.

Recent research has identified that these workers face particular risks related to the temporary nature of their employment; these include difficult and crowded living conditions, demanding and sometimes dangerous working conditions, and prolonged and repeated separations from families (Hennebry, McLaughlin, and Preibisch 2016; McLaughlin, Hennebry, and Haines 2014; McLaughlin et al. 2017). Additional social determinants of health issues—such as low income, education, and social status; poor literacy and/or lack of knowledge of the dominant language in the areas in which individuals live and work; lack of social support and integration in Canadian communities; visible minority status; and lack of citizenship rights—compound these risks (McLaughlin 2009). The minority of women migrant workers face distinct health issues and vulnerabilities (Edmunds et al. 2011).

Further, agriculture is already an industry in which labour rights are restricted. In Ontario, where the majority of migrants are employed, agricultural workers are excluded from the Labour Relations Act (and therefore denied collective bargaining rights) as well as some components of the Employment Standards Act (McLaughlin, Hennebry, and Haines 2014). Contracts in which workers' rights to both work and reside in Canada are bound to their employers place workers in an extremely precarious position. They fear that complaining about negative conditions, or even becoming ill or injured, could compromise their current or future abilities to work in Canada, upon which they rely for needed income for their families (Basok 2002; McLaughlin and Hennebry 2013; Wells et al. 2014).

In this context, workers experience a variety of health issues, many of which relate to occupational health. They also may have existing health issues such as diabetes or hypertension, the same as any working population (DiCostanzo 2014). Agricultural work is physically demanding, involving long working hours with exposure to harsh climatic conditions (e.g. extreme cold or heat, sun, rain, lightning), as well as dust, plant material, and pesticides, which contribute to dermatological, ocular, and respiratory concerns. Ocular issues include conjunctivitis and symptoms of irritation, as well as a high prevalence of pterygium. Repetitive bending and lifting, as well as exposure to machines and blades often without sufficient training or protective equipment, lead to both chronic and acute musculoskeletal injuries (McLaughlin, Hennebry, and Haines 2014). Gastrointestinal (GI) issues, sometimes related to changes in diet or to the challenges of maintaining a healthy diet given the demands of work, as well as limited cooking and food storage conditions, present additional challenges. For example, some reported cases of GI illness were due to consuming food that had spoiled due to lack of fridge space in communal kitchens (Weiler, McLaughlin, and Cole 2017). Mental and emotional health, as well as sexual and reproductive health issues, are also areas of concern for migrants who endure prolonged and painful family separations (Narushima, McLaughlin, and Barrett-Greene 2016; Mysyk, England, and Avila Gallegos 2008; McLaughlin et al. 2017).

These workers come here to work. If their health is compromised, whether it is due to working conditions or otherwise, not only is their productivity impacted, but also their ability to stay in Canada and support their families back home. Thus, their health and work are inherently interrelated.

Migrant agricultural workers generally have legal access to provincial health care plans, but they face numerous practical barriers. These include long hours of work and limited clinic hours in rural areas, lack of transportation, delays in receiving health cards, lack of information about and integration into the local health care system, and language and literacy barriers (Hennebry, McLaughlin, and Preibisch 2016; McLaughlin 2009; Preibisch and Otero 2014; Pysklywec et al. 2011). Access to supplementary benefits and prescription drug coverage remain inconsistent and insufficient for many workers.

Perhaps the most unique and problematic access barrier is these migrants' dependence on employers to facilitate health care access. Workers may require employers' assistance to receive time off work and access transportation, information about clinics, and/or informal translation services. Even when employers are willing to facilitate health care access, which is variable, their involvement compromises workers' confidentiality and privacy. Of particular concern to workers it that their employer may view their health issues negatively, which could impact future employment (Hennebry, McLaughlin, and Preibisch 2016; Preibisch and Otero 2014). Applying for workers' compensation programs presents similar challenges, particularly because workers are reluctant to admit workplace injuries and risk disappointing or angering employers by missing work and/or causing their insurance premiums to rise (McLaughlin et al. 2014). For these reasons, many sick or injured workers fail to access the services that are available to them, or they access them only partially (e.g., by failing to return for recommended follow-up testing, treatment, or interventions).

As our research began to uncover some of these systemic access issues, we sought to find opportunities for intervention. In 2006, the Occupational Health Clinics for Ontario Workers (OHCOW) began to assess migrant agricultural workers with work-related conditions. To overcome some of the aforementioned barriers to accessing health care, clinics were held at several accessible locations with high migrant worker density at times when workers were off duty; they could often be accessed by workers when they came to town to shop. As well, translators were available. While up to 60 percent of health issues were

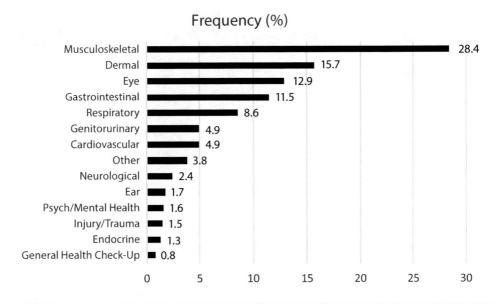

Figure 19.2: Frequency of Health Conditions of Migrant Agricultural Workers by System (*N* = 1460, 2007–2016)

Source: Occupational Health Clinics for Ontario Workers (Hamilton) data.

work related, many of the presenting conditions had a broad primary care focus (see figure 19.2 for a summary of issues). In many instances, these clinics were the only opportunities workers had to access care. From a prevention perspective, interventions were developed to address the most prevalent health problems seen. For example, an eye health care program provided an educational workshop on eye hazards, prevention interventions, general eye care, and provision of safety glasses or guidance on selection and sourcing them.

While a few community health centres (CHCs) and family health teams in Southern Ontario provided targeted services to migrant populations, access to services remained elusive for many workers. As a result of community engagement, stakeholder meetings, and lobbying, pilot funding was provided by the Local Health Integration Network for specific migrant agricultural worker primary care services through two CHCs in the regions of Niagara and Haldimand-Norfolk. The first season of this pilot project, held in 2014, proved to be immensely successful, with over seven hundred worker visits. Clinics were held when workers had time off—Thursday and Friday evenings in Simcoe and Sunday afternoons in Niagara—and in locations that were centrally accessible, with additional supports, such as the provision of transportation and translation services. No health cards or payments were required. Clinic services offered episodic care and follow-up when needed, resulting in treatment, education, investigations, and referral for specialist care. Of all visits, 35 percent were repeats, often for a new health issue, indicating ongoing needs and workers' confidence in the service. A survey of workers who attended the clinics (*N* = 86), focusing

> ### Personal Story: Pablo
>
> Pablo is a worker from Mexico who has been coming to Canada for 15 seasons and has been with the same employer for the last 10 years. He is trained as a pesticide sprayer, and he is proud of this specialized job. He has been having some breathing issues for the past few weeks and is concerned that it may be from the pesticides. He drives a tractor with an enclosed cab, but it seems that the cab may not be well sealed. There is also a lot of dust when he is working. He has to wait until the weekly shopping trip to town to see a doctor, as he doesn't want his employer to know he has symptoms. Luckily, there is a new clinic open for migrant workers, where they have translators. The doctor wishes to order some follow-up tests to assess Pablo's respiratory status and the source of his symptoms, but he refuses. The clinician also suggests that Pablo mention the leaky cab to his employer, but he does not wish to do that either. He does not want to jeopardize his higher-paying job and the status that it brings. It is the end of the spraying season, and he is encouraged to follow up with the clinic should his symptoms return this or next season.

on issues of access and patient satisfaction, found 100 percent of workers satisfied or very satisfied with their care (Mayell, McLaughlin, and Tew 2015). Health promotion activities, such as cooking classes and sexual health seminars, were also offered. As of 2018, the clinics are still operating; they have expanded various services and locations and continue to attract high volumes of workers.

Despite these advances, even with services that are established with migrant workers' specific needs in mind, additional challenges are encountered.

In Pablo's case (see box above), as in many others, clinicians may be limited in the treatments or solutions they can propose due to workers' structurally precarious immigration and employment status. In a precarious system in which being fired also leads to deportation, many workers are willing to sacrifice their health to secure their jobs (Orkin et al. 2014). Only broader policy changes that promote workers' empowerment can address these vulnerabilities. Some of the changes that have been recommended include the following: more education to both employers and workers about workers' rights; proactive (not only reactive) workplace inspections; access to an impartial appeals process prior to being fired and deported; rights to collectively bargain; the provision of open rather than tied work permits; and access to permanent residency (Faraday 2012; McLaughlin, Hennebry, and Haines 2014; McLaughlin et al. 2014).

In our experience, however, even within the current structural restrictions, clinicians who make their practices accessible to workers can make a significant difference in their health trajectories, providing high quality care to a population that has often gone without. To truly make care accessible for migrant workers, health care barriers should be anticipated and addressed in a proactive manner (see table 19.1). The efforts mentioned above

Table 19.1. Barriers to Health Care Access and Strategies to Address Them

Barriers to Health Care Access	Strategies
• Communication and language difficulties including low literacy	• Provide translation services • Utilize practitioners with knowledge of the population • Provide culturally and linguistically appropriate patient resources with illustrations
• Distance and lack of transportation • Limited availability to access services due to loss of income, work demands, or fear of disappointing employer • Lack of access to primary care practitioners and long wait times • Employer reluctance to facilitate care	• Locate clinics at a time and place when/where migrant agricultural workers will be available (e.g., in town when getting groceries, during periods off work) • Partner with community groups to assist with transportation • Educate and inform employers of service availability; negotiate access time with employer
• Lack of health insurance card (Ontario Health Insurance Plan [OHIP])	• Utilize community health centres (CHCs) and other clinics that do not require OHIP cards • Provide workers with proof of OHIP registration • Check OHIP to see if service has been activated
• Lack of confidentiality	• Provide accessible services independent of employer • Assure workers that employers will not be contacted
• Lack of knowledge of health care services • Difficulties with contacting and accessing allied health and test services	• Educate workers on health services and how to access them • Assist with arranging investigative service and allied health service access (e.g., diagnostic testing)
• Difficulties with follow-up	• Offer regularly scheduled and advertised clinic services • Use electronic medical records • Negotiate availability of advanced care services (e.g., surgery)
• Cultural differences and financial barriers	• Educate practitioners • Leverage community and corporate goodwill

could easily be replicated elsewhere, so long as proper funding and support are provided. Although general principles, such as providing Spanish-speaking translators and office hours when workers are off duty, may be universally applicable, each community must adapt to its specific circumstances. For example, depending on the harvest considerations, regional layouts, and local migrant population, additional supports such as bus transportation to clinics or translators of other languages, such as Thai, may be required. Access to follow-up treatment or investigative services may be challenging, and assisting workers with service navigation and attainment (e.g., ascertaining how workers would get testing, providing hours and locations for labs, providing aids for getting treatment items from pharmacy, and booking follow-up appointments) may be necessary. Given their limited access to treatment options, providing resources that workers can review on their own (e.g., illustrated, multilingual patient handouts) is beneficial. Being cognizant of the fact that workers' health status determines their ability to stay in Canada, clinicians may need to be flexible or creative with work-related restrictions. While covered by workers' compensation, many workers are reluctant to initiate claims for fear of losing their jobs. Clinicians can help by providing good documentation in the clinical record of work-related health problems and their origins, as this may prove valuable should the worker have ongoing health issues and need to make a later claim.

Almost every major migrant-employing community has now established a number of community groups that work with migrant workers (see Hennebry 2012), and such groups can be major assets in planning appropriate services, assisting with translation, and linking workers to the community. Seeking and engaging interested clinicians such as pharmacists, optometrists, and physiotherapists, as well as family physicians, will create increased accessibility to needed allied health services. While migrant workers do not easily fit into pre-existing health care models, clinicians, health promoters, and planners can make services accessible by considering outreach or alternative care models, learning from established initiatives, and partnering with locally based migrants and their advocates.

CRITICAL THINKING QUESTIONS

1. Given that the demand for migrant agricultural workers has only expanded over the past 50 years, and that the need for agricultural labourers is permanent, why do you think Canada continues to deny workers the chance to immigrate? Do you think workers should receive this right?
2. This chapter describes how, for fear of losing their jobs, many workers prefer not to modify their working conditions or report their health conditions to workers' compensation. What policies and practices could be modified to ensure workers feel more empowered to protect their health and access their rights?
3. In this chapter, we explain how specialized health care efforts have sought to overcome barriers to health care access for migrant workers in select regions, but not every community can provide specialized clinics. In what ways can every community work to more meaningfully integrate migrant populations into pre-existing health and social services? How can migrants be integrated into the community to address isolation and social stress?

ADDITIONAL RESOURCES

Migrant Worker Health Project: http://www.migrantworkerhealth.ca
> This website offers a wealth of resources, contacts, and information about migrant health risks and needs, health care, and compensation for migrant agricultural workers. While most of the information is based in Ontario, much of it will be relevant to contexts across the country.

OHCOW Migrant Farm Worker Program: http://www.ohcow.on.ca/migrant-farm-worker-program.html
> This website includes resources for farm workers, employers, and clinicians concerning a variety of occupational health issues. Current projects are described, and proceedings are available from annual stakeholder Migrant Farm Worker Health Forums. Consultation services are free.

Migrant Dreams Documentary: http://tvo.org/video/documentaries/migrant-dreams-feature-version
> In this 2016 documentary by Min Sook Lee, viewers get a glimpse into the difficult realities facing a group of primarily women Indonesian migrant agricultural workers in Ontario, who enter Canada through the low-wage stream of the Temporary Foreign Worker Program.

Matices Documentary: https://www.youtube.com/watch?v=9UntNX_uDzs
> This bilingual 2006 documentary by Mexican filmmaker Aaraón Díaz Mendiburo features the varying perspectives of Mexican migrant workers, community members, advocates, employers, health providers, and government officials involved in the Seasonal Agricultural Worker Program.

Farmworker Clinical Care Resource for Occupational Health: http://www.farmworkerclinicians-manual.com
> As many health issues are related to work in this population, this website is extremely useful for clinicians in diagnosis and assessment and includes guidelines for realistic management and educational material as well. Most education material is in Spanish and English. While it originates in the United States, the conditions and management are fairly universal.

TEDx Talk: "Working Together to Support Migrant Worker Health": https://www.youtube.com/watch?v=JURD_BlcnRY
> In this TEDx Talk, chapter author Janet McLaughlin describes community initiatives to support migrant worker health care in Ontario, including those explained in this chapter.

REFERENCES

Basok, Tanya. 2002. *Tortillas and Tomatoes*. Montreal: McGill-Queen's University Press.

Curry, Bill. 2014. "Everything You Need to Know about Temporary Foreign Workers." *Globe and Mail*, May 2. http://www.theglobeandmail.com/news/politics/temporary-foreign-workers-everything-you-need-to-know/article18363279/.

DiCostanzo, Melissa. 2014. "Harvesting Good Health." *Registered Nurse Journal* (July/August): 12–16.

Edmunds, Kathryn, Helene Berman, Tanya Basok, Marilyn Ford-Gilboe, and Cheryl Forchuk. 2011. "The Health of Women Temporary Agricultural Workers in Canada: A Critical Review of the Literature." *Canadian Journal of Nursing Research* 43: 68–91.

Employment and Social Development Canada (ESDC). 2016. "Annual Labour Market Impact Assessment Statistics 2008–2015: Primary Agriculture Stream." Last modified August 2. https://www.canada.ca/en/employment-social-development/services/foreign-workers/reports/2014/lmia-annual-statistics/agricultural.html.

Faraday, Fay. 2012. *Made in Canada: How the Law Constructs Migrant Workers' Insecurity*. Toronto: Metcalf Foundation.

Government of Canada. 2015. "Facts & Figures 2015: Immigration Overview—Temporary Residents—Annual IRCC Updates." July 31. http://open.canada.ca/data/en/dataset/052642bb-3fd9-4828-b608-c81dff7e539c.

Hennebry, Jenna. 2012. "Permanently Temporary? Agricultural Migrant Workers and Their Integration in Canada." Institute for Research on Public Policy Paper, February 28. http://irpp.org/research-studies/study-no26/.

Hennebry, Jenna, Janet McLaughlin, and Kerry Preibisch. 2016. "'Out of the Loop': Improving Access to Health Services for Migrant Farm Workers in Canada." *Journal of International Migration and Integration* 17: 521–38.

Mayell, Stephanie, Janet McLaughlin, and Michelle Tew. 2015. *Migrant Farmworker Health in Ontario: Evaluating a Provincial Pilot Initiative to Increase Access to Primary Health Care*. Report Prepared for the Quest and Grand River Community Health Centres.

McLaughlin, Janet. 2009. "Trouble in Our Fields: Health and Human Rights among Canada's Foreign Migrant Agricultural Workers." PhD diss., University of Toronto.

McLaughlin, Janet, and Jenna Hennebry. 2013. "Pathways to Precarity: Structural Vulnerabilities and Lived Consequences for Migrant Farmworkers in Canada." In *Producing and Negotiating Non-citizenship: Precarious Legal Status in Canada*, edited by Luin Goldring and Patricia Landolt, 175–94. Toronto: University of Toronto Press.

McLaughlin, Janet, Jenna Hennebry, Donald Cole, and Gabriel Williams. 2014. "The Migrant Farmworker Health Journey: Stages and Strategies." IMRC Policy Points VI, April. Waterloo, ON: International Migration Research Centre. http://imrc.ca/wp-content/uploads/2013/10/IMRC-Policy-Points-VI.pdf.

McLaughlin, Janet, Jenna Hennebry, and Ted Haines. 2014. "Paper versus Practice: Occupational Health and Safety Protections and Realities for Temporary Foreign

Agricultural Workers in Ontario." *Pistes: Interdisciplinary Journal of Work and Health* 16 (2). https://doi.org/10.4000/pistes.3844.

McLaughlin, Janet, Don Wells, Aaraón Díaz Mendiburo, André Lyn, and Biljana Vasilevska. 2017. "'Temporary Workers,' Temporary Fathers: Transnational Family Impacts of Canada's Seasonal Agricultural Workers' Program." *Relations Industrielles* 72 (4): 682–709.

Mysyk, Avis, Margaret England, and Juan Arturo Avila Gallegos. 2008. "Nerves as Embodied Metaphor in the Canada/Mexico Seasonal Agricultural Worker Program." *Medical Anthropology* 27: 383–404.

Narushima, Miya, Janet McLaughlin, and Jackie Barett-Greene. 2016. "Needs and Risks in Sexual Health among Temporary Foreign Migrant Farmworkers in Canada: A Pilot Study with Mexican and Caribbean Workers." *Journal of Immigrant and Minority Health* 18 (2): 374–81.

Orkin, Aaron, Morgan Lay, Janet McLaughlin, Michael Schwandt, and Donald Cole. 2014. "Medical Repatriation of Migrant Farm Workers in Ontario: Coding and Descriptive Analysis." *Canadian Medical Association Journal* 2: E192–8.

Preibisch, Kerry, and Gerardo Otero. 2014. "Does Citizenship Status Matter in Canadian Agriculture? Workplace Health and Safety for Migrant and Immigrant Laborers." *Rural Sociology* 79 (2): 174–99.

Pysklywec, Mike, Janet McLaughlin, Michelle Tew, and Ted Haines. 2011. "Doctors *within* Borders: Meeting the Health Care Needs of Migrant Farm Workers in Canada." *Canadian Medical Association Journal* 18: 1039–43.

Weiler, Anelyse, Janet McLaughlin, and Donald Cole. 2017. "Food Security at Whose Expense? A Critique of the Canadian Temporary Farm Labour Migration Regime and Proposals for Change." *International Migration* 55 (4): 48–63.

Wells, Don, Janet McLaughlin, André Lyn, and Aaraón Díaz Mendiburo. 2014. "Sustaining North-South Migrant Precarity: Remittances and Transnational Families in Canada's Seasonal Agricultural Program." *Just Labour* 22: 144–67.

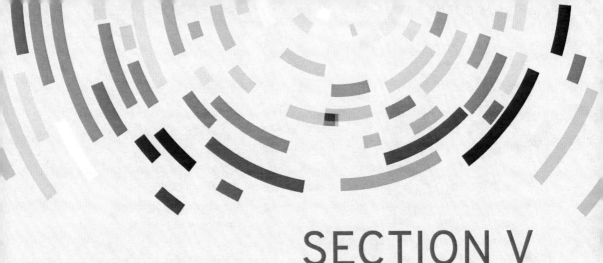

SECTION V

RESEARCH FOR UNDER-SERVED POPULATIONS

SECTION INTRODUCTION BY THOMAS PIGGOTT AND NEIL ARYA

Whether or not you are planning on a career in research, considering ethics and practical approaches to research may still be relevant to you. You might rely on research for policy development, for practice, or for education; in any case, understanding roots and biases of research, on which your field depends, will be important. The pieces we have included address research in diverse environments with varied populations, from the Arctic to inner-city Hamilton, from Indigenous communities to refugees in Vancouver; these chapters present principles that may be applied more broadly.

With respect to each population, issues related to participation and informed consent are explored. Under-served populations may face multiple barriers—of which life trajectory, education, economics, and literacy are but a few—and these populations can experience further marginalization by the research process itself if careful consideration to proper approaches is not taken. For all, having a common understanding, appreciating cultural needs, and developing research questions that are most meaningful to populations affected is essential. For under-served populations, particularly Indigenous populations as described by Healey in Chapter 20, different ways of knowing may create tensions in research question prioritization and methodological preference. Humility is important when approaching each population. Flexibility and appreciation of different lenses, frequently lacking in rigid biomedical ethics boards, is also required.

Central to all research is the researcher-participant dyad. Guba and Lincoln (1994) discuss two theories, a critical lens theory and constructivism, relevant to vulnerable populations addressed in this volume, each of which addresses this important dyad and each of which considers the environment or context. A critical lens theory recognizes that reality exists as influenced by social, political, economic, cultural, and gender factors; that research findings are mediated by values; and that the transactional nature of research necessitates a dialogue between the investigator and participants in the inquiry. *Constructivism* considers multiple socially constructed realities influenced by social, cultural, and historical contexts where findings are inseparable from the relationship of researcher and participant.

Throughout this volume, we have attempted to emphasize the resilience of our populations; in research, they are often vulnerable for reasons of language, education, and socioeconomic status. Sometimes, members of these populations are victims of direct deception, such as in Tuskegee syphilis studies, where relevant information about their diagnoses and therapeutic options were withheld from participants in order to achieve better understanding of the progression of disease—for "the greater good." At other times, with the appearance of funds, an entire industry may develop around the "needs" of the marginalized. As with other aspects of relationships with under-served populations, we must not ignore historical echoes—the collective memory of trauma—lest we be condemned to repeat such mistakes as research marches forward.

REFERENCE

Guba, E. G., and Y. S. Lincoln. 1994. "Competing Paradigms in Qualitative Research." In *Handbook of Qualitative Research*, edited by E. G. Guba and Y. S. Lincoln, 105–17. Thousand Oaks, CA: Sage.

CHAPTER 20

Indigenous Health Research: Lessons from Life in the Arctic

Gwen K. Healey

LEARNING OBJECTIVES

After reading this chapter, you should be able to:

1. Identify important research concepts related to epistemology and methodology.
2. Appreciate some Indigenous research perspectives.
3. Recognize the value of exploring different theories and approaches to answering research questions.

BACKGROUND

In recent years, the Arctic has received increasing attention, not just in terms of exploration and resource development but also in media and research. Among this research is that concerning health and Canada's Inuit. Little health and social science literature has previously explored Indigenous views on health, society, and the relationships between people therein. In the education field, however, Indigenous knowledge and research epistemologies have been the focus of discussions in Western and Indigenous research theory (Deloria 1995; Kovach 2010; Wilson 2008; Battiste and Henderson 2000; Barnhardt and Kawagley 2005; Battiste 2002; Alfred and Corntassel 2005; Walters, Simoni, and Evans-Campbell 2002). This literature contributes perspectives on the assumptions implicit in different research approaches and provides models for doing or interpreting research based on Indigenous world views. Although significant advances have been made to *engage* Indigenous communities in research, there remains a need for research models that are *born from* Indigenous perspectives on research—from the underlying assumptions, to the research questions, to how to find the answers (Prior 2006; Kovach 2009; Wilson

2008). In the past, the vulnerability of Indigenous communities made them easy targets for exploitation by researchers who wished to advance their own interests (Nickels, Shirley, and Laidler 2006; NTI 2013; Dosseter 2005; Wachowich et al. 1999). Community-based participatory research, as described by Salsberg et al. in Chapter 23 in this volume, has been a method that has been promoted to counter this exploitation. However, a number of Inuit organizations and research collaborators have identified ongoing challenges with levelling the power imbalance that continues to exist between academic researchers and Inuit communities (Nickels, Shirley, and Laidler 2006; Healey 2006; NTI 2013). In a 2013 report by Nunavut Tunngavik Inc., the organization highlighted that there is still "tension between research as an occupation that directly benefits researchers and the need for Inuit to participate in research in order to understand the needs of our communities more completely" (NTI 2013, 29).

The guide from Inuit Tapiriit Kanatami (Nickels, Shirley, and Laidler 2006) was written to help researchers understand some community concerns and expectations in relation to research projects, as well as to determine appropriate levels of community involvement in various research stages. Concurrently, a growing body of literature in academic circles has focused on articulating Indigenous knowledge and research epistemologies, leading the way for greater discussion of Western and Indigenous research approaches

Inuit Tapiriit Kanatami: Guide for Researchers Working in Inuit Communities

Many Inuit regard scientific research as a valuable tool to protect public well-being, generate wealth, and advance knowledge (for the benefit of communities and society at large). Researchers are recognized as experts who possess specialized skills and knowledge and who can help provide the information and assessment needed by Inuit for sound decision-making and planning areas such as land use management, environmental assessment, mineral exploration, wildlife management, community health, infrastructure, and so on. Research projects are also perceived as an important source of direct employment and revenues, a source for local training and professional experience (particularly for young people), and, occasionally, a tool to support community advocacy and empowerment (e.g., by providing scientific evidence to support community claims in the national and international arenas). Across the Arctic, community members are increasingly seeking help from researchers to design and conduct their own studies that address local questions and concerns. Research collaborations and partnerships between Inuit and the scientific community are increasing. Inuit are by-and-large not opposed to pure scientific research; however, they would like the opportunity to share their valuable knowledge and to assist scientists in designing and conducting scientific studies (even if the phenomena under investigation are not of immediate local relevance).

and contributing to more meaningful research (Deloria 1995; Kovach 2010; Wilson 2008; Battiste and Henderson 2000; Barnhardt and Kawagley 2005; Alfred and Corntassel 2005). This chapter adds to this body of literature by providing Inuit perspectives on health-related research epistemologies and methodologies with the intent that it may inform health research approaches in Arctic communities.

WAYS OF KNOWING

Epistemology is the theory of knowledge that questions what knowledge is, how it is acquired, and the extent to which a given subject can be known (Thayer-Bacon 2003, 18). It is the investigation of what distinguishes justified belief from opinion, particularly with regard to methods, validity, and scope. It is the starting point upon which we build our theoretical assumptions. What do we know and how do we know it? Do we know it individually or collectively? Is there more than one way to know something? Do we possess knowledge, or do we engage with it? Or both? Epistemology is the space in which these questions are posed and explored.

Indigenous Ways of Knowing

A growing segment of the academic community is focused on explaining and understanding Indigenous knowledge and ways of knowing. This group recognizes that such knowledge is perceived, collected, and shared in ways that are unique to these communities. Battiste (2002) states that the recognition and intellectual activation of Indigenous knowledge today is an act of empowerment by Indigenous peoples. Indigenous peoples throughout the world have sustained unique world views and associated knowledge systems for millennia, even while going through social upheavals as a result of transformative forces beyond their control. Many of the core values, beliefs, and practices associated with these world views have survived and are beginning to be recognized as being just as valid for today's generations as they were for generations past. The depth of Indigenous knowledge rooted in the long inhabitation of a particular place offers lessons that can benefit everyone, from educators to scientists (Barnhardt and Kawagley 2005).

In Eurocentric thought, Indigenous knowledge has often been represented by the term *traditional* knowledge, which suggests a body of considerably old data that has been handed down generation to generation relatively unchanged (Battiste 2002). Grenier (1998) offers that Indigenous knowledge embodies certain characteristics, which are not mutually exclusive, such as the following: 1) Indigenous knowledge is accumulative and represents generations of experiences, careful observations, and trial and error experiments; 2) Indigenous knowledge is dynamic, with new knowledge continuously added and external knowledge adapted to suit local situations; 3) all members of the community—that is, elders, women, men, and children—have Indigenous knowledge; 4) the quantity and quality of Indigenous knowledge that an individual processes will vary according to age, gender, socioeconomic status, daily experiences, roles and responsibilities in the home and the community, and so on; 5) Indigenous knowledge is stored in the memories and activities of the people and is expressed in stories, songs, folklore, proverbs, dances, myths, cultural values, beliefs, rituals, cultural community, laws, local language, artifacts, forms of communication, and organization; and 6) Indigenous knowledge is shared and communicated orally and by specific example and through cultural practices such as dance and rituals (Grenier 1998). In addition, Battiste (2002) also describes Indigenous knowledge as embodying a web of relationships within a specific ecological context; containing linguistic categories, rules, and relationships unique to each knowledge system; having localized content and meaning; having established customs with respect to acquiring and sharing of knowledge; and implying responsibilities for possessing various types of knowledge.

Knowledge can be viewed as something people develop as they have experiences with each other and with the world around them (Thayer-Bacon 2003). Ideas are shared, changed, and improved upon through the development of understanding and meaning that is derived from experience. Fundamentally, this knowledge is rooted in a relational epistemology—a foundation for knowing that is based on the formulation of relationships among the members of the community of knowers (Thayer-Bacon 2003, 73–98). Through these relationships, knowledge is created and shared.

Relational Epistemology

Chilisa (2012) states that "knowing is something that is socially constructed by people who have relationships and connections with each other, the living and the non-living and the environment. Knowers are seen as beings with connections to other beings, the spirits of the ancestors, and the world around them that inform what they know and how they can know it" (116). A relational epistemology draws our attentions to relational forms of knowing. This differs from the common Western practice of focusing on individual descriptions of knowing. Knowing is informed by the multiple connections of knowers with other beings and the environment, by participating in events and observing nature, such as the birds, animals, rivers, and mountains (Thayer-Bacon 2003, 183). Wilson (2008) and Getty (2010) identify that knowledge comes from the people's histories, stories, observations of the environment, visions, and spiritual insights. Each of these relationships has implications for how research is conducted.

Relations with People

Relation building is an essential aspect of everyday life experience for Indigenous communities in Canada and around the world. Greeting becomes a way of building relationships and rapport among participants and researchers—and readers. From the moment of the first greeting, we are inevitably placed in a relationship, through mutual friends or through knowledge, with certain landmarks and events. We become part of the circles of relations that are connected to one another and *to which we are also accountable* (Deloria 1995). From a relational perspective, the development of a relationship with a colleague or research participant is part of establishing trust and accountability (Kovach 2009; Wilson 2008), which then feeds into the entire research method, from establishing rigour to respecting an ethical Indigenous knowledge framework to sharing and disseminating the results of a study.

Relations with the Land/Environment

Many Indigenous peoples have a physical, emotional, and spiritual connection with the land, the environment, and the creatures who share this space. The relationship with the environment/land also has implications for the way research is conducted. The construction of knowledge has to be done in a manner that builds and sustains relationships with the land/environment and is respectful of the environment (Chilisa 2012; Getty 2010; Barnhardt and Kawagley 2005). In this context, knowledge is embodied in a connection with the land and the environment. When interviews are used as a technique for gathering data, they are best conducted in a setting that is familiar to the research participant and relevant to the topic of the research (such as in their home, on the land, or in a comfortable community space). This enables the researcher to make connections with the environment and the space where the construction of knowledge takes place.

Relations with the Spirit

Spirituality may include one's personal connection to a higher being, or humanity, or the environment (Wilson 2008). Spirituality can be viewed as a connection or exercise that builds otherworldly relationships that are ceremonial in nature. Recognizing spirituality allows researchers to explore the interconnections between sacred and practical aspects of research. Understanding comes through factual and oral history that connects to ancestral spirits (Chilisa 2012) and/or through dreams (Wilson 2008). Knowledge is also regarded as a sacred object, and seeking knowledge is a spiritual quest that may begin with a ceremony (Wilson 2008). Knowing can come through prayer or dreams as a way people connect themselves with those around them, the living and the non-living, and the ancestral spirits. In this way, the mind, body, and spirit are involved in the gathering of information and understanding of the world.

PILIRIQATIGIINNIQ

Piliriqatigiinniq is the concept for working in a collaborative way for the common good.

The Piliriqatigiinniq Model for Community Health Research

The Qaujigiartiit[1] Health Research Centre has developed a model for how research should be conducted both within the centre and by the researchers with whom the centre engages. Qaujigiartiit developed the Piliriqatigiinniq Partnership Model for Community Health

Research in the centre's formative years (Healey 2008). This model was developed in response to the community-identified need for health research that explores topics of concern to Nunavummiut and is collected, analyzed, and disseminated in a holistic and collaborative way.

The Piliriqatigiinniq model is a visual representation of the web of relationships we have with each other and is built upon the principle that anyone can be involved in health research in some capacity if we are all working for the common good. Multidisciplinary collaboration strengthens research projects, enriches data analysis with additional perspectives, and fosters greater sharing of knowledge and implementation of findings across sectors. While there may not be a representative from every sector involved in every project, the model serves as a reminder to look beyond the scope of what is commonly defined as *health* and *research* to include knowledge holders and stakeholders from other disciplines and walks of life. This model was developed to provide practical organizational and methodological guidance; the foundations, however, run much deeper.

The model shown in figure 20.1 originated from a dialogue about health and the history of health research in Nunavut communities. It was derived from the stories and

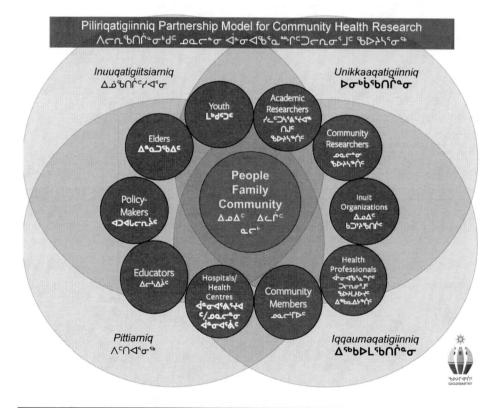

Figure 20.1: The Piliriqatigiinniq Partnership Model for Community Health Research

Source: Qaujigiartiit Health Research Centre (2013).

voices of people across Nunavut who attended community engagement sessions held between 2006 and 2008 (Healey 2006, 2008). While the model originated from a health perspective, the underlying principle is cross-cutting and interdisciplinary. The model is structured on the relational aspects of life in Nunavut communities—the relationships that are shared are the foundation from which we move forward to achieve wellness. Those relationships can be with anyone from any walk of life and with anything from any environment. The knowledge that is shared and created in this space is helpful for everyone. The motivations with which one engages in the project are the same: coming together for the common good and the betterment of health and wellness. The group is accountable to each other, to the relationships they have formed and/or will form together, and to the relationships they have with others in their community. In essence, this is a model for an Inuit epistemology in action because it arises from the relational perspective and is built on what was known, what is known, and what will come to be known in Inuit communities. Its development is predicated on the past, present, and future experiences of Nunavummiut.[2]

From this epistemological perspective, ethics, accountability, methodology, knowledge, understanding, and our relationships with each other as human beings and our environments are part of the same space. And this is, in our opinion, the essence of an Inuit epistemological perspective.

The Qaujigiartiit Health Research Centre promotes the idea that research must be used as a tool for action—that when one understands the scope and breadth of the issue, one is better equipped to move forward and take action on it. Multi-sectoral collaboration strengthens research projects, contributes added perspective to data analysis, and contributes to greater dissemination and implementation of findings across sectors. Therefore, this approach can be considered one that promotes active engagement, the sharing of knowledge, advocacy, and action.

It is particularly important in Inuit communities that research projects be collaborative and inclusive. The historical context of research in the North, including harmful and unethical research practices, have led to an environment of mistrust and displeasure with researchers in many communities (Healey 2006, 2008; NTI 2013; Nickels, Shirley, and Laidler 2006; Gearheard and Shirley 2007). When we lead our own research projects, we are able to focus on answering our own questions and incorporate methods that are reflective of what we know about wellness and how we know it. This view underscores the right of colonized, Indigenous peoples to construct knowledge in accordance with the self-determined definitions of what they want to know and how they want to know it.

CONCLUSION

Health research should answer the questions of the people, and such research should be collaborative. Being collaborative necessitates a participatory research approach as described by Salsberg et al. in Chapter 23; however, it also requires a commitment on the part of the researcher to learning and immersion to better appreciate Indigenous perspectives and ways of knowing. We recognize that not all projects can incorporate the methods outlined in this chapter, and variations exist depending on the approach incorporated in any given project. With this chapter it has been our intent to share epistemological considerations for northern community health researchers. This chapter is a beginning of a dialogue, and we look forward to engagement with the expansion of this literature in the future.

CRITICAL THINKING QUESTIONS

1. Reflect upon your personal experiences with research. Have you participated in a research study? In a telemarketing survey? Did you know the people who were studying you? Do you know where the information went or how it was used? How did it make you feel?
2. How does the content of this chapter expand your understanding of Indigenous research methods?
3. Reflect upon the types of questions you have about health and how you would approach answering them. Does it involve a collective or people, a partnership, or a group effort? In what ways can you draw on different types of expertise to answer the questions you have?

ACKNOWLEDGEMENTS

The growth development of this model and the centre over time has been a group effort. Valuable guidance, feedback, and support has been provided by Shirley Tagalik, Janet Tamalik McGrath, and Jamal Shirley in the development of this chapter.

NOTES

1. *Qaujigiartiit* is the Inuktitut word for "looking for knowledge."
2. *Nunavummiut* is the Inuktitut word for "people of Nunavut."

REFERENCES

Alfred, T., and J. Corntassel. 2005. "Being Indigenous: Resurgences against Contemporary Colonialism." *Government and Opposition* 40 (4): 597–614. https://doi.org/10.1111/j.1477-7053.2005.00166.x.

Barnhardt, R., and A. O. Kawagley. 2005. "Indigenous Knowledge Systems and Alaska Native Ways of Knowing." *Anthropology and Education Quarterly* 36 (1): 8–23.

Battiste, M. 2002. *Indigenous Knowledge and Pedagogy in First Nations Education: A Literature Review with Recommendations*. Ottawa: Government of Canada, Department of Indian and Northern Affairs (INAC).

Battiste, M., and J. Y. Henderson. 2000. *Protecting Indigenous Knowledge and Heritage: A Global Challenge*. Saskatoon, SK: Purich.

Chilisa, B. 2012. "Postcolonial Indigenous Research Paradigms." In *Indigenous Research Methodologies*, edited by B. Chilisa, 98–127. Thousand Oaks, CA: Sage.

Deloria, V. 1995. *Red Earth, White Lies: Native Americans and the Myth of Scientific Fact*. New York: Scribner.

Dosseter, J.B. 2005. *Beyond the Hippocratic Oath: A Memoir on the Rise of Modern Medical Ethics*. Edmonton: University of Alberta Press.

Egan, C. 1998. "Points of View: Inuit Women's Perceptions of Pollution." *International Journal of Circumpolar Health* 57 (suppl 1): 550–4.

Gearheard, S., and J. Shirley. 2007. "Challenges in Community-Research Relationships: Learning from Natural Science in Nunavut." *Arctic* 60 (1): 62–74.

Getty, G. A. 2010. "The Journey between Western and Indigenous Research Paradigms." *Journal of Transcultural Nursing* 21 (1): 35–39.

Grenier, L. 1998. *Working with Indigenous Knowledge: A Guide for Researchers*. Ottawa: International Development Research Centre.

Healey, G. 2006. *Report on Health Research Ethics Workshop and Community Consultation in Iqaluit, Nunavut*. Iqaluit, NU: Qaujigiartiit/Arctic Health Research Network—Nunavut.

Healey, G. 2008. *Piliriqatigiinniq Partnership Model for Community Health Research. Position Statement*. Iqaluit, NU: Qaujigiartiit Health Research Centre.

Kovach, M. 2009. *Indigenous Methodologies: Characteristics, Conversations, and Contexts*. Toronto: University of Toronto Press.

Kovach, M. 2010. "Conversational Method in Indigenous Research." *First Peoples Child and Family Review* 5 (1): 40–48.

Nickels, S., J. Shirley, and G. Laidler, eds. 2006. *Negotiating Research Relationships with Inuit Communities: A Guide for Researchers*. Ottawa, ON/Iqaluit, NU: Inuit Tapiriit Kanatami/Nunavut Research Institute. http://www.nri.nu.ca/sites/default/files/public/files/06-068%20ITK%20NRR%20booklet.pdf.

Nunavut Tunngavik Inc. (NTI). 2013. *Annual Report on the State of Inuit Culture and Society: Inuit Health Survey*. Iqaluit, NU: NTI.

Prior, D. 2006. "Decolonizing Research: A Shift toward Reconciliation." *Nursing Inquiry* 14 (2): 162–8.

Qaujigiartiit Health Research Centre. 2013. Piliriqatigiinniq Model (figure). Iqaluit: Qaujigiartiit Health Research Centre.

Thayer-Bacon, B. 2003. *Relational Epistemologies*. New York: Peter Lang.

Wachowich, N., A. A. Awa, R. K. Katsak, and S. P. Katsak. 1999. *Saqiyuq: Three Stories of the Lives of Inuit Women*. Montreal: McGill-Queen's University Press.

Walters, K., J. Simoni, and T. Evans-Campbell. 2002. "Substance Use among American Indians and Alaska Natives: Incorporating Culture in an 'Indigenist' Stress-Coping Paradigm." *Public Health Reports* 117 (suppl 1): S104–17.

Wilson, S. 2008. *Research is Ceremony: Indigenous Research Methods*. Blackpoint, NS: Fernwood.

CHAPTER 21

Overcoming Challenges of Conducting Longitudinal Research in Stigmatized Urban Neighbourhoods

Biljana Vasilevska, Angela Di Nello, Erin Bryce, and James R. Dunn

---

LEARNING OBJECTIVES

After reading this chapter, you should be able to:

1. Enumerate several ways that recruitment activities can be adapted to support participant retention for longitudinal studies.
2. Appreciate why some people from marginalized communities would have a difficult relationship with research and researchers.
3. Critically consider ways of demonstrating reciprocity in the relationship of researchers with study participants.

It can be challenging to recruit and retain marginalized populations residing in stigmatized neighbourhoods into longitudinal studies. The most common ways rely on the mail, phone calls, and the Internet, which, given residential instability, intermittent phone service, and poor access to the Internet, may pose challenges when working with such populations. As such, researchers may face low recruitment rates and poor retention in longitudinal studies because standard forms of communication and engagement are not successful with all populations. Failure to recruit hard-to-reach populations can bias research and lead to inaccurate results (Odierna and Schmidt 2009). Recruitment is a common focus in research with marginalized populations, but retention is less frequently discussed. Successfully retaining participants from marginalized populations within longitudinal studies requires challenging traditional forms of communication and engagement at every point of contact between researcher and participants throughout the life of the study.

Our team has conducted longitudinal research with low-income tenants of subsidized housing and with residents of urban neighbourhoods that have been stigmatized in the local media (Dunn et al. 2015; Dunn et al. 2014). The two large-scale studies we refer to in this chapter investigate the changes in the health of individuals and in communities that occur as a result of changes to their environment, rather than their characteristics, at any one point in time. Both studies take place in Southern Ontario, a region where the loss of manufacturing jobs in the past two decades has had a negative effect on incomes and mobility and, in some cities, has been coupled with rising housing prices.

The Greater Toronto Area (GTA) West Housing and Health Study has surveyed over five hundred adults in four municipalities that form the western portion of the GTA: the cities of Toronto and Hamilton and the regions of Peel and Halton. This study investigates the extent to which low-income individuals may experience a change in their health if they move into subsidized housing.

The Hamilton Neighbourhoods Study investigates changes in healthy behaviours and chronic illness in 2,100 randomly selected residents living in a subset of neighbourhoods in Hamilton, Ontario. Hamilton is a city at the western edge of Lake Ontario with approximately 500,000 residents. As a result of the largest employment opportunities shifting from heavy industry (and in particular the production of steel) to health care, education, and service sector employment, the city has seen a profound shift in its labour market and culture. The residents who have been surveyed live in neighbourhoods that are part of a multi-year community development initiative.

Both of these studies use a combination of in-person and telephone surveys, depending on the stage of the study. We place great emphasis on creating a relationship with participants, both in order to retain them throughout the life of the study and to build goodwill to overcome any negative perception of research. In this chapter, we share some of the obstacles we have encountered when conducting longitudinal studies with stigmatized urban populations and the strategies we have used to overcome them.

PRIVACY AND COLLABORATION WITH PARTNERS

As with many studies involving marginalized populations, and as elaborated by Salsberg et al. in Chapter 23 regarding participatory research, our studies have involved close collaboration with community partners and intermediary agencies, particularly during the recruitment stage, in order to have community members as active participants in the research process. Our partners have included municipalities, social service agencies, and agencies that manage the applications for subsidized housing. Partnering agencies can offer a great deal of support in the recruitment and retention of study participants. The role they play will depend on the study, and it is to be expected that the nature of their involvement will change over the course of the study. One role that partners can fulfill is to provide "research brokers" to actively recruit participants. Brokers are individuals who have an ongoing, trusting relationship with the population being studied, and who may themselves be, or have been, members of that same population, and for that reason are sometimes referred to as "cultural brokers" and

> ## The Hamilton Neighbourhoods Study
>
> The Hamilton Neighbourhoods Study (HNS) investigates the health impact of the City of Hamilton's multi-year Neighbourhood Action Strategy (NAS). The NAS is a community development initiative created by the City of Hamilton and the Hamilton Community Foundation. It was implemented in 12 neighbourhoods that were identified in a local media report as having poor health outcomes.
>
> The NAS is a response both to residents' concerns about the stigmatizing manner in which their neighbourhoods have been portrayed, and a way of collaborating with residents and local agencies to support residents' goals for neighbourhood improvement.
>
> The HNS has conducted surveys with 2,100 participants in six intervention neighbourhoods and a matched cohort of comparison households. Baseline surveys were conducted when the participating neighbourhoods were beginning to define goals and actions for neighbourhood improvement, and follow-up surveys are conducted at two-year intervals. Prior to beginning recruitment, research staff attended the six neighbourhoods' monthly planning team meetings. The research team used a participatory research approach to come to know the regular attendees of these community meetings and the staff supporting the NAS, and consulted them extensively on how to conduct recruitment in each neighbourhood (for more details on participatory research, see Salsberg et al., Chapter 23 in this volume). By having regular physical presence at community meetings, residents were able to informally ask questions of the research staff. Notices about the study findings were prepared for resident groups, who were presented with the findings before they were published. The research team also supported the local planning teams by, for example, buying advertising space in their community newspapers to inform residents that researchers would be in their neighbourhood or to disseminate summaries of the research findings.
>
> The research team also participated in local events outside of the somewhat formal planning team meetings—summer barbecues in the park, for example. By being a presence in the life of the community, the study team was able to demonstrate a shared commitment to the success of the NAS. Through providing feedback on study design and how to share research findings, community members were essential to the research process.

"language brokers." Brokers are often an integral component of action research and are important study partners for research with specific marginalized urban populations, including minority ethnic groups; lesbian, gay, bisexual, and transgender communities; recent refugees; sex workers; and homeless people. Brokers may be employees or volunteers at a partnering agency, and they have important insights and experiences to contribute on how to approach potential research participants, and how to address research questions that may be particularly sensitive—for example, questions that may be a trigger for psychological trauma.

The use of brokers is not appropriate or relevant to all studies. For our longitudinal surveys, we have aimed to recruit a random sample of residents in urban neighbourhoods that have been stigmatized in the local media and of applicants to subsidized housing. Our partnering agencies have not fulfilled a brokering function in terms of direct recruitment, but they have supported recruitment through sharing information that has allowed our team to recruit participants ourselves, thereby ensuring the randomization that is important to the design of our studies. Two potential challenges to the use of brokers relate to the principle of non-coercion and to privacy and anonymity. There is sometimes a question of how freely participants have volunteered to be in a study if they have been recruited by an individual with whom they have an ongoing relationship. A person who is already marginalized in some way, and one who has few supporting people in their life, may feel an obligation to participate in a study, particularly if the broker also provides some service to them and it has not been made clear that participating in a study would have no influence on the service they are receiving. Additionally, because brokers may be employed by a partnering agency, they may find themselves in conflict with the privacy norms of their agency and those expected by the academic research community.

Every institution has its own privacy and anonymity norms and is governed by relevant legislation. These norms and the interpretation of such legislation may occasionally be in tension with those of other institutions in the research partnership, such as academic research ethics boards. For example, the GTA West Housing and Health Study, which tracked applicants to rent-geared-to-income subsidized housing, involved six institutions in total (two academic research institutions and four municipal housing agencies), creating a number of challenges. In both studies, before any recruitment could begin, processes needed to be established among the partners that would allow every institution to maintain their privacy standards, yet still allow for information sharing. In some cases, the resulting recruitment process involved 11 different steps and took up to 6 weeks from beginning to end (see Dunn et al. 2014 for full details). It took numerous iterations of study protocols with the partners to achieve all of the following simultaneous goals: maximize recruitment, retention, and study rigour; protect participant privacy; achieve voluntary participation and comprehensibility; and uphold research ethics and institutional privacy standards. These logistical hurdles were solved through maintaining strong relationships with our partner institutions and demonstrating creativity, patience, and a determination for the research to proceed.

HIRING AND SENSITIVITY

An often underappreciated aspect of conducting studies with marginalized populations in stigmatized neighbourhoods concerns hiring decisions. In some instances, it may be appropriate to hire peer researchers from the target communities for the research so that these communities can benefit from the economic activity provided by the research and some individuals can benefit from the job skills and other training they receive as part of their employment. In our studies, we have not explicitly attempted to hire peer researchers because of issues concerning transportation to distant research sites (households spread across a metropolitan area) and because of the sensitive information we ask from participants (health information). We wanted to avoid the possibility of a participant's social network intersecting with the person interviewing them. Others attempt to hire staff who reflect their target population in terms of gender, age, ethnicity, language, and so on. Instead, we elected to provide interpretation to address language issues and be as inclusive as possible in our hiring, without employing any specific quotas or targets for particular groups. Ultimately, we have hired research assistants who have demonstrated an awareness of the potential power imbalances between themselves and the participants, as well as an understanding of the kinds of challenges faced by participants, and who are capable of responding professionally yet sympathetically under difficult circumstances.

Because research staff may be interacting with participants who are living with adversity and may have experienced traumatic events, we provide staff with a high level of training on how to deal with difficult situations, whether in person or over the phone. We also encourage staff to formally debrief with peers and supervisors during weekly meetings, and informally after an encounter; during these debriefings, they are welcome to speak with colleagues, a supervisor, or non-staff members about the experience, or simply sit or write in a quiet room, as they wish.

Our surveys ask potentially sensitive and personal questions about the participants' lives and their emotional well-being, and about the availability and accessibility of resources to meet their needs. When participants are not aware of resources, it is common for them to ask the research assistant if they are aware of any. For this reason, we have created resource guides listing agencies, community groups, and support services available in the area. These guides are postcard-sized, written in plain language, and distributed to every participant with whom we conduct an in-person survey. Surveys over the phone are necessarily handled differently. When a telephone interviewer senses that a participant is becoming upset, he or she follows a protocol that begins with asking the participant if they have accessed any resources. If the person has used support services, the interviewer validates the participant; if they have not used support services, the interviewer asks the participant for permission to tell them about resources. At the end of this exchange, the interviewer thanks the participant for talking and sharing their experiences. If this exchange has happened in the middle of the survey, the participant is asked if they would like to continue with the survey or if they would prefer to finish it at another time or stop doing the survey altogether.

Since our research assistants are "front-line" staff, possibly providing the only interaction that participants have with our studies, they are important ambassadors for the work being done, and the quality of their interactions may influence participant attrition rates. Selecting and training staff takes time, effort, and money. The high quality and trustworthiness of our staff has had a positive effect on the quality of our studies overall, because our staff have taken the initiative to report on those recruitment and communication strategies that have not been successful and have suggested improvements to our processes and communications. Consistency in staffing (e.g., a participant doing all of the interviews with the same staff person) is also a desirable goal, since study participants are more likely to trust staff members they have met multiple times.

OVERCOMING NEGATIVE PERCEPTIONS OF RESEARCH

Many socially marginalized individuals have limited experience with research, or they may possess negative preconceived notions of research (McKenzie et al. 1999). Research is not necessarily well understood and valued, or its value may be questioned by some participants, especially those living in areas that are frequently the subject of research. Some participants might have felt exploited by research and researchers in the past, both as individuals and as members of a community that may have received a great deal of attention from researcher. Contemporary research within academic settings operates within a framework of codified research ethics—for example, in Canada, it is the *Tri-Council Policy Statement: Ethical Conduct on Research Involving Humans* (CIHR, NSERC, and SSHRC 2014). Many institutions and disciplines also have their own standards of ethical conduct. Strict adherence to some of the practices set out in these and other documents may inadvertently discourage some people—those from marginalized populations in particular—from participating in research. While it is not appropriate to generalize about all participants in all studies, we have found certain characteristics to be common in our work with low-income tenants and with residents of stigmatized neighbourhoods. Knowing these characteristics helps with planning similar studies and, in particular, with retention strategies for the follow-up stages.

As is common with research hosted by universities and their affiliates, there is standard language that we must use on recruitment and consent forms, resulting in forms that, depending on the study, can stretch to six pages in length. This documentation is a potential barrier to participation in the research, to participants giving meaningful consent, and to building a relationship with participants. Individuals with lower literacy skills, or for whom English is not their primary language, may be intimidated or upset by such forms. Even for those who do have very strong English language literacy, the request to read and sign such a form can be a lengthy, awkward intrusion in what might develop into a strong, positive encounter. Such practical issues have required our negotiation with research ethics boards. Because we never assume that a participant will read any of the study's documentation, no matter the length, research staff always ask the participant if they would like to have the content of the documents summarized. In addition to the full consent forms, many studies use a single-page, plain-language summary.

Similarly, certain protocols around maintaining "neutrality" are culturally specific and may be given a different meaning by participants than what is intended by researchers and their institutions. An offer of an honorarium could be seen by some institutions as potentially coercive and as nullifying the principle of voluntary consent. On the other hand, an honorarium can be considered fair compensation for an individual's time and the sharing of their perspective. Our studies offer honoraria at all stages of participation; as well, research staff preface every survey by reiterating the voluntary nature of participation, and that refusing to answer questions or withdrawing from the study is always an option. Another common challenge that we have faced regards the requirement to refuse participants' offers of food or drink. The participant may feel that offering refreshments is a polite (or obligatory) exchange when someone has come into their home, and indeed may be part of the relationship that we hope to build.

Beyond the day-to-day encounters, there are important considerations for how the study is framed and how the results are communicated. An entire study or a series of questions that focus on negative experiences may evoke strong reactions and demonstrate a lack of sensitivity. Individuals who are marginalized in some way do have positive experiences to share, and it is potentially a threat to the quality of the data, as well as to the relationship with the individual participant and the population, not to consider the many dimensions of their experience.

MAINTAINING COMMUNICATION AND PARTICIPANT INTERACTION

The ability to keep track of our participants over time is both crucial to the success of our longitudinal studies and one of our primary challenges. A great deal of effort has gone into creating processes and infrastructure to ensure that we either know how to contact a participant or can get this information in as few steps as possible. Because we did not use research brokers in these studies, all contact information and efforts to follow up with participants resided with the study team.

Many of our participants are highly mobile, moving as need dictates. Some have little or inconsistent access to the Internet; many are unable to maintain mobile or landline phone services consistently, so their phone numbers may be in service one month but not the next. To manage costs, many people keep their mobile phones off and turn them on only to make an outgoing call or if they are expecting a call. Using postal mail to reach participants may be problematic, as high residential mobility means participants may have moved, often leaving no forwarding address.

Participants in our studies have been unlikely to follow up on our mailed requests to update their contact information themselves, be it by phone, mail, or a website. Language barriers, lack of access to computers, low digital literacy, and the effort involved have all served to make this option very poorly used, even when we attempted to make these options time- and cost-efficient (e.g., by providing postage-paid business reply envelopes addressed to our office, offering grocery store gift cards as an incentive to update, or having simple forms on our website where participants can update their contact information). In addition, participants may forget that they are involved in a study and not appreciate the request being made of them. Therefore, we have become very proactive in recording participant details, and we contact them regularly to update their contact information ourselves, a practice demonstrated to increase the odds of completing follow-up interviews (Gilmore and Kuperminc 2014). We use multiple methods to keep in contact with participants and prioritize means that are least likely to cost them time or money.

Our record-keeping has evolved to facilitate such contact. Early in our studies, we used spreadsheets for such information, but we needed to develop a database to record more details, which could be queried for each participant. For example, when we contact a participant, we begin by reminding them that they did a survey on a particular date with a particular individual. We have found that most participants remember the research staff member they spoke with, and that person is their trigger for recalling that they are participating in a study. The database also prompts us to make phone calls at certain times and serves as a record of each call, so that we are not phoning someone too often.

In order to minimize the number of participants who we deem to be "lost to follow-up," we confirm or update the contact information of the participant at every data collection point, and we also ask them to give us the contact information of one or two people who are close to them and will likely know their whereabouts (usually a friend or relative). One study has demonstrated that sisters and grandmothers are more likely to know how to contact a participant than brothers or any other relative (Farrall et al. 2015). Because we are requesting information of a close friend or relative, the importance of a trusting relationship with the research staff is critical. Research staff are trained to discern "soft" refusals for any request made of participants, including requests to provide follow-up contact information. Staff are permitted to exercise their own judgment in how assertively they may ask for such information, bearing in mind the importance of voluntariness of participation in the study and the importance of maintaining a strong relationship with participants.

We only resort to contacting a friend or family member after we have been unable to locate the participant after mailing them, visiting their last known address in person, and phoning or texting them on different days of the week and different times of day. One challenge with asking friends and family about a participant's current phone number or whereabouts is that the act of participation in a research study needs to remain confidential. However, the friends and relatives we are contacting are entitled to know why a stranger is asking for this information. We are not able to disclose that their friend or relative is participating in a study, but we do whatever we can to allay their concerns. We use a script that begins with our research assistant introducing themselves, and stating that they are calling from McMaster University, and were given this contact information by the participant (whom we refer to by name) in case we could not contact them. The research assistant then reads the contact information on file for the participant and asks if they have different or updated information. If the person we are calling does not feel comfortable disclosing the updated contact information, the research assistant will ask him or her to write down the caller's name, our study phone number, and the study email address to give to the participant. Remaining ambiguous about why the participant is being sought may make someone unnecessarily suspicious and concerned for the participant's well-being, but being too open about the content of the study could also be harmful and a threat both to the research relationship and to the relations between the participant and the person who has been contacted.

For the surveys that we conduct over the phone, which may take up to 30 minutes, we offer participants additional funds to defray their telephone costs if they have been using a mobile phone, which is particularly appreciated by those on "pay-as-you-go" plans. If data collection is done at intervals of one year or longer, we initiate a "check-in" phone call approximately every six months; when data collection is every six months, the check-in call is every three months. The check-in calls serve a number of purposes, including verifying or updating contact information; reminding participants about the study; informing or reminding participants of any information that was mailed to them (usually a plain-language summary of the study's findings to date); and telling them all the ways they can keep in contact with us, including by phone, email, and social media. These practices have been demonstrated to improve retention (Leonard et al. 2014).

In response to the challenge of following up with participants when they have not given us the contact information of a friend or relative, and whom we were not able to contact by mail or in-person visits, we began using social media to "friend" or "follow" participants as a way to keep in contact with them and to facilitate booking future surveys. This mid-course correction required additional work—in seeking out the correct person and requesting that they connect with us. Social media proved to be a valuable means of sharing our study results, both with participants and the broader community. If we were to do similar studies in the future, we would plan for these options during the recruitment phase and would incorporate a social media strategy into the overall retention and communications plan, understanding that social media is a common part of many people's lives and thus can serve to facilitate recruitment and build rapport with researchers (Lunnay et al. 2015).

Regular contact has the additional benefit of promoting a relationship with the project. We try to incorporate reciprocity in these ongoing research relationships, not only asking for data, since doing so risks perpetuating power inequities and any negative perceptions participants may have to the idea of research. We use a number of tactics, including distributing information sheets we have created for each neighbourhood, which indicate specific community resources that are relevant to the study (such as community health centres and drop-in programs); creating plain-language research summaries that are mailed to participants; advertising our studies in community newspapers; presenting at community events; and posting reports through and having a presence on social media. We have found it helpful to create a strong and consistent visual identity through all of these communications for the study. This visual identity includes a professionally designed logo, a clear and simple name for the study ("GTA West Housing and Health" and "Hamilton Neighbourhoods Study"), and colour and branding standards that incorporate the colour scheme of our university. Use of plain language and a strong visual identity for our study materials helps to ensure that they are seen and understood by as broad an audience as possible and serves as a reminder for the (hopefully positive) experience they are having, thereby building goodwill both for the study and for research in general.

CONCLUSION

Traditional methods of recruitment and retention in research may not be successful when the population is culturally diverse, vulnerable, or marginalized. Lower-income individuals and people whose housing is precarious present challenges throughout the research process; however, their inclusion is critically important for comprehensive research findings. While there is no single formula for successful research with such populations, practices that we have found effective include using multiple methods to initiate and remain in contact with participants, as well as maintaining a presence in the lives of both the participants and the community where we are conducting the research. Disseminating the results of a study is part of the research relationship, and we strive to do so in ways that are welcomed by and accessible to participants. Attention to ethical conduct must continue throughout the life cycle of the study, and not just at the point of signing a consent form. Ethical conduct includes acknowledging different forms of communication and building them into all phases of a study. Planning for and overcoming obstacles to recruitment and retention in low-income individuals or residents of stigmatized urban neighbourhoods helps facilitate research that can then be used to benefit members of these populations.

CRITICAL THINKING QUESTIONS

1. Why is reciprocity important in social research, particularly when working with marginalized populations? Think of three examples of reciprocity in practice.
2. Why might there be more than one definition of *ethics* and *ethical conduct* in research? What are some ways that researchers may negotiate these different definitions?
3. What are some of the challenges with using research brokers when working with marginalized populations? Conversely, how can brokers be a benefit? What steps might you take to minimize problems with the use of research brokers and maximize benefit?

ACKNOWLEDGEMENTS

The authors would like to acknowledge the valuable contributions of former members of the research team. In particular, we thank Hilary Gibson-Wood, Madeleine Cahuas, and Paula Smith for their leadership, and the research assistants whose on-the-ground experiences and problem-solving supported the success of these studies.

REFERENCES

Canadian Institutes of Health Research (CIHR), Natural Sciences and Engineering Research Council of Canada (NSERC), and Social Sciences and Humanities Research Council of

Canada (SSHRC). 2014. *Tri-Council Policy Statement: Ethical Conduct for Research Involving Humans.* (RR4-2/2014E-PDF). Ottawa: Her Majesty the Queen in Right of Canada.

Dunn, J. R., A. Di Nello, H. Gibson-Wood, and B. Vasilevska. 2015. "Recruitment and Retention of Survey Participants in Marginalized Neighbourhoods." *SAGE Research Methods Cases.* https://doi.org/10.4135/978144627305014557922.

Dunn, J. R., P. Smith, H. Gibson-Wood, A. Di Nello, T. Dowbor, and B. Vasilevska. 2014. "Institutional Ethics, Privacy, and Recruitment for a Multi-site, Longitudinal Study on Social Housing." *SAGE Research Methods Cases.* https://doi.org/10.4135/978144627305014539106.

Farrall, S., B. Hunter, G. Sharpe, and A. Calverley. 2015. "What 'Works' when Retracing Sample Members in a Qualitative Longitudinal Study?" *International Journal of Social Research Methodology* 19 (3): 287–300. https://doi.org/10.1080/13645579.2014.993839.

Gilmore, D., and G. P. Kuperminc. 2014. "Testing a Model of Participant Retention in Longitudinal Substance Abuse Research." *American Journal of Evaluation* 35 (4): 467–84. https://doi.org/10.1177/1098214014523822.

Leonard, A., M. Hutchesson, A. Patterson, K. Chalmers, and C. Collins. 2014. "Recruitment and Retention of Young Women into Nutrition Research Studies: Practical Considerations." *Trials* 15 (1): 23. https://doi.org/10.1186/1745-6215-15-23.

Lunnay, B., J. Borlagdan, D. McNaughton, and P. Ward. 2015. "Ethical Use of Social Media to Facilitate Qualitative Research." *Qualitative Health Research* 25 (1): 99–109. https://doi.org/doi:10.1177/1049732314549031.

McKenzie, M., J. P. Tulsky, H. L. Long, M. Chesney, and A. Moss. 1999. "Tracking and Follow-Up of Marginalized Populations: A Review." *Journal of Health Care for the Poor and Underserved* 10 (4): 409–29. https://doi.org/10.1353/hpu.2010.0697.

Odierna, D. H., and L. A. Schmidt. 2009. "The Effects of Failing to Include Hard-to-Reach Respondents in Longitudinal Surveys." *American Journal of Public Health* 99 (8): 1515–21.

CHAPTER 22

Practical and Ethical Considerations for Health Research with Refugees

Patricia Gabriel

LEARNING OBJECTIVES

After reading this chapter, you should be able to:

1. Appreciate key ethical challenges to conducting research with refugees.
2. Appreciate key practical challenges to conducting research with refugees.
3. Identify strategies for conducting research with refugees that will facilitate participation in an ethical manner.

BACKGROUND

Conducting health research with vulnerable populations can be ethically challenging, and the protection of research subjects is of paramount importance. At the same time, ensuring that an appropriate representation of the population participates in the study is necessary to achieve valid results and consider generalization of findings. This chapter will explore both methodological and ethical challenges in health research for vulnerable populations focusing on recruitment and the informed consent process with refugees in Canada from which lessons may be learned for application more broadly.

ETHICAL CHALLENGES IN HEALTH RESEARCH WITH REFUGEES

Health research conducted in many Western countries has a dark history. Beyond the prominent examples of the Tuskegee syphilis studies and Nazi human experimentation during World War II, there are numerous accounts of exploitation of research participants across the globe, particularly among vulnerable populations (Lott 2005). Migrant populations in Canada, particularly refugees, are examples of vulnerable groups that pose unique ethical challenges and require conscientious ethical consideration (Campbell-Page and Shaw-Ridley 2013; Lott 2005; Merry et al. 2014). Ethical concerns can occur because of language and cultural barriers, low levels of education, financial burdens, perceived lack of rights, dependency on host country governments, endemic hostility, and a history of physical or emotional distress (Lott 2005; Ellis et al. 2007). These factors can create power imbalances between researchers and participants (Ogilvie, Burgess-Pinto, and Caufield 2008). Consequently, some refugees may be at risk of engaging in research without understanding its voluntary nature, engaging despite known risks because of a lack of perceived alternatives or, at worst, being coerced to participate.

Several scholarly frameworks have been created to guide ethical engagement with all research participants (see table 22.1).

A particularly practical and contemporary article, "What Makes Clinical Research Ethical?" (Emanuel, Wendler, and Grady 2000), outlines seven essential requirements to guide researchers in conducting clinical health research ethically in any setting. In 2007, Ellis applied this framework to specifically consider research with refugees (Ellis et al. 2007). The first of the seven requirements posits that the research must be of social or scientific value and that the research findings should be disseminated so that the knowledge can be put to use. In the refugee setting, Ellis notes the importance and challenge of disseminating findings within refugee communities themselves. Second, research must have scientific validity to avoid potential harm from false conclusions necessitating careful attention to methodological challenges that are more common in refugee research. Third, fair subject selection must focus on the need to recruit subjects on scientific merit, not convenience. This is pertinent in refugee health, given that refugees are often excluded from research aimed at studies of the general population due to challenges with recruitment. For research specifically with refugees, certain individuals may also be excluded due to inadvertent exclusion of minority subgroups. Fourth, there must be a favourable risk/benefit ratio for those participating in the research. Assessing risk and benefit in refugee populations should include an understanding of what specifically may make the refugee group vulnerable and how the participants and community might find the research to be valuable. The fifth principle is the need for independent review of research proposals, typically conducted by institutional review boards or funding agencies in North America. In refugee research, additional review by community members is suggested to contribute to the achievement of the prior five principles. The sixth principle is respect for participants, which requires trust and understanding of participants' perspectives in addition to effective communication and negotiation that addresses underlying power disparities.

The remaining seventh principle, informed consent, attempts to ensure that an individual is participating autonomously. Autonomy in research entails that individuals are capable of deliberation and can act under their own direction without obstruction (National Commission for the Protection of Human Subjects of Biomedical and Behavioral Research

Table 22.1. Ethical Research Frameworks

Framework	Year of Publication	Key Points
The Nuremberg Code	1947	• emerged from the Nuremberg Trial after World War II • research ethics principles for human experimentation • includes principles of informed consent, absence of coercion, and beneficence
Declaration of Helsinki	1964	• created by the World Medical Association • has undergone seven revisions, the most recent in 2013 • focuses on human research ethics
The Belmont Report	1979	• prompted by concerns arising from the Tuskegee Syphilis study • created in the United States by the National Commission for the Protection of Human Services of Bio-medical and Behavioral Research • Three core principles: respect for persons, beneficence, and justice • Three applications: informed consent, assessment of risks and benefits, and selection of subjects
International Ethical Guidelines for Biomedical Research Involving Human Subjects	1982	• by the Council for International Organizations of Medical Sciences • updated in 2002 • contains 21 guidelines with commentary
Canadian Tri-Council Policy Statement: Ethical Conduct of Research Involving Humans	1998	• a joint policy of Canada's three federal research agencies: the Canadian Institutes of Health Research (CIHR), the Natural Sciences and Engineering Research Council of Canada (NSERC), and the Social Sciences and Humanities Research Council of Canada (SSHRC)

1979) and is perhaps the foundation of Western medical ethics. Yet it is the most challenging to address in the refugee context due to language, education, and the cultural context of self-determination, particularly in collectively oriented communities. For Western researchers, the creation of an informed consent process has become a convenient tool where ethical considerations are summarized. For research ethics boards, a study's ethical merit is often scrutinized through analysis of the informed consent form. For better or for worse, informed consent processes have become a proxy for "research ethics" and as such deserve particular attention. However, there is a paucity of empirical evidence (Ellis et al. 2007) directly studying the informed consent process with refugees or assessing refugees' perspectives.

RECRUITMENT CHALLENGES IN HEALTH RESEARCH WITH REFUGEES

In addition to ethical challenges, for those with a history of institutional discrimination, injustice, or trauma, attitudes of distrust, fear, and suspicion (Johnson, Ali, and Shipp 2009) may be more prevalent and may cause individuals to be unduly wary of participation (Dingoyan, Schulz, and Mosko 2012). Refugees have complex migration histories leading to health concerns prior to, during, and after settlement in their new host countries. For many refugees, there may be obvious challenges in recruitment due to communication difficulties as a result of language and cultural barriers (Strohschein et al. 2010), and in the case of some subgroups of refugees, rates of illiteracy are higher (Halabi 2005). Additionally, refugees may be more difficult to recruit due to being a highly mobile, "socially invisible" (Sulaiman-Hill and Thompson 2011), and difficult-to-reach population (Dhanani et al. 2002). For all these reasons, standard Western recruitment strategies may need to be modified.

In response to the lack of research about both informed consent and recruitment with refugees, a 2012 Canadian research study on ethical and practical challenges in health research with refugees was undertaken. This chapter will focus on this research as a case study to further elucidate theoretical and practical issues in research with refugees.

Case Study: Canadian Qualitative Research Study

In 2012, qualitative focus groups were conducted in British Columbia with four government-assisted refugee (GAR) language groups, including Arabic- (Iraqi), Dari- (Afghan), Karen- (Burmese), and Somali- (Somali) speaking refugees to study the success of various recruitment strategies with refugees and to assess refugees' attitudes towards research participation and the informed consent process. Inclusion criteria for the focus groups included GARs who had been in Canada for fewer than five years and were older than 19. Recruitment of refugees was facilitated by hiring four language-concordant research assistants with varying degrees of connectedness to their respective refugee communities. To allow for comparisons of the appropriateness and effectiveness of different strategies, we analyzed five different recruitment methods, including in-person recruitment at a health care clinic, cold calls from a health care clinic, in-person recruitment at a community centre, invitations to research assistants' personal contacts, and snowball sampling of participant contacts. Participants were offered lunch, child care, a transportation reimbursement of 5 dollars, and an honorarium of 20 dollars. The language-concordant focus groups examined participant perspectives on practical and ethical issues of conducting research with refugees, seeking, in particular, to identify factors affecting willingness to participate in research and attitudes towards five traditional components of informed consent. Last, we empirically observed how participants interacted with the three different informed consent process options.

FINDINGS

Factors Affecting Willingness to Participate

Analysis of the four focus groups identified 23 factors influencing refugees' willingness to engage in research (see table 22.2). The findings about refugees were in line with previous findings about the perspectives of ethnic minorities more generally (Dingoyan, Schulz, and Mosko 2012; Levkoff and Sanchez 2003; Ruppenthal, Tuck, and Gagnon 2005); however, new variables were also identified.

Of note, three factors were identified that enhanced the efficacy of recruitment but with ethical concerns. First, if refugees were being recruited into a research study shortly after arrival in their host country, participants predicted that this would result in either lower participation rates due to confusion, fear, and feeling overwhelmed, or higher participation rates due to misconceptions about participation being obligatory or fear of the consequences of refusal. One Karen male stated, "When he first came [he] is confused and he does not want to participate"; a Somali female stated, "For me, if a researcher came on my first day with an interpreter, I would probably cooperate more. But after a week, chances are people have told me so many things, and they have warned me a lot and planted so much fear in me that I will not cooperate." In both circumstances, there are ethical concerns due to the risk of exclusion, on one hand, and of coercion, lack of comprehension, and involuntary participation on the other. As a result, researchers should try to avoid research recruitment shortly after refugees' arrival in the country of resettlement.

Second, if refugees perceive that participation in research is mandatory, they are more likely to participate. The perception of mandatory participation seemed most likely to occur if research activities appeared to be related to government activities. One Afghan female said, "I would find if it is necessary by the government to participate … then I would participate." Consequently, researchers need to pay particular attention to the power dynamics and the perceptions that may occur as a result of any stated or assumed research affiliations. The voluntary nature of participation must be clearly stated and understood.

Third, participants indicated that a refugee's fear of consequences of not participating may also inappropriately increase a participant's willingness to participate at any time. A Somali male commented that "he might take part because he fears if he doesn't they will not help him. So he might even sign the papers without knowing what he is signing." Researchers should be aware of this possibility and make special efforts to inform participants that their health and opportunities will not be affected by refusing to participate.

Recruitment Rates

The overall recruitment rate across all four groups was 66 percent. This rate was consistent with a 2011 systematic literature review of recruitment strategies of focus group research with minority populations in the United States, which showed recruitment rates

Table 22.2. Factors Influencing Willingness to Participate in Research

Research Design Factors		Individual Factors	
Recruitment Factors		**Demographic Variables**	
Financial incentives	Financial incentives increase willingness to participate.	Education level	Low education level may decrease willingness to participate for some, but not all, participants.
Timing	Shorter duration of time in Canada decreases willingness to participate, or increases willingness, but only due to fear and sense of necessity.	Exposure to war	Exposure to war decreases willingness to participate.
Language	Language-concordant research sessions, documents, and research staff or the presence of an interpreter increase willingness to participate.	Lack of local language	Lack of comfort with the local language decreases willingness to participate.
Informed consent	Improved disclosure and enhanced comprehension increase willingness to participate.	Religious beliefs	Religious beliefs generally do not impact willingness to participate in research.
Perception of mandatory participation	If patient perceives research to be mandatory, they are more likely to participate.	Gender of participant	The gender of the participant has variable impact on willingness to participate, from no impact, to females being more likely to participate, to females being less likely to participate.
Research Team Factors		**Participant Attitudes**	
Gender of the researcher	The gender of the researcher generally doesn't matter, but some participants prefer same-gender researchers, particularly for sensitive topics.	Positive attitudes towards research	Positive attitudes towards research increase willingness to participate.
Nationality of the researcher	The nationality of the researcher generally doesn't matter, but it may for refugees with certain political contexts.	Negative attitudes towards research	Fear and suspicion decrease willingness to participate.

continued

Personally knowing the researcher	Personally knowing the researcher increases willingness to participate.		Fear of loss of confidentiality decreases willingness to participate.
Personal qualities of the researcher	Good personal qualities of the researcher, such as friendliness, increase willingness to participate.		Fear of consequences of refusing to participate might increase willingness to participate.
Affiliations or occupation of the researcher	Researcher affiliations with health or settlement organizations, or researchers with trustworthy occupations, increase willingness to participate.		
Research Study Factors		**Participant Knowledge and Experience with Research**	
Expected outcomes of the study	Opportunities that might benefit participants or others, acquiring of knowledge, and a belief that the purpose of the study is meaningful increase willingness to participate.	Previous knowledge and experience with research	Participant knowledge and experience with research did not impact willingness to participate in research.
Logistical factors	A practical location and the availability of child care increase willingness to participate. Time constraints can decrease willingness to participate. Beyond practicality, the location of the research does not seem to matter.		
Safety concerns	Any research that puts participants at risk decreases the likelihood of participation.		

ranging from 43 to 87 percent across 21 studies (Ndumele et al. 2011). Recruitment rates within refugee subgroups for this study ranged from 50 to 82 percent based on language group and from 52 to 89 percent based on method of recruitment (tables 22.3 and 22.4). The most effective recruitment strategy was an invitation from somebody in a familiar community organization, from a research assistant who was already a friend or acquaintance, or from someone else who was already planning on participating. These rates were higher than the two recruitment rates at the health clinic. This finding suggests that being invited to participate by a familiar contact might increase the likelihood of participation, and recruitment through health care workers or a health care clinic might decrease the likelihood of participation.

The language groups with the most effective recruitment rates utilized research assistants that shared similar demographic characteristics with the target population. In this study, the highest recruitment rate was 82 percent in the Arabic group, where the assistant was a refugee from the same country as participants. He was also a physician in his home country, where his occupation was considered a position of respect and authority. The next highest recruitment rates were in the Somali and Karen groups at 69 percent and 65 percent, respectively. Both assistants were refugees sharing the same language and culture with the focus group participants. The language group with the lowest recruitment rate was the Farsi/Dari group at 50 percent. The Farsi-speaking assistant was an immigrant from Iran, while her focus group was primarily composed of refugees from Afghanistan. This finding suggests that research team members with shared demographic features to the target population may have higher recruitment rates.

Table 22.3. Recruitment Rates by Language Group

Language Group	Invited (*N*)	Attended (*N*)	Attended (%)
Farsi	20	10	50
Karen	20	13	65
Somali	16	11	69
Arabic	17	14	82
Total	73	48	66

Table 22.4. Recruitment Rates by Method of Recruitment

Method of Recruitment	Invited (*N*)	Attended (*N*)	Attended (%)
Health clinic in-person	23	12	52
Health clinic cold call	8	5	62
Friend of participant	25	17	68
Friend of researcher	8	6	75
Community centre	9	8	89
Total	73	48	66

FINDINGS ABOUT THE FIVE PRINCIPLES OF INFORMED CONSENT

Disclosure and Comprehension

Disclosure—that is, ensuring that participants are adequately informed—is known to often be complicated by language barriers (Johnson, Ali, and Shipp 2009) and by insufficiently trained research assistants (Nakkash, Makhoul, and Afifi 2009). Inappropriate translation of research materials and a lack of professional interpretation of verbal interactions can result in the inaccurate exchange of information. Research personnel who lack appropriate cultural competency or familiarity with endemic concepts of health and research may be unable to convey information appropriately or accurately to participants, thus preventing them from being truly informed.

Comprehension refers to a participant's ability to understand the purpose of the research and the implications of participating in the research. Comprehension can be compromised in refugee populations. Participants may struggle with understanding due to illiteracy, low levels of formal education, and lack of familiarity with research (Nakkash, Makhoul, and Afifi 2009). If there is a power differential, assessing comprehension can be difficult if participants are unwilling or unable to disclose a lack of understanding due to fear, embarrassment, or a desire to please. As a result, for refugees, there is a higher risk of consent without understanding their rights, and a higher risk of refusal to participate due to a lack of understanding of the rationale or objectives of the proposed research (Lott 2005; Wong-Kim and Song 2007).

Assessment of the informed consent process in this case study showed that disclosure and comprehension were facilitated by training research assistants (RAs) and recruitment team members, providing language-concordant written and oral information, and repeating information on numerous occasions. Insufficient disclosure and comprehension were noted to occur when relying on word-of-mouth recruitment strategies and when informing participants with limited literacy and low formal education.

Analysis of the focus group transcripts identified marked cross-cultural consensus about the importance of ensuring disclosure and comprehension. The ability to ask questions was highlighted by participants as a means of achieving comprehension, and comfort with the language of engagement was a key determinant for a participant's likelihood of feeling comfortable to do so. Comprehension was highly valued, and participants indicated that if they did not understand the purpose of the study, they would not participate. One Arabic male captured this concisely, stating, "For me, I wouldn't agree to participate in any research if I didn't understand."

Capacity

Capacity broadly implies an individual's ability to reason and make his or her own decisions. In refugees, as in any population, capacity can be affected by age and mental ability.

With certain vulnerable migrants, capacity can also be impacted by real or perceived extraneous cultural or political circumstances that may limit an individual's liberty (Nakkash, Makhoul, and Afifi 2009). Practically, an individual's ability to participate in research may be impacted by language barriers or by illiteracy.

Capacity was addressed by having an age cut-off of 19 years, and health care workers and RAs were asked to consider the appropriateness of inviting anyone with known decreased mental capacity. Knowing that language and illiteracy could impair a participant's capacity, we designed all parts of the study to be accessible to those without any English language skills or literacy.

Observationally, we did not witness any overt examples where a participant was incapable of deciding whether or not to participate independently. However, assistance in signing consent forms or documenting responses on questionnaires was often sought from fellow participants; thus, we were no longer able to ensure a participant's autonomy or confidentiality in documenting their opinion.

From our qualitative findings, insufficient language skill was mentioned as a barrier that might result in declining participation. A history of exposure to war was thought to negatively impact a refugee's ability, not just willingness, to participate in research. Education and literacy were also mentioned as factors influencing a participant's ability to participate, mostly as potential barriers, but participants rejected this notion in some cases. This was captured most clearly by a Somali woman who reflected on uneducated participants being able to partake in research, stating, "because you still have a brain, and if you put your mind to it, you can change something."

Case Study: Informed Consent?

A bilingual university student working as a research assistant was trained to facilitate the focus group session with a group of mostly illiterate Somali women. After reading his own translation of the English consent form out loud in Somali, he asked if there were any questions. After answering questions, he asked the women to sign the consent form if they felt comfortable participating. If they did not sign, but still wished to participate, they did not have to sign the form—they could stay, and their consent would be inferred by any participation in the conversation. Women could also choose to leave if they did not want to participate. About half the women signed their own forms. It became clear that some women did not know how to sign their own name. One women showed her neighbour how to make and X on the consent line. Another pair of women huddled over the consent form and one women signed her neighbour's form on her behalf. Some forms were left unsigned. The focus group continued without anyone leaving, and all women participated in the conversation.

Voluntariness

Voluntariness means that an individual agrees to participate in research under conditions that are free of undue influence and coercion. In research with refugees, voluntariness can be impacted by a power imbalance between researchers and participants (Mkandawire-Valhmu, Rice, and Bathum 2009). Refugees may also be influenced by a desire to please or to act altruistically (Ellis et al. 2007). Reimbursements or promises of reward might be unreasonably persuasive in the context of refugees who often live in poverty, and this may lead to coercion (Nakkash, Makhoul, and Afifi 2009). Refugees from sociopolitical environments that violate human rights may not trust that an invitation to participate in research is truly voluntary and may fear negative consequences to declining to participate, such as deportation or loss of legal status (Ellis et al. 2007). In collectivist-oriented cultures, individuals may be influenced by the desires of their family or community, or may even defer the decision to participate in research to another individual (Ellis et al. 2007). The Western construct of voluntariness may not be valid in all ethnocultural contexts.

In our study design, we tried to facilitate voluntary participation by informing participants at each stage of the process that participation was voluntary. For those being recruited at the health clinic, we specifically indicated that their ability to receive ongoing health care would not be impacted by their decision to participate. While food and a financial reimbursement were offered, we felt that these were not out of proportion to the participant's contribution of time, and participants were also informed that they were welcome to leave after lunch and that they would still receive their reimbursement.

Evidence of voluntary participation was apparent in all four groups. Most participants contributed eagerly during the focus groups sessions and for the most part were in no rush to leave at the end of the session. One Karen male concluded the session by saying, "On behalf of us, we are very happy to participate in this research study and thank you for doing a research and we would like you to do more research study in the future."

Despite our efforts to inform participants of the voluntary nature of the study, there was a possibility that some of the participation was involuntary. For example, all patients approached at the health clinic agreed to receive a follow-up phone call from an RA. While this high rate of agreement may have been truly voluntary, only half ultimately attended the focus group sessions. This suggests that patients may have had difficulty saying no to a member of their health care team.

There may have also been involuntary participation resulting from our snowball sampling approach. Parents and spouses often volunteered to bring their family members, and the research assistant did not necessarily speak to these family members independently. The level and type of persuasion utilized within families is unknown, but the potential for involuntary participation did exist, as we had five participants bring a spouse, and six other participants brought their adult children, of which at least two noticeably participated very little in the focus group session.

In the focus groups, while many participants agreed that participation would often be voluntary, many comments indicated a likelihood of involuntary participation due to compliance with authority, a fear of the consequences of not participating, a desire to reciprocate a favour, or their decision having been made by a family member. One Somali female said, "When I was new and I came, someone comes to me, they already welcomed me, I really don't know them that well yet, so I will do whatever they tell me to do."

DOCUMENTATION OF CONSENT

The final step in ensuring the principle of autonomy involves the act of giving consent, where an individual indicates that they are willing to participate. This typically takes place with the signing of a written consent form. Obtaining written consent can be negatively impacted by a participant's literacy level or by their suspiciousness of signing "official" documents (Karwalajtys et al. 2010). Oral-based cultures may prefer oral or implied consent (Ellis et al. 2007). However, these methods introduce potential challenges and may encounter resistance from ethics review boards.

In our study, we created three options for participants to indicate their consent to participate. These included signing a language-concordant consent form, implied consent by handing in signed or unsigned questionnaires, and implied consent by participation in the focus group session.

Observation of consent rates across three methods revealed a high rate of signed consent (92 percent). Of note, the informed consent process took up to 25 minutes in the most illiterate group—some participants did not know how to sign their name and asked a neighbour to sign. Further, over 30 percent of the signed consent forms had some degree of "error," such as not being dated. Implied consent as demonstrated by handing in questionnaires voluntarily was 98 percent and by participation in the focus groups was 100 percent.

From the focus groups, most participants were comfortable with documentation of consent with a signature and preferred this method. However, in the Somali group, there was no consensus: some preferred no documentation while another strongly indicated a preference for documentation. There was concern about arousing suspicion for both recording consent in writing and verbally. In regard to written consent forms, participants preferred shorter forms, so long as they sufficiently conveyed necessary information, and there was a strong preference for forms to be written in participants' own language.

RECOMMENDATIONS FOR HEALTH RESEARCH WITH REFUGEES

To improve recruitment rates, investigators should consider logistical factors such as selecting convenient times and locations, providing child care, and considering the provision of reasonable financial reimbursement for participants' time. With respect to communication factors, we recommend ensuring that all research materials and in-person communications are available in the participants' own languages, providing clear information about the purpose of the research, and ensuring comprehension. With respect to the timing of recruitment, researchers should be cautious about recruiting refugees for research in the first several months after their arrival.

Further recommendations include engaging RAs who speak participants' language and who are good communicators with strong interpersonal skills. For sensitive research topics, consider using RAs who are the same gender as the target population. Engaging RAs who are personally acquainted with potential participants or who are affiliated with health or settlement services may also enhance recruitment; however, one must be cautious that this does not result in coercion or the perception of involuntary participation. Further, researchers must consider the impact on the community members serving as part of the research team and the ethical dilemmas that they might face (Molyneux, Kamuya, and Marsh 2010; Stapleton, Murphy, and Kildea 2015), balancing the objectives of recruitment with their role in the community.

Researchers should be aware of the characteristics of refugee subgroups that may be associated with recruitment challenges and corresponding strategies that may aid in engaging these groups. Refugees who have lower levels of education or who are illiterate may have more trouble participating in research. This can be addressed by using appropriate terminology and aiding in reading written materials. Refugees who have been exposed to war may also be reluctant to engage in research. Researchers should consider the ethical appropriateness of recruiting this population and consider the benefits and harms of participation for these individuals. Refugees who for various reasons may have negative attitudes towards research, such as suspicion of research and fear of loss of confidentiality, are less likely to engage in research. To address this, researchers can ensure transparency of research procedures, adequate disclosure, opportunities for questions, and diligent attention to maintaining confidentiality. With respect to gender, some female refugee subgroups may be shy or fear shame. This may be addressed by utilizing female RAs. As for males, they may have more concerns about financial and occupation commitments that could be affected by participating in research. This can be addressed by planning appropriate times for research activities and providing financial reimbursements.

Beyond recruitment challenges, there are additional practical challenges in refugee research, such as managing multilingual data, using interpreters, using methods of translating data, adapting research tools, and retaining participants for long-term studies (Arriaza et al. 2015; McMichael et al. 2014; Formea et al. 2014). Current recommendations for addressing methodological challenges share features with the above suggestions for recruitment, such as consulting with refugee communities (Riggs et al. 2015), utilizing participatory research approaches (Makhoul et al. 2014), and formally training community members as RAs (Hawley et al. 2014; Formea et al. 2014; Stapleton, Murphy, and Kildea 2015). Additional recommendations exist that are specific to qualitative methods (Arriaza et al. 2015) and longitudinal cohort studies (McMichael et al. 2014).

Recommendations for ethical conduct of research starts with ensuring adequate disclosure and comprehension by providing language-appropriate oral and written information, with additional time, in an environment where participants are comfortable asking questions, particularly for participants from populations with low literacy and education levels. We recommend pilot testing all research materials with members of the target population.

To address factors that might impact capacity to give consent, such as low education, illiteracy, and previous exposure to war, researchers should consult with members of the target community to identify appropriate ways to empower refugees with these characteristics so that they may have the opportunity to participate if desired.

To facilitate voluntary participation, we recommend informing participants at each stage of the process that participation is voluntary. For those being recruited at a health clinic, it should be specifically indicated that refugees' ability to receive ongoing health care will not be affected by their decision to participate. Keep in mind that refugees may have difficulty saying no to a member of their health care team; try to create a recruitment strategy that will empower a potential participant to feel comfortable declining. If food or financial reimbursement are offered, consider that these are not out of proportion to the participant's contribution of time to prevent an incentive being unduly persuasive. If using a snowball sampling approach, consider that parents and spouses may volunteer to bring their family members without their explicit consent and that the level and type of persuasion that might be utilized is unknown. Efforts should be made to contact these individuals independently to ensure that they have adequate comprehension.

Voluntariness can be affected by utilizing a familiar person in recruitment. On one hand, it can address the traditional power imbalance between researchers and participants (Ogilvie, Burgess-Pinto, and Caufield 2008). In ideal circumstances, utilizing a familiar person may help interested but otherwise fearful or shy potential participants engage in an opportunity; at the same time, it may foster autonomy by enhancing comprehension and empowering participants to comfortably decline to participate. However, using a familiar person may result in feelings of obligation or a desire to please. How to address this complexity is unclear, and a broader vision may be needed to consider what is ethical and voluntary in the context of the refugee populations' ethical paradigm.

Last, for documentation of consent, multiple options for oral, verbal, and implied consent should be considered based on community consultation. With written consent, language-concordant and local language options should be available, and consent forms should be concise yet sufficient to include necessary information.

Additional challenges are prevalent in addressing the other key ethical principles of justice, beneficence, and non-malfeasance in refugee health research. A review of these, along with valuable recommendations, are summarized by Merry and colleagues (2014) and serve as a useful tool for any Canadian researchers involved in refugee health research.

CONCLUSION

This chapter draws on a literature review and analysis of novel research on recruitment and the informed consent process in refugees. It identifies recruitment strategies, research design factors, and participant factors associated with recruitment success. It also articulates how to facilitate participant autonomy through the informed consent process. The recommendations in this chapter should be considered by researchers and ethics boards across Canada and other culturally similar countries that receive refugees. Refugees face similar challenges to engaging in research with some other minority and under-served populations. Consequently, the findings and suggestions for research with refugees may be carefully extrapolated for consideration in other vulnerable populations.

CRITICAL THINKING QUESTIONS

1. In Western bioethics, participant autonomy is prioritized over other ethical principles such as benefit to a participant or to a community. In collectivist cultures, participant autonomy may be seen as secondary to the goals and values of a community. For example, in some cultures, it might be expected that the male head of household or a community leader be consulted prior to an individual consenting to participate in a research study. How might such a request be addressed for research occurring in Canada?
2. Research with refugees often requires assistance from bilingual members of the refugee community working with the research team. What types of ethical dilemmas may arise for these community-based research team members?
3. How might community-based participatory research methods address practical and ethical challenges to doing research with refugees?

RECOMMENDED READINGS

1. For a concise review of the seven essential requirements to guide researchers in conducting clinical health research ethically with refugees, the following peer-reviewed article is recommended:
   Ellis, B. H., M. Kia-Keating, S. A. Yusuf, A. Lincoln, and A. Nur. 2007. "Ethical Research in Refugee Communities and the Use of Community Participatory Methods." *Transcultural Psychiatry* 44 (3): 459–81.

2. For further details on factors that affect refugees' willingness to participate in research and details of the study covered in this chapter, a concise review can be found in the following peer-reviewed article:
   Gabriel, Patricia, Janusz Kaczorowski, and Nicole Berry. 2017. "Recruitment of Refugees for Health Research: A Qualitative Study to Add Refugees' Perspectives." *International Journal of Environmental Research and Public Health* 14 (2): 125.

3. For a comprehensive review of practical and ethical issues in conducting health research with refugees, consider referring to Patricia Gabriel's full master's thesis on this topic:

Gabriel, Patricia. 2013. "Practical and Ethical Issues in Conducting Health Research with Refugees." MA thesis, Faculty of Health Sciences, Simon Fraser University. http://summit.sfu.ca/item/13738.

REFERENCES

Arriaza, P., F. Nedjat-Haiem, H. Y. Lee, and S. S. Martin. 2015. "Guidelines for Conducting Rigorous Health Care Psychosocial Cross-Cultural/Language Qualitative Research." *Social Work in Public Health* 30 (1): 75–87.

Campbell-Page, R. M., and M. Shaw-Ridley. 2013. "Managing Ethical Dilemmas in Community-Based Participatory Research with Vulnerable Populations." *Health Promotion Practice* 14 (4): 485–90.

Dhanani, S., J. Damron-Rodriguez, M. Leung, V. Villa, D. L. Washington, T. Makinodan, and N. Harada. 2002. "Community-Based Strategies for Focus Group Recruitment of Minority Veterans." *Military Medicine* 167 (6): 501–5.

Dingoyan, D., H. Schulz, and M. Mosko. 2012. "The Willingness to Participate in Health Research Studies of Individuals with Turkish Migration Backgrounds: Barriers and Resources." *European Psychiatry: The Journal of the Association of European Psychiatrists* 27 (suppl 2): S4–9.

Ellis, B. H., M. Kia-Keating, S. A. Yusuf, A. Lincoln, and A. Nur. 2007. "Ethical Research in Refugee Communities and the Use of Community Participatory Methods." *Transcultural Psychiatry* 44 (3): 459–81.

Emanuel, E. J., D. Wendler, and C. Grady. 2000. "What Makes Clinical Research Ethical?" *JAMA: The Journal of the American Medical Association* 283 (20): 2701–11.

Formea, C. M., A. A. Mohamed, A. Hassan, A. Osman, J. A. Weis, I. G. Sia, and M. L. Wieland. 2014. "Lessons Learned: Cultural and Linguistic Enhancement of Surveys through Community-Based Participatory Research." *Progress in Community Health Partnerships: Research, Education, and Action* 8 (3): 331–6.

Halabi, J. O. 2005. "Nursing Research with Refugee Clients: A Call for More Qualitative Approaches." *International Nursing Review* 52 (4): 270–5.

Hawley, N. C., M. L. Wieland, J. A. Weis, and I. G. Sia. 2014. "Perceived Impact of Human Subjects Protection Training on Community Partners in Community-Based Participatory Research." *Progress in Community Health Partnerships: Research, Education, and Action* 8 (2): 241–8.

Johnson, C. E., S. A. Ali, and M. P. Shipp. 2009. "Building Community-Based Participatory Research Partnerships with a Somali Refugee Community." *American Journal of Preventive Medicine* 37 (6 suppl 1): S230–6.

Karwalajtys, T. L., L. J. Redwood-Campbell, N. C. Fowler, L. H. Lohfeld, M. Howard, J. A. Kaczorowski, and A. Lytwyn. 2010. "Conducting Qualitative Research on Cervical Cancer Screening among Diverse Groups of Immigrant Women: Research Reflections: Challenges and Solutions." *Canadian Family Physician / Medecin De Famille Canadien* 56 (4): e130–5.

Levkoff, S., and H. Sanchez. 2003. "Lessons Learned about Minority Recruitment and Retention from the Centers on Minority Aging and Health Promotion." *Gerontologist* 43 (1): 18–26.

Lott, J. P. 2005. "Module Three: Vulnerable/Special Participant Populations." *Developing World Bioethics* 5 (1): 30–54.

Makhoul, J., R. Nakkash, T. Harpham, and Y. Qutteina. 2014. "Community-Based Participatory Research in Complex Settings: Clean Mind—Dirty Hands." *Health Promotion International* 29 (3): 510–17.

McMichael, C., C. Nunn, S. M. Gifford, and I. Correa-Velez. 2014. "Studying Refugee Settlement through Longitudinal Research: Methodological and Ethical Insights from the Good Starts Study." *Journal of Refugee Studies* 28 (2): 238–57.

Merry, L., A. Low, F. Carnevale, and A. J. Gagnon. 2014. "Participation of Childbearing International Migrant Women in Research: The Ethical Balance." *Nursing Ethics* 23 (1): 61–78.

Mkandawire-Valhmu, L., E. Rice, and M. E. Bathum. 2009. "Promoting an Egalitarian Approach to Research with Vulnerable Populations of Women." *Journal of Advanced Nursing* 65 (8): 1725–34.

Molyneux, S., D. Kamuya, and V. Marsh. 2010. "Community Members Employed on Research Projects Face Crucial, Often Under-Recognized, Ethical Dilemmas." *American Journal of Bioethics: AJOB* 10 (3): 24–26.

Nakkash, R., J. Makhoul, and R. Afifi. 2009. "Obtaining Informed Consent: Observations from Community Research with Refugee and Impoverished Youth." *Journal of Medical Ethics* 35 (10): 638–43.

National Commission for the Protection of Human Subjects of Biomedical and Behavioral Research. 1979. *Belmont Report: Ethical Principles and Guidelines for the Protection of Human Subjects of Research.* Washington, DC: US Department of Health, Education and Welfare.

Ndumele, C. D., G. Ableman, B. E. Russell, E. Gurrola, and L. S. Hicks. 2011. "Publication of Recruitment Methods in Focus Group Research of Minority Populations with Chronic Disease: A Systematic Review." *Journal of Health Care for the Poor and Underserved* 22 (1): 5–23.

Ogilvie, L. D., E. Burgess-Pinto, and C. Caufield. 2008. "Challenges and Approaches to Newcomer Health Research." *Journal of Transcultural Nursing* 19 (1): 64–73.

Riggs, E., J. Yelland, J. Szwarc, S. Casey, D. Chesters, P. Duell-Piening, S. Wahidi, F. Fouladi, and S. Brown. 2015. "Promoting the Inclusion of Afghan Women and Men in Research: Reflections from Research and Community Partners Involved in Implementing a 'Proof of Concept' Project." *International Journal for Equity in Health* 14 (1): 13.

Ruppenthal, L., J. Tuck, and A. J. Gagnon. 2005. "Enhancing Research with Migrant Women through Focus Groups." *Western Journal of Nursing Research* 27 (6): 735–54.

Stapleton, H. M. R., R. Murphy, and S. V. Kildea. 2015. "Insiders as Outsiders: Bicultural Research Assistants Describe Their Participation in the Evaluation of an Antenatal Clinic for Women from Refugee Backgrounds." *Qualitative Social Work* 14 (2): 275–92.

Strohschein, F. J., L. Merry, J. Thomas, and A. J. Gagnon. 2010. "Strengthening Data Quality in Studies of Migrants Not Fluent in Host Languages: A Canadian Example with Reproductive Health Questionnaires." *Research in Nursing & Health* 33 (4): 369–79.

Sulaiman-Hill, C. M., and S. C. Thompson. 2011. "Sampling Challenges in a Study Examining Refugee Resettlement." *BMC International Health and Human Rights* 11: 2.

Wong-Kim, E., and Y. Song. 2007. "Obtaining Informed Consent for Research on Immigrant Populations." *Journal of Empirical Research on Human Research Ethics: JERHRE* 2 (1): 83–84.

CHAPTER 23

Engaging Communities to Identify Needs and Develop Solutions: Participatory Research Incorporates Community Voice in All Aspects of Health Research Decision-Making

Jon Salsberg, Soultana Macridis, Treena Delormier, Richard Hovey, Neil Andersson, Alex M. McComber, and Ann C. Macaulay

---

LEARNING OBJECTIVES

After reading this chapter, you should be able to:

1. Summarize principles of participatory research and distinguish between traditional research and participatory research.
2. Describe and understand the benefits and value, as well as the challenges, of participatory research for community and for the research process.
3. Describe how participatory research underpins knowledge translation.
4. Appreciate who is community, how community is represented, and the ethical implications surrounding community.
5. Provide examples of how participatory research has been incorporated into various research designs (such as randomized control trials).

BACKGROUND

Participatory research (PR) is an approach to research that fosters equity and self-determination through engaging individuals and communities to contribute their knowledge and expertise in shaping scientific inquiry—and so it gives voice to marginalized or underserved populations. PR builds research partnerships *with* communities for the goals of incorporating local expertise to identify community issues and develop the evidence and interventions. This contrasts with top-down research *on* or *about* communities and interventions developed *for* communities by external *experts*, including policy-makers, health officials, health professionals, and researchers. PR is the systematic co-creation of new knowledge by researchers working in equitable partnerships with those affected by the issue under study, or those who will benefit from it or ultimately act on its results (Green et al. 1995; Israel et al. 1998; Macaulay et al. 1999). Partners can include communities, patients, health care providers, and policy-makers. PR encompasses any research design and is not a methodology but rather an approach to equitable co–decision-making. Thus, PR promotes social justice, self-determination, and knowledge utilization (Cargo and Mercer 2008) by increasing communities' capacity to identify and address their own issues and increasing decision-makers' and service providers' abilities to mobilize resources and improve policies and professional practices (Gaventa and Cornwall 2006; Macaulay et al. 1999; Minkler and Wallerstein 2008).

PR also integrates *knowledge translation* by including appropriate end-user partners in decision-making throughout the research. Partners should be offered full engagement, but they may choose not to be involved in every stage, such as the development of tools or the collection and analysis of data. Significantly, partners should be involved in finalizing the research questions, interpreting results, and disseminating and applying findings (Macaulay et al. 1999; Minkler and Wallerstein 2008; Parry, Salsberg, and Macaulay 2009; Salsberg, Macaulay, and Parry 2014). *Integrated knowledge translation* is the preferred means of co-creating action-oriented knowledge to assure that contextual factors are always central to knowledge production, thus improving relevance and knowledge uptake (Salsberg, Macaulay, and Parry 2014; Straus, Tetroe, and Graham 2009).

PR builds on the existing strengths of individuals and communities. Community members, including those in marginalized or under-served communities, know best how to approach problems, and they have an intimate understanding of their social environments and ways to build on existing resilience (Kirmayer et al. 2011).

It Doesn't Matter Who Asks Whom to Dance

Some researchers are concerned that their project cannot be truly participatory if the question did not originate from their knowledge-user partners. While it is certainly true that if the research question comes from the end-user group, you can guarantee that the group has an interest in the project and the results, this is not the only way to get there. The impetus can just as easily arise from the researcher, and can be successful, as long as it resonates meaningfully with the knowledge users. Sometimes researchers, familiar with the current state of their field, are better situated to identify an issue as needing investigation, and can bring this to the attention of those who may need to know.

CASE STUDY 1—HEALTH PROFESSIONAL INITIATION

A nurse is very concerned that many patients, especially those from various ethnic and Indigenous communities, are not completing their treatment for tuberculosis (TB). She explains her concern to a researcher who suggests partnering with representatives from

continued

these communities. The end result is a research team, including research associates from seven ethnic communities and three Indigenous communities, with goals to identify and understand sociocultural factors and improve practices for prevention and treatment of TB. The team developed guiding foundation principles, and the community partners helped finalize the questions, interview their community members, interpret the results, and disseminate the findings back to their communities. Outcomes included six single-page information sheets in the languages of participating communities, which were also printed in local newspapers and featured on a local radio call-in show; an educational video; and a nurse educator who would visit high-risk communities with new research-based knowledge and community-specific TB prevention strategies. The trained community research associates gained new skills useful for further employment (Gibson et al. 2005).

CASE STUDY 2—RESEARCHER INITIATION

A researcher wishes to conduct a systematic review of *the benefits of using participatory research*. She first assembled a team of co-investigators, including experts in all the areas needed to strengthen the review. The team then imagines the possible end-users of the knowledge they hope to produce and forms a list of possible decision-maker partners, including funding agencies, university ethics review boards, public health agencies, and organizations dedicated to promoting participatory research with both community and academic members. These partners are approached, and one stakeholder from each of these domains agrees to join the project. As partners, they then contribute to refining and finalizing the study design for the grant application and commit themselves to partnering on the research and disseminating and applying results within their organizations (Jagosh et al. 2011).

CASE STUDY 3—COMMUNITY INITIATION

An Indigenous physician in a family medicine resident training program undertakes a chart review in his community hospital and determines that the prevalence of type 2 diabetes among adult members of his community is twice as high as the national population. Beside publishing these results in a mainstream clinical journal, the resident and his supervisor present these results to community members and political leaders who, naturally, find these rates alarming. They are particularly concerned that their children, grandchildren, and the *seventh generation* going forward do not have to bear this same burden, so they ask the family doctors to "*do something about it.*" The doctors reply that they are not sure what they could do but would seek advice from research colleagues at the university. This community prompting led to a long-standing community-based participatory research project (see the Kahnawake Schools Diabetes Prevention Project [KSDPP] case study further down in this chapter) (Macaulay et al. 1997).

COMMUNITY

Who represents community? This is an age-old question (Green and Mercer 2001). Classically, communities form community advisory boards (CABs) or committees to partner with researchers. CAB members are frequently those whose lives are affected by the issue under study, community leaders, representatives of community organizations, and interested individuals. Depending on specific goals, CABs may also include health professionals, service managers, and policy-makers (Malus et al. 2011). At the beginning, the important question is, "Who is in a position to use the results to effect change?" If decision-makers are included from the beginning, they will be well placed to trust the results and use their positions to speed knowledge uptake. Guidelines exist for assessing the appropriateness of partnerships and their level of engagement (Mercer et al. 2008).

THE EVIDENCE FOR PR BENEFITS

A systematic review of PR partnerships with high levels of community engagement, co–decision-making, and co-governance (Jagosh et al. 2012) documented multiple benefits. PR generates (1) culturally and logistically appropriate research characteristics for shaping the scope of research, developing and implementing program and research protocols, interpreting data, and disseminating findings; (2) the capacity to recruit community members to advisory boards, for implementation, and as program recipients (intervention enrolment); (3) the capacity of both community and research partners; (4) conflict between partners that, when resolved, leads to positive outcomes for subsequent programming; (5) the accumulation of partnership synergy through repeated successful experiences, thus increasing the quality of outcomes over time; (6) sustained goals beyond initial funding and during funding gaps; and (7) systems change and new unanticipated projects and activity. Interviews with researchers and community members showed that implementing and maintaining trust was a key element, with projects evolving through *ripple effects*, where outcomes of one stage formed the context for the next stage (Jagosh et al. 2015).

PRACTICAL STAGES IN PR

PR may start with a community-identified action need, or a researcher-identified knowledge gap. Whichever its origins, what is important is that all partners agree on the relevance of the issue. While researchers provide methodological know-how, partners provide expert knowledge on context, history, and setting. PR is an exercise in trust building, particularly in cases where partners have been ill-served or harmed by past research. Community members should have opportunities to fully understand the knowledge-creation process, including opportunities for collecting and analyzing data.

Community partners *must* be involved in interpreting the results, as they know best what findings mean within their context (Macaulay et al. 2007), and they must have a full voice in crafting messages both for their peers and the larger academic and practice communities. This strengthens the messaging and mitigates stigmatizing language, which has frequently harmed communities (Katz and Martin 1997).

PR CHALLENGES

What can be challenging for researchers is learning how to work as members of a team, learning how to respect other viewpoints, sharing power and authority, developing positive relationships, understanding different agendas and time frames, developing the flexibility required to accommodate unexpected events, building trust, and finding mutually beneficial solutions (Salsberg, Macaulay, and Parry 2014). Community partners face similar challenges, including the need to understand the importance of research rigour and university time frames. To overcome these barriers, researchers need to develop skills that include active listening, lay communication, nominal group processes, negotiation and conflict resolution, the ability to work in multicultural environments (including multidisciplinary cultures), self-reflection, and the ability to admit one's errors. Most importantly, researchers must develop humility: a willingness to learn from community—to recognize that others have knowledge and experiences that, though very different than their own, will make valuable contributions (Mercer et al. 2008; Salsberg, Macaulay, and Parry 2014).

ETHICAL GUIDELINES

All research requires adherence to mandated bioethical regulations. Beyond individual informed consent, partnership research *additionally* requires obtaining community consent. In Canada, this is outlined in the second edition of the *Tri-Council Policy Statement: Ethical Conduct for Research Involving Humans* (TCPS2) (Panel on Research Ethics 2014). In addition, researchers must adhere to setting-specific ethics (see Healey, Chapter 20 in this volume, and the KSDPP case study below).

Important PR ethical considerations include the following: Who represents the community, and do they have a legitimate voice recognized by the community members implicated in the research? Who owns the data and the results? A useful data ownership framework is OCAP® (*ownership, control, access,* and *possession*), developed by the National Aboriginal Health Organization (NAHO 2007). Also, does your institutional ethical review board allow for prior or parallel community review? TCPS2 requires that in certain circumstances, the ethical review board include community representatives; however, separate prior or parallel review by a community board allows for a stronger community voice and greater community protection.

COMMUNITY-LED RANDOMIZED CONTROL TRIALS

PR has a long heritage of use with small localized groups of people, geographical communities (e.g., Indigenous communities), people sharing a common experience (e.g., people with HIV/AIDS, refugees), and urban ethnic communities. However, PR can be multi-centred, national or international in scope, and now includes large-scale community-led randomized control trials (RCTs).

RCTs are often upheld as the gold standard for determining effectiveness and are necessary to generate the evidence to sway policy-makers to allocate resources. Therefore, we should merge the evidence-generating power of RCTs with the community empowerment and action power of PR.

Rebuilding from Resilience was a partnership of 12 Indigenous women's shelters across Canada, and the first Indigenous, completely community-run clustered RCT. This tested the impact and cost implications of evidence-based community-led initiatives to decrease domestic violence (Andersson et al. 2010). For the women's shelters, randomization was a fair way of working out whose turn was next to receive the available resources. At a design meeting, each shelter director drew a number out of a hat, indicating whether their shelter would join the first wave or the second wave. The comparison between the first wave and a second wave provided the "control" comparison—that is, the second-wave baseline provided an unexposed contrast for the follow-up study of the first wave after two years of interventions.

In another community-led trial conducted in Mexico and Nicaragua, communities were engaged to discuss evidence on dengue in their region, local volunteers received training, and communities selected and implemented their own dengue prevention strategies (Andersson et al. 2015). Both trials were examples of how communities reduced gender violence and dengue infections; they were not about externally developed, silver-bullet behaviour-change interventions (Iwama et al. 2009).

CASE STUDY: THE KAHNAWAKE SCHOOLS DIABETES PREVENTION PROJECT

The Kahnawake Schools Diabetes Prevention Project (KSDPP) is a long-established PR partnership between the Kanien'kehá:ka (Mohawk) community of Kahnawà:ke (Quebec) and university-based researchers. For two decades, KSDPP has undertaken numerous PR projects focusing on intervention and policy programming for the primary prevention of type 2 diabetes (see http://www.ksdpp.org and http://pram.mcgill.ca/ksdpp_pubs.php for all KSDPP scientific publications). All research is overseen by the community advisory board (CAB) and follows the *KSDPP Code of Research Ethics* (KSDPP 2007; Macaulay et al. 1998)—jointly developed principles emphasizing community self-determination and Kanien'kehá:ka world view. Thus, KSDPP assures that all research addresses community-identified needs and combines scientific rigour with Kanien'kehá:ka traditional values and decision-making. This exemplifies *two-eyed seeing* (Hatcher et al. 2009; Iwama et al. 2009), incorporating both Western and Indigenous knowledge frameworks.

Social-Relational Understandings of Health and Well-Being from an Indigenous Perspective

In response to a discussion regarding increasing community programming for diabetes prevention, a project was established to examine how well-being was understood within Kahnawà:ke (Hovey, Delormier, and McComber 2014). The researchers employed philosophical hermeneutics (Davey 2006; Gadamer 1989, 1996; Hovey 2014) with Haudenosaunee (Iroquois) world view and ways of knowing to value Kanien'kehá:ka concepts of holistic well-being, while respecting the unique social and historical context of Kahnawà:ke to achieve a decolonized research approach. This approach structured the collection, analysis, and interpretation of interviews conducted with key community stakeholders. Findings revealed that the *social* conditions created by external Western influences on culture, language, and epistemologies are strongly connected to the *relational* conditions that continue to influence the health and well-being of individuals, families, and the community—a sentiment echoed in other Indigenous communities (see Healey, Chapter 20 in this volume). In Kahnawà:ke, well-being was closely related to being *Onkwehón:we* ("real human beings who live with spirit"), to the roles and responsibilities of families as nurturers of health-promoting relationships, and to processes promoting the healing of multi-generational traumas rooted in colonization. Developing a shared understanding of what is required to effectively prevent type 2 diabetes while simultaneously fostering the sense of being Onkwehón:we is a new approach to health promotion within Kahnawà:ke. This may have relevance in other Indigenous communities with health issues rooted in similar historical and social-relational conditions.

Influencing Policy

KSDPP and two community elementary schools partnered to develop and implement a School Wellness Policy to promote healthy nutrition and physical activity (Hogan et al. 2014). This policy includes the community-identified need to develop school active transportation (AT) to increase physical activity through walking or biking to school (Active Healthy Kids Canada 2014; Buliung et al. 2011). With KSDPP and school support, a doctoral student, with expertise in school AT, initiated a School Travel Planning (STP) project (Macridis 2015; Macridis et al. 2016; Salsberg et al. 2017). The student recruited an STP committee comprising teachers, parents, school administrators, transportation management, a community protection representative, and KSDPP intervention staff, who met monthly from January 2013 to August 2014.

Engagement and Knowledge Co-creation

Following the *KSDPP Code of Research Ethics* (KSDPP 2007), the research was jointly developed, and data were jointly collected, analyzed, and interpreted, which contributed to a context-specific and evidence-informed STP Action Plan for the elementary schools. The first eight months were spent building trust, designing the research, and planning data collection activities, timelines, and terms of reference. All committee members participated in one or more data collection activities based on discussions of Active and Safe Routes to School (Green Communities Canada 2012), including on-site traffic observations, walkability assessments, and in-class mapping by elementary school children (Macridis 2015; Macridis et al. 2016; Salsberg et al. 2017). Involvement in data collection and providing feedback on analysis afforded members first-hand research experience.

Integrating Knowledge Translation Activities

Committee members combined their expertise with baseline findings and translated these into actions for each school. General goals included reducing traffic congestion, increasing

Insights from Community Stakeholders

The participatory nature of the STP project allowed for community stakeholders to share and learn about their unique experiences and perspectives, both personally and professionally. Before the project began, a community stakeholder stated, "there [were] a few things we knew about ahead of time. First and foremost, it was the safety aspect of it. Ya know, parents are extremely over protective." Through involvement in the STP project, members were able to validate preconceptions and learn about newer issues and ideas: "When we get the information about rolling stops, the amount of kids that walk to school, where they live in comparison to their school, like in terms of the whole logistical map and all. I think it's extremely informative" (community stakeholder). Upon further reflection, a community stakeholder stated,

> Well, overall it's been a good experience and I like to share my input and hear others' input in this.... Ideas are sometimes things I haven't thought of. Sometimes a simple sentence from somebody and my wheels start to turn.... When you're in a group setting, and listening to other people elaborate on something, it's ... you're hearing different perspectives. It's something we need more of, ya know? Like in communications, so it's umm ... I think it's been good.

Source: Macridis (2015).

traffic-pedestrian safety, and increasing the number of children using AT. Over the entire STP project, the PhD student fostered community ownership over the research and AT program (Salsberg, Macridis, et al. 2015; Salsberg, Parry, et al. 2015; Macridis et al. 2016; Salsberg et al. 2017), including encouraging an open research environment, building trust, contributing to other community events outside of the immediate project, building research capacity, planning project goals and products relevant for committee members—both within the STP project and their day jobs—and reminding committee members that this was *their* project to run after the student departed (Salsberg, Macridis, et al. 2015). These actions successfully fostered project ownership among key committee members (Salsberg, Parry, et al. 2015; Salsberg, Macridis et al. 2015; Macridis et al. 2016; Salsberg et al. 2017). Community ownership is important for long-term sustained program maintenance and impact, particularly when an outside researcher initiates the project (Salsberg, Macaulay, and Parry 2014). The STP project contributed evidence to promote active living. Moreover, examining community participation in this project provided insights on building community ownership and self-determination.

CONCLUSION

Participatory research meaningfully engages community stakeholders in partnerships to create and apply new knowledge to address identified needs. By definition, PR is action-oriented, and such approaches promote social justice and community self-determination. By fostering environments where communities identify their needs and develop their own solutions, PR redresses a history of often ill-fitting solutions imposed by mostly well-meaning outside research. Today, PR philosophy and engagement have been scaled up to generate high-value evidence serving local needs while being generalizable to other settings. PR creates knowledge and interventions that come from pragmatic, real-world contexts, and are thus deemed more appropriate and easily translatable in community settings. PR approaches are highly recommended for all community-based, action-oriented evidence creation, notably for under-served populations.

CRITICAL THINKING QUESTIONS

1. Is it possible for a community to "research itself"?
2. What additional ethical issues, beyond those in all research, must be considered in participatory research?
3. How can participatory research make evidence more relevant and *usable*?
4. How can mutual trust act as a key mechanism in change?

RECOMMENDED READING

Minkler, M., and N. Wallerstein., eds. 2011. *Community-Based Participatory Research for Health: From Process to Outcomes.* Hoboken, NJ: John Wiley & Sons.

This classic community-based participatory research (CBPR) textbook, now in its third edition, provides the perfect primer for those new to participatory research; it also serves as a rich source of insight for seasoned practitioners. The text provides history, background, and philosophy of CBPR alongside exemplary chapters from various application contexts.

Jagosh, J., A. C. Macaulay, P. Pluye, J. Salsberg, P. L. Bush, J. Henderson, E. Sirett, et al. 2012. "Uncovering the Benefits of Participatory Research: Implications of a Realist Review for Health Research and Practice." *Milbank Quarterly* 90 (2): 311–46.

This systematic review of CBPR takes a critical realist approach to unpacking the mechanisms that underlie effective and impactful engaged research. It was the first study to identify the added benefits of long-term partnerships, as well as the value of *productive conflict* within partnerships.

Denzin, N. K., Y. S. Lincoln, and L. T. Smith, eds. 2008. *Handbook of Critical and Indigenous Methodologies*. Thousand Oaks, CA: Sage.

This textbook serves as the perfect reader for critically approaching the methodological and epistemological divide from the perspective of those whose world views have historically been drowned out by the Western gaze. It contains both theoretical and practical guidance, along with examples from various global contexts.

Parry, D., J. Salsberg, and A. C. Macaulay. 2009. *A Guide to Researcher and Knowledge-User Collaboration in Health Research*. Ottawa: Canadian Institutes of Health Research (CIHR). http://www.cihr-irsc.gc.ca/e/44954.html.

These CIHR Knowledge Translation Learning Modules teach researchers the pragmatics of co-producing knowledge with those who must ultimately use the results of their research. The modules cover all areas of participatory research, including finding research partners, maintaining partnerships over time, overcoming barriers, co-designing research, and disseminating and navigating ethical considerations. Examples and cases are presented throughout.

REFERENCES

Active Healthy Kids Canada. 2014. *Is Canada in the Running? How Does Canada Stack Up against 14 Other Countries on Physical Activity for Children and Youth?* Toronto: Active Healthy Kids Canada.

Andersson, Neil, Elizabeth Nava-Aguilera, Jorge Arostegui, Arcadio Morales-Perez, Harold Suazo-Laguna, José Legorreta-Soberanis, Carlos Hernandez-Alvarez, Ildefonso Fernandez-Salas, Sergio Paredes-Solís, and Angel Balmaseda. 2015. "Evidence Based Community Mobilization for Dengue Prevention in Nicaragua and Mexico (*Camino Verde*, the Green Way): Cluster Randomized Controlled Trial." *British Medical Journal* 351: h3267. https://doi.org/10.1136/bmj.h3267.

Andersson, Neil, Beverley Shea, Carol Amaratunga, Patricia McGuire, and Georges Sioui. 2010. "Rebuilding from Resilience: Research Framework for a Randomized Controlled Trial of Community-Led Interventions to Prevent Domestic Violence in Aboriginal Communities." *Pimatisiwin* 8 (2): 61–88.

Buliung, R., G. Faulkner, T. Beesley, and J. Kennedy. 2011. "School Travel Planning: Mobilizing School and Community Resources to Encourage Active School Transportation." *Journal of School Health* 81 (11): 704–12. https://doi.org/10.1111/j.1746-1561.2011.00647.x.

Cargo, M., and S. L. Mercer. 2008. "The Value and Challenges of Participatory Research: Strengthening Its Practice." *Annual Review of Public Health* 29: 325–50. https://doi.org/10.1146/annurev.publhealth.29.091307.083824.

Davey, Nicholas. 2006. *Unquiet Understanding: Gadamer's Philosophical Hermeneutics*. Albany: State University of New York Press.

Gadamer, Hans-Georg. 1989. *Truth and Method*. Translated by J. Weinsheimer and D. G. Marshall. New York: Continuum.

Gadamer, Hans-Georg. 1996. *The Enigma of Health: The Art of Healing in a Scientific Age*. Translated by J. Gaiger and N. Walker. Cambridge: Polity Press.

Gaventa, J., and A. Cornwall. 2006. "Challenging the Boundaries of the Possible: Participation, Knowledge and Power." *IDS Bulletin* 37 (6): 122–8.

Gibson, N., A. Cave, D. Doering, L. Ortiz, and P. Harms. 2005. "Socio-cultural Factors Influencing Prevention and Treatment of Tuberculosis in Immigrant and Aboriginal Communities in Canada." *Social Science & Medicine* 61 (5): 931–42. https://doi.org/10.1016/j.socscimed.2004.10.026.

Graham, I. D., and J. Tetroe. 2007. "How to Translate Health Research Knowledge into Effective Health Care Action." *Healthcare Quarterly* 10 (3): 20–2.

Green Communities Canada. 2012. *Canadian School Travel Planning Facilitator Guide*. Peterborough, ON: Green Communities Canada. http://www.saferoutestoschool.ca/wp-content/uploads/2017/09/STP-Guide-2017_update.pdf.

Green, L. W., A. George, M. Daniel, C. J. Frankish, C. P. Herbert, W. R. Bowie, and M. O'Neill. 1995. *Study of Participatory Research in Health Promotion: Review and Recommendations for the Development of Participatory Research in Health Promotion in Canada*. Ottawa: Royal Society of Canada.

Green, L. W., and S. L. Mercer. 2001. "Can Public Health Researchers and Agencies Reconcile the Push from Funding Bodies and the Pull from Communities?" *American Journal of Public Health* 91 (12): 1926–9.

Hatcher, Annamarie, Cheryl Bartlett, Albert Marshall, and Murdena Marshall. 2009. "Two-Eyed Seeing in the Classroom Environment: Concepts, Approaches, and Challenges." *Canadian Journal of Science, Mathematics and Technology Education* 9 (3): 141–53.

Hogan, L., E. G. Bengoechea, J. Salsberg, J. Jacobs, M. King, and A. C. Macaulay. 2014. "Using a Participatory Approach to the Development of a School-Based Physical Activity Policy in an Indigenous Community." *Journal of School Health* 84 (12): 786–92. https://doi.org/10.1111/josh.12214.

Hovey, Richard B. 2014. "Where the Word Breaks Off, No Thing May Be: Testimony, Research and Hermeneutics." *Intima: A Journal of Narrative Medicine* (Spring). http://www.researchgate.net/publication/271842297_Where_the_word_breaks_off_no_thing_may_be_Testimony_Research_and_Hermeneutics.

Hovey, Richard B, Treena Delormier, and Alex McComber. 2014. "Social-Relational Understandings of Health and Well-Being from an Indigenous Perspective." *International Journal of Indigenous Health* 10 (1): 35–54. https://doi.org/10.18357/ijih.101201513195.

Israel, B. A., A. J. Schulz, E. A. Parker, and A. B. Becker. 1998. "Review of Community-Based Research: Assessing Partnership Approaches to Improve Public Health." *Annual Review of Public Health* 19: 173–202.

Iwama, Marilyn, Murdena Marshall, Albert Marshall, and Cheryl Bartlett. 2009. "Two-Eyed Seeing and the Language of Healing in Community-Based Research." *Canadian Journal of Native Education* 32 (2): 3–23.

Jagosh, J., A. C. Macaulay, P. Pluye, J. Salsberg, P. L. Bush, J. Henderson, E. Sirett, et al. 2012. "Uncovering the Benefits of Participatory Research: Implications of a Realist Review for Health Research and Practice." *Milbank Quarterly* 90 (2): 311–46. https://doi.org/10.1111/j.1468-0009.2012.00665.x.

Jagosh, J., P. Pluye, A. C. Macaulay, J. Salsberg, J. Henderson, E. Sirett, P. L. Bush, et al. 2011. "Assessing the Outcomes of Participatory Research: Protocol for Identifying, Selecting, Appraising and Synthesizing the Literature for Realist Review." *Implementation Science* 6: 24. https://doi.org/10.1186/1748-5908-6-24.

Jagosh, Justin, Paula L. Bush, Jon Salsberg, Ann C. Macaulay, Trish Greenhalgh, Geoff Wong, Margaret Cargo, Lawrence W. Green, Carol P. Herbert, and Pierre Pluye. 2015. "A Realist Evaluation of Community-Based Participatory Research: Partnership Synergy, Trust Building and Related Ripple Effects." *BMC Public Health* 15 (1): 725.

Kahnawake Schools Diabetes Prevention Project (KSDPP). 2007. *Kahnawake Schools Diabetes Prevention Project (KSDPP) Code of Research Ethics*. Kahnawake, QC: KSDPP. https://www.ksdpp.org/elder/code_ethics.php.

Katz, J. Sylvan, and Ben R. Martin. 1997. "What Is Research Collaboration?" *Research Policy* 26 (1): 1–18.

Kirmayer, Laurence J., Stéphane Dandeneau, Elizabeth Marshall, Morgan Kahentonni Phillips, and Karla Jessen Williamson. 2011. "Rethinking Resilience from Indigenous Perspectives." *Canadian Journal of Psychiatry* 56 (2): 84–91.

Macaulay, A. C., L. E. Commanda, W. L. Freeman, N. Gibson, M. L. McCabe, C. M. Robbins, and P. L. Twohig. 1999. "Participatory Research Maximises Community and Lay Involvement. North American Primary Care Research Group." *British Medical Journal* 319 (7212): 774–8.

Macaulay, A. C., T. Delormier, E. J. Cross, L. Potvin, G. Paradis, R. Kirby, S. Desrosiers, and A. McComber. 1998. "Participatory Research with the Native Community of Kahnawake Creates Innovative Code of Research Ethics." *Canadian Journal of Public Health* 89: 105–8.

Macaulay, A. C., A. Ing, J. Salsberg, A. McGregor, J. Rice, L. Montour, and K. Gray-Donald. 2007. "Community-Based Participatory Research: Sharing Results with the Community.

An Example of Knowledge Translation from the Kahnawake Schools Diabetes Prevention Project." *Progress in Community Health Partnerships: Research, Education, and Action* 1 (2): 143–52.

Macaulay, A. C., G. Paradis, L. Potvin, E. J. Cross, C. Saad-Haddad, A. McComber, S. Desrosiers, et al. 1997. "The Kahnawake Schools Diabetes Prevention Project: Intervention, Evaluation, and Baseline Results of a Diabetes Primary Prevention Program with a Native Community in Canada." *Preventive Medicine* 26 (6): 779–90. https://doi.org/10.1006/pmed.1997.0241.

Macridis, S. 2015. "An Ethnographic Evaluation of a Community-Based Participatory Research Project: Understanding Community Mobilization & Participation in School Active Transportation Initiatives in the Kanien'kehá:ka Community of Kahnawake, QC." PhD diss., McGill University.

Macridis, S., E. Garcia Bengoechea, A. M. McComber, J. Jacobs, and A. C. Macaulay. 2016. "Active Transportation to Support Diabetes Prevention: Expanding School Health Promotion Programming in an Indigenous Community." *Evaluation and Program Planning* 56: 99–108. https://doi.org/10.1016/j.evalprogplan.2016.02.003.

Malus, Michael, Michael Shulha, Vera Granikov, Janique Johnson-Lafleur, Vinita d'Souza, Michaela Knot, Christina Holcroft, Kenneth Hung, Isabel Pereira, and Carmelina Ricciuto. 2011. "A Participatory Approach to Understanding and Measuring Patient Satisfaction in a Primary Care Teaching Setting." *Progress in Community Health Partnerships: Research, Education, and Action* 5 (4): 417–24.

Mercer, S. L., L. W. Green, M. Cargo, A. Potter, M. Daniel, R. S. Olds, and E. Reed-Gross. 2008. "Reliability-Tested Guidelines for Assessing Participatory Research Projects." In *Community-Based Participatory Research for Health: From Process to Outcome*, edited by M. Minkler and N. Wallerstein, 407–18. San Francisco: Jossey-Bass.

Minkler, M., and N. Wallerstein. 2008. *Community-Based Participatory Research for Health: From Process to Outcome.* 2nd ed. San Francisco: Jossey-Bass.

National Aboriginal Health Organization (NAHO). 2007. *OCAP: Ownership, Control, Access and Possession.* Ottawa: NAHO.

Panel on Research Ethics. 2014. *TCPS 2 (2014)—Tri-Council Policy Statement: Ethical Conduct for Research Involving Humans.* Ottawa: Panel on Research Ethics, Government of Canada. http://www.pre.ethics.gc.ca/eng/policy-politique/initiatives/tcps2-eptc2/Default/.

Parry, D., J. Salsberg, and A. C. Macaulay. 2009. *A Guide to Researcher and Knowledge-User Collaboration in Health Research.* Ottawa: Canadian Institutes of Health Research.

Salsberg, J., A. C. Macaulay, and D. Parry. 2014. "Guide to Integrated Knowledge Translation Research." In *Turning Knowledge into Action: Practical Guidance on How to Do Integrated Knowledge Translation Research*, edited by I. D. Graham, J. Tetroe, and A. Pearson, 176–82. Adelaide: Wolters Kluwer-Lippincott-JBI.

Salsberg, J., S. Macridis, E. Garcia Bengoechea, A. C. Macaulay, S. Moore, and Members of the Kahnawake Schools Diabetes Prevention Project—School Travel Planning Committee.

2017. "Engagement Strategies that Foster Community Self-Determination in Participatory Research: Insider Ownership Through Outsider Championship." *Family Practice* 34 (3): 336–40. https://doi.org/10.1093/fampra/cmx001.

Salsberg, J., S. Macridis, E. Garcia Bengoechea, A. C. Macaulay, S. Moore, and Members of the KSDPP School Travel Planning Committee. 2015. "Engaging Community Stakeholders for School-Based Physical Activity Intervention." *Retos: Nuevas Tendencias en Educación Física, Deporte y Recreación* 28: 225–31.

Salsberg, J., D. Parry, P. Pluye, S. Macridis, C. Herbert, and A. C. Macaulay. 2015. "Successful Strategies to Engage Research Partners for Translating Evidence into Action in Community Health: A Critical Review." *Journal of Environmental and Public Health* 2015: 191856. https://doi.org/10.1155/2015/191856.

Straus, S. E., J. Tetroe, and I. Graham. 2009. "Defining Knowledge Translation." *Canadian Medical Association Journal* 181 (3–4): 165–8. https://doi.org/10.1503/cmaj.081229.

SECTION VI

MAKING CHANGE—EDUCATION, ADVOCACY, AND SYSTEM CHANGE

SECTION INTRODUCTION BY NEIL ARYA AND THOMAS PIGGOTT

In this final section of the book, we move to making lasting change for under-served populations. Previous chapters have presented approaches and solutions to specific populations and issues. These have included cultural safety for and reconciliation with Indigenous populations; social policy and public health strategies to address the health of those who are marginalized, living in poverty, and experiencing homelessness; and delivering culturally safe and effective health care for refugees arriving to and living in Canada. Building on such strategies, we will now begin this last section of the book addressing the *process* of making change for under-served populations through education, advocacy, and policy.

Evidence is important and should be a necessary prerequisite in changing public policy to improve the health of under-served populations—but sparking political will takes more than just evidence. Sometimes governments will act quickly, where general principles are known, but concrete evidence for specific interventions are sparser (e.g., minimum wage); sometimes there is a need to develop evidence, such as for guaranteed income projects; sometimes intense consultation and rollout are involved (e.g., decriminalizing marijuana possession, or legalizing soft drugs or safe injection sites).

But when is studying or committee work enough? And when do we take the plunge? Prochaska and DiClemente's (1983) (see also Chapter 12, Koivu and Piggot) incremental Transtheoretical Stages of Change model describes the phases of precontemplation, contemplation, preparation, action, and maintenance. This model, developed to apply to behaviour change in individuals, might also be applied to societies. However, societies may also change quickly in response to a changing environment.

But what moves us to move from precontemplation to action—is it merely getting evidence into the hands of decision-makers? And who are the decision-makers? Why is it that after seemingly bumping our heads against a wall that the wall suddenly gives in—whether we think of gay marriage or smoking cessation, from pot legalization to safe injection sites? The answers to these questions are complex, but we hope that this section helps you in a search to make change.

When do we use our voices? For those without a voice or political power to make change on their own, as is often the case for under-served and marginalized populations, the need to push for inclusion of that voice is all the more critical. This must not be done as merely speaking "for" these populations but, where possible, amplifying their own voice—rendering service, not charity.

With certain activities, this requires reflecting on the motivations of making change and ensuring that self-aggrandizing aspirations are not involved. This necessitates questioning the assumptions of good intentions and recognizing them as insufficient. Sometimes, we have to consider competing goals (e.g., the pedagogical value of student-run clinics) while ensuring individual-level ethics. The benefits of sensitizing future physicians for future generations needs to be trumped, for example, by true informed consent, beneficence, and non-maleficence.

This section reviews two ends of the spectrum of change: education, where long-term change can be promoted and capacity can be built, and advocacy, where more immediate change is sought. In Chapter 24, Cooper, Arya, Negoita, and Pham describe the evidence on strategies to improve education regarding under-served populations. In Chapter 25 and 26, Meili, Piggott, and Andermann discuss re-orienting health systems and public health to improve health equity for under-served populations and to create a healthy society. Finally, as described by Berger and colleagues in Chapter 27 and Arya in Chapter 28, "taking to the streets" to garner political and public attention for key health issues may sometimes be necessary.

Lasting change comes not from a few loud voices; rather, it comes from intersectoral collaboration. Yet, as Margaret Mead said, "Never doubt that a small group of thoughtful, committed citizens can change the world; indeed, it's the only thing that ever has."

REFERENCE

Prochaska, J., and C. DiClemente. 1983. "Stages and Processes of Self-Change in Smoking: Toward an Integrative Model of Change." *Journal of Consulting and Clinical Psychology* 5: 390–5.

CHAPTER 24

Educating Health Professionals to Care for Vulnerable and Marginalized Populations

Lesley Cooper, Neil Arya, Mona Negoita, and Ngan Pham

LEARNING OBJECTIVES

After reading this chapter, you should be able to:

1. Recognize the important challenges faced by educators teaching about working with marginalized populations.
2. Reflect on the impact of the teacher's stance when discussing and working with marginalized populations.
3. Identify the voice of and learn from marginalized groups in the health care system.
4. Compare traditional health care delivery experience of the mainstream community with that of disadvantaged and marginalized groups and formulate alternative approaches.

BACKGROUND

In 2010, the *Lancet* sought expert advice on better ways to prepare health professionals for a global and independent world (Frenk et al. 2010). With the outcome of transformative education in mind, the panel proposed reforms to instructional design, adopting competency approaches as criteria for classification of health professional that would be more responsive to changing local conditions. Competencies were promoted as criteria for classification of health professionals. Important for marginalized populations were recommendations for a common set of values underlying social accountability of health professionals.

Interprofessional education and practice with marginalized populations is highlighted in the *Lancet* report. This contrasts with traditional professional education in isolated silos with little sharing of expertise, classes, or curricula. Educators of professionals in the academy need to both discuss and use the strengths and capabilities of other professions to improve the well-being of all.

The *Lancet* noted that health care is distributed inequitably within, and between, nations (Frenk et al. 2010). There is both a shortage and maldistribution of health professionals. In order for health practitioners to work effectively with marginalized and/or socially diverse populations, Frenk and colleagues suggest that their education must create opportunities for mutual learning and greater cooperation, resulting in graduate outcomes that provide skills needed to meet the needs of all people.

The social accountability theme is evident in a review on medical education for the twenty-first century titled *Global Consensus for Social Accountability of Medical Schools* (2010). This marked a significant aspirational change in promoting action for future medical education at the global level but does not necessarily mean any commitment to this direction. Charles Boelen, co-chair of the above committee, later differentiated between socially responsible action with a commitment to the welfare of society; socially responsive actions directing education and research to the welfare of society; and socially accountable actions, which are specific and done in collaboration with patients and stakeholders to provide a positive impact and evidence of effectiveness (Boelen, Dharamsi, and Gibbs 2012).

In 2012 the Association of Faculties of Medicine of Canada (AFMC) et al. (2012) recommended changes to medical education ranging from student admissions to faculty leadership recognizing the economic and health disparities between various Canadian populations and regions, noting the need to confront health issues in rural, remote, and Indigenous communities. Of particular interest are recommendations relating to social responsibility, promotion, and prevention in public health; the importance of diverse learning contexts; and re-valuing generalist practice. Two specific recommendations stand out, however. Canadian health educators were urged to devise programmes to better equip trainees for work in poorly resourced and under-served communities, offering generalist and specialist care to diverse populations in these communities, whether these were regional, national, or international. Educators were also asked to examine and reflect on the *hidden curriculum* operating in medical education.

This hidden curriculum, "a set of influences that function at the level of organizational structure and culture" (Hafferty 1998, 404), which implicitly transmits specific values and attitudes and is embedded in the teaching processes, organizational arrangements, or the values espoused by teaching staff, may well conflict with the stated institutional educational mission. Addressing tacit attitudes requires reflection and critical reflection for teachers and students and culturally safe ways to expose this hidden curriculum.

The AFMC suggested a need for diversification of learning contexts and training. As part of this, student and patient safety remain critical. Training and preparation for commencing work in these communities, together with academic support throughout the learning process, is core. Consultation with community stakeholders and other professionals is a central feature of this direction.

RETHINKING LEARNING AND TEACHING APPROACHES AND CONTEXTS

Two key themes influence the following discussion: transformative education and social accountability for work with marginalized and under-served populations. Transformative education, which comes from Mezirow (1991) and recently Cranton (2010), requires changing student perspectives by exploring the frames of reference evident in our thoughts, feelings, and actions; understanding ourselves and our social locations; and appreciating the impact of power and its intersection with race, gender, and class. Through this exploration, alternative approaches based on concepts of social justice are possible.

Traditional forms of learning are often classroom-based, with an active teacher, passive students, rote learning, and drills. The instructor aims to fill gaps in students' knowledge, resulting in students using surface learning approaches and regurgitating material in multiple-choice questions and other forms of examination. Student-centred teaching approaches have the teacher as facilitator so that students control their learning and use experiences to construct new forms of knowledge.

It has been argued that an understanding of the complexities associated with the access, delivery, and practice of twenty-first century health care is enhanced when students work interprofessionally with marginalized communities.

Learning contexts vary geographically, socioeconomically, and culturally, from remote Indigenous communities through urban refugee populations to inner-city homeless and mentally ill—all with multiple forms of deprivation, disadvantage, and marginalization. Working with isolated individuals in a mainstream health care setting does not necessarily prepare practitioners for work with marginalized populations in place with families, neighbours, and community. These wider contexts allow students to engage with service users whose knowledge and experience of health care and chronic diseases contrast with the socioeconomic values and cultural experiences of many students and their teachers. Working with varied populations gives practitioners different forms of knowledge in addition to awareness of perceptions and ability to engage with such people.

KNOWLEDGE: SOCIAL JUSTICE AND EQUITY

Social justice is at the core of international health policy and professional missions. Commitment to social justice has multiple meanings. In a broader policy context, social justice is expressed as a human right, which enhances physical and mental health and allows citizens to exercise other rights. It also refers to social accountability and resource redistribution from those better off to those living in poverty and suffering from ill health.

Social justice is evident in discussions of equity. Discussions on *equity* and other terminology related to under-served populations were elaborated at length in Chapter 1 by Piggott and Orkin. Equity principles underpin social accountability and commitment to under-served populations. If practitioners are to serve marginalized populations, then appreciating access to and need for health services is necessary.

The starting point for this understanding is inequity and the complementary concepts of horizontal and vertical equity (Starfield 2011). Inequity represents systemic but potentially remedial differences between populations with diverse geographic, socioeconomic, or cultural statuses. Horizontal inequity occurs when individuals with similar needs do not have access to the same health care resources. Vertical inequity happens when people with greater needs do not have access to greater resources. Understanding concepts of inequity enables practitioners to think beyond individual and illness paradigms to a health model with a focus on person and population and the disadvantage. This implies a new way of thinking about the focus of learning. Understanding equity and its application to health care alone is insufficient, as *enacting* equity in our actions, behaviours, and relationships with others is required. Enacting means doing and engaging in social practices that contribute to the well-being of all.

Many health professions (social work, medicine, and nursing) express commitment to social justice and equity in health care. Mill and colleagues (2010) argue that global citizenship is a critical component of the roles and responsibilities of professional nurses; however,

> despite a long tradition of the involvement of nurses in the advancement of social justice issues, the integration of knowledge related to social justice into the education of undergraduate nurses and the practice of professional nurses is inconsistent in the North American context. (E2)

Leaders in nursing argue that conceptualization of social justice is ambiguous and not enacted in practice, as opposed to in social work, where social justice is a core component of both academic and practice curricula. Nursing discourse remains grounded in individualism, which precludes collective commitment to injustices and their expression in homelessness, stigma, and discrimination based on racial grounds (Bekemeier and Butterfield 2005, 152; Kirkham and Browne 2006, 333).

PERSPECTIVE: WHAT WE SEE AND HOW WE INTERPRET

When learning to work with those we seek to serve, it is essential to start with understanding the perspective we bring, our social location, and how these influence our interactions with others. According to Mezirow (1991), this change in perspective is critical to the learning process. Students come to professional education with a ready-made package of personal experiences, views about social issues, and a tacit understanding of their social and cultural location in society. These views and our "taken-for-granted" assumptions about the world and relationships are determined by our gender, (dis)abilities, sexual orientation, class, race, religion, and cultural background. Their individual backgrounds afford students particular opportunities and experiences that privilege (or marginalize) and enhance short and long-term status and influence what a person sees and interprets. These views may not be helpful in working with people who do not share their views. Grappling with the consequences of our social and cultural positions and their impact on people and communities is core to learning about working with marginalized populations. The starting point for this learning is awareness of the origins of a person's values and attitudes and their impact, as this will assist in appreciating service users' and carers' views about health care.

A growing movement is seeking the views of service users and carers internationally. These people have particular knowledge of inclusion and exclusion and the ways in which domination and privilege operate in health care. While many readers have been service users or consumers, the disadvantaged and marginalized are the "outsiders within." It is in the best interests of those who are marginalized to understand the dominant perspectives. The marginalized are uniquely positioned to offer their unique understanding of health care, challenging existing operational paradigms. The conceptual framework underpinning this is standpoint theory (Harding 2009). Our standpoint represents who we listen to and who we ignore, affecting which concepts are intelligible and salient, and which features are important to us. Listening to the voices of the marginalized, the stakeholders, and the service users and carers allows us to challenge our ways of thinking, behaving, and being. Their stories about initial involvement and engagement with the health care system provides us with views about how the system is regarded, as well as insights into our behaviour.

Evidence of the service user and carer movement can be found in the consultation with users of health care conducted by Mount Sinai Hospital (Lam n.d.). This study and a subsequent report specifying equity competencies for health care professionals outline what is important to marginalized groups and provides recommendations for health care providers and the hospital. Importantly, the views of service users provide a basis to explore privilege and difference, enabling us to challenge the dominant system of privilege underlying the status quo.

VALUES

Awareness of different value perspectives and thoughtful enacting of values in day-to-day practice is essential in working with marginalized populations. There is general agreement about core values across the health sector. These core values have been expressed in a variety of ways and include warmth, empathy, genuineness, respect, acceptance, and positive regard. What is less evident is enactment of these values in our social and professional behaviour. Enacting values is more challenging, demanding a level of introspection and critical reflection on our practice. Actively seeking feedback from patients, colleagues, and community can enhance our self-awareness and ultimately our practice.

Values enable us to mediate oppression and provide more thoughtful and engaged health care. Some populations are very clear about core practice values. Mount Sinai Hospital in Toronto chose to solicit community feedback by surveying different groups, asking, "What are the values, attitudes, knowledge and skills that health care providers need to have to be able to serve you in a culturally-appropriate manner?" (Lam n.d.). The stakeholders consulted wanted hospitals to provide more tailored care and supports, such as more specialists, better access to interpreters, and the capacity to hire staff to advocate for at-risk communities. There was one core message: patients want health care providers to look beyond stereotypes and labels and treat them as individuals. All too often, what "stands out" as a different characteristic provides a label, which becomes the only thing that providers perceive. People object to labels and want to be treated as individuals for the condition for which they are seeking medical attention.

This consultation revealed clear values: the importance of respect and dignity, regardless of personal circumstances, and the worth of insight into oppressive practices. Participants also outlined how these values are expressed. For example, they suggested responding to them with a smile or a nod, seeking their input into health care plans, and allowing longer appointments as ways of enacting key values. In addition, participants detailed recommendations for a range of enacted values. Similar values are echoed by Pinto and Upshur (2009), who cite humility, introspection, solidarity, and social justice as essential core components of global health education. Unfortunately, these authors do not elaborate how these values may be enacted or assessed in practice.

PRIVILEGE, RACISM, AND CULTURE

In 1988, Peggy McIntosh wrote her classic paper entitled "White Privilege and Male Privilege: A Personal Account of Coming to See Correspondences through Work in Women's Studies." She argued that white people are taught from an early age not to recognize the advantages that accrue as a result of being white: "I have come to see white privilege as an invisible package of unearned assets which I can count on cashing in each day, but about which I was 'meant' to remain oblivious. White privilege is like an invisible weightless knapsack of special provisions, maps, passports, codebooks, visas, clothes, tools and blank checks" (McIntosh 1988, 1–2).

Describing white privilege makes one newly accountable. As a feminist, McIntosh's starting point was the observation that males were not taught to recognize their male privilege and dominance, even though they talked about the extent to which women are disadvantaged. In the process of defining white privilege, McIntosh started with a personal examination of how this played out in her own life by asking herself many penetrating questions. One question included whether we can go to a supermarket and buy the staple foods that fit with our cultural traditions. As a white person, privilege is tacit and taken for granted. Understanding privilege is important, but the challenges are, *inter alia*, recognition of our actions and their consequences in the complexities of patient care; consideration of our emotional readiness to confront our oppressive behaviours and practices; and relinquishment of our power and privilege. Beyond this, health professionals require strategic thinking about how best to discuss the powerful and unexamined policies and procedures within organizations where systems of privilege are taken for granted.

Indigenous populations discuss cultural safety in a similar and related manner. At the heart of cultural safety is the capacity to communicate competently in the patient's cultural, spiritual, social, and economic realm; to challenge inequalities in order to improve access and care for marginalized populations; and to reflect on the way the provider's culture impacts on health care (Baba 2013). This is preferable to the professional approach. The concept of *cultural safety* has origins in nursing in New Zealand. With its bicultural recognition embedded in the Treaty of Waitangi, New Zealand has focused on equality between Maori and the white population. Bicultural practices and systems transformation provided justification for discussion of cultural safety among nurses.

In the early eighties, Maori people were experiencing poor health outcomes resulting from racism and culturally inappropriate health care (Papps and Ramsden 1996). The concept of treating everyone in the same way was disputed, as it was evident that this did not happen in practice. The Nightingale Oath, a commitment to people *regardless* of their colour or creed, was reworded to be *regardful* of both colour and creed when caring for a person from another culture. Nurses were subsequently required to explore the impact of their own culture on their patients as an essential element in improving quality of care. They were subsequently encouraged to focus on their knowledge, skills, and attitudes; understand the power in therapeutic relationships; reflect on their actions; and use these insights to improve both their relationships with and the empowerment of their patients. Since the 1980s, the concept of culture has expanded from race and ethnicity to take further into account the intersection of gender, sexual orientation, (dis)ability, and social class.

Underpinning cultural safety are cultural awareness, cultural sensitivity, and cultural competence, the latter being a set of behaviours that combine to enable practitioners to work in culturally appropriate ways. Cultural safety also means that practitioners directly address racism, discrimination, and prejudice, and their manifestations in unequal therapeutic relationships and access to timely health care and treatment. In a Canadian context, graduating students are expected to demonstrate competence in cultural safety through post-colonial understanding, communication skills that demonstrate culturally safe practice, their inclusivity and a willingness to engage in dialogue, and effective relationship building with First Nations peoples. Graduating students are expected to enact respect by identifying communities at risk and acting to rectify deficits (Baba 2013, 10).

EMPATHY

Good therapeutic relationships and communication depend on the capacity to convey empathy. The starting point is being able to put oneself in the shoes of another person and understand their experiences, emotions, experiences, behaviours, and the meanings attached to these. Empathy is "trying to understand as carefully and sensitively as possible, the nature of another person's experience, their unique point of view, and what meaning this carries for that individual" (Trevithick 2012, 194). There are many dimensions to empathy: commitment to appreciate the needs of others; affective capacity to subjectively experience the feelings of others; cognitive ability to explain objectively subjective dimensions; openness and willingness to reflect on the complex interactions of motivations, feelings, and actions; and the sensitivity to communicate this understanding to the other (Mercer and Reynolds 2002).

Understanding empathy, to put into words the feelings and emotions of others in a respectful and caring manner, is challenging, but what is important is our willingness to try. The most important aspect is acting on our understanding in a helpful way. This should be at the core of the healing professions. These strategies with patients, families, and communities create confidence and understanding and ultimately improve patient outcomes. While there have been concerns about the hardening of empathic responses of medical students over their training (Newton et al. 2008), particularly as they enter the clinical years (Hojat et al. 2009), studies have shown that this was fostered over time due to an intimidating educational environment, negative educational experiences, perceptions of "belittlement and harassment," and partial sleep deprivation. Strategies proposed by health educators to enhance empathy in clinical training include a patient-centred interview (Benbassat and Baumal 2004).

PEDAGOGICAL STRATEGIES

The *Lancet* Commissions called for transformative learning in health care (Frenk et al. 2010). Three successive levels of learning were noted—the informative, the formative, and the transformative:

> As a valued outcome, transformative learning involves three fundamental shifts: from fact memorisation to searching, analysis, and synthesis of information for decision making; from seeking professional credentials to achieving core competencies for effective teamwork in health systems; and from non-critical adoption of educational models to creative adaptation of global resources to address local priorities. (Frenk et al. 2010, 6)

Informative learning is about acquisition of knowledge and skills with the goal of producing experts. Formative learning is socializing students about their values with the goal of creating professionals. Transformative learning aims to develop graduates who engage in self-examination, critically assessing their assumptions, and demonstrate options for new ways of acting, thereby acquiring knowledge and skills for new roles (Cranton 2010). In other words, an enlightened professional is able to execute changes embedded in emancipation and social justice and apply these changes in work with patients and communities.

Pedagogical strategies facilitating transformative learning are the responsibilities of teachers. Giving students the skills to continue learning as practitioners is important. Some of the core skills emerging from the discussion in the previous section include the ability to think critically and reflect, participation in partnerships with others, and practical real-world knowledge. Of special importance is the willingness to challenge our values, attitudes, and stances towards marginalized populations and health care and to be challenged by others at the same time.

There are diverse pedagogical approaches that include discovery learning, practical learning in the "real world" with peers and in various organizations external to the university, simulations, case studies, and a variety of practical skills. In the section that follows, illustrations of transformative approaches will be discussed.

EXPERIENTIAL LEARNING

This form of learning is an active process of learning through experience. Kolb (1984) outlined the stages as follows: having a concrete experience, reflection on and observation of experiences, active conceptualization, and, finally, active experimentation. Active engagement and experimentation are at the core as the following example suggests.

Godkin and Savageau (2001) provided students in preclinical years the opportunity to learn and improve skills in the language of people newly arrived in the United States, and to improve their sensitivity to people as a result of these experiences. Students had the opportunity to work with a local immigrant family using that family's language in order to appreciate their personal attitudes to health care. This was followed by the opportunity to live in a new country to learn the language, cultural beliefs, and health care practices. For the final experience, students participated in a domestic community-service project that included a soup kitchen, an HIV health education activity, and work as a family support worker. All students attended concurrent seminars. The evaluation indicated that the students exposed to these experiences were more comfortable than their peers with patients from other cultural groups and that they developed linguistic and cultural competence (Godkin and Savageau 2001).

CLINICAL ELECTIVE

Various electives in clinical settings have been set up for different professions. One unique approach to understanding marginalization was a marginalized community elective at Western University designed by the author (NA). It involved medical students working in a variety of settings, including refugee health clinics, Indigenous health clinics, prisons, methadone clinics, downtown community health centres, and public health, during a four-week block. This variety was important logistically in order not to place a major burden on providers or clients given the time required to adapt to be useful at a medical school level, as well as the sporadic nature of such services and the amount of time given by individual providers; however, it also allowed for an appreciation of the commonality of issues affecting different populations in different settings. This approach was recognized by *Corporate Knights* as one of the most innovative in the country (Lappano 2011).

SIMULATIONS

Simulations are real-world processes carefully designed to allow practitioners the opportunity to respond to complex situations without harming participants, to learn skills, to communicate effectively, and to work in teams. Poverty simulations are an effective tool to increase understanding of barriers faced by populations challenged by minimal income and resources. In a study by Strasser et al. (2013), public health students were assigned roles of family members with minimal income and were asked to pay for rent, food, utilities, and other basic needs. In post-testing, participants indicated increased empathy with low-income populations, especially in their understanding of the barriers faced by these groups. As a result of the simulation, they had greater confidence in their ability to understand poverty and factors contributing to poverty. The result was an increased confidence in participants' abilities to empathize with those suffering financial hardships.

LEARNER-CENTRED PORTFOLIOS

Portfolios are tools that provide multiple learning opportunities, depending on the way in which they are introduced, integrated, assessed, and supported. They are valuable instruments as teaching moves away from information-giving and acquisitive approaches and towards a competency-based approach to learning. Students use portfolios in a variety of ways, including as descriptive accounts of actual work experiences, whether describing practice processes, interactions, a practice dilemma such as a critical incident, some personal reflective writing, or other forms of art expressing work experiences. Using these encounters, students can analyze and reflect on their experiences, track their progress, and evaluate competencies acquired in practice. The tool is at its best when teachers and students are able to use the portfolio's content to deepen conversations about actual practice and reflect on such concepts as marginalization, oppression, or discrimination. The value of using portfolios depends on assessment criteria and integration with other subjects in the curriculum. While there are claims that portfolios enable reflective, self-directed learning, their effectiveness requires clear guidelines and supportive mentors to stimulate critical reflection and strategies for deep learning (Driessen et al. 2007).

SERVICE LEARNING

Service learning combines experiential learning and strong elements of social accountability. Many definitions provide a particular emphasis—for example, the accent may be on a subject, the structure of learning, a course-based educational experience, or the value of service to the learner or to those being served. The term *service learning* has been challenged, particularly the use of the word *service*, as it suggests service *for* people rather than service *with* people. Some writers prefer *civic engagement* or *community-based learning*. Whatever the terminology, learners deliberately engage with their community in a

Case Study: Student-Run Health Clinics (by Neil Arya)

"Student-run" clinics have the potential to be the epitome of community service learning, providing opportunities to experience practice, gain first-hand knowledge of responsibility and professionalism, acquire professional skills, and challenge values, all while serving communities. Clinics to deal with the needs of under-served populations, each associated with a medical school, have been set up across Canada, including CHIUS in Vancouver, SHINE in Edmonton, CDIRC in Calgary, SWITCH in Saskatoon, SEARCH in Regina, WISH in Winnipeg, and IMAGINE in Toronto (Holmqvist et al. 2012; SWITCH n.d.). Such clinics are frequently transdisciplinary or interprofessional, sometimes including non-professional undergraduate students.

The concept of free clinics serving the uninsured and marginally housed has roots in the United States, and has been immortalized by Patch Adams and the eponymously named movie starring Robin Williams. These clinics address mental health and substance abuse issues, engage clients in prevention manoeuvres, and assist chronic disease management, monitoring, and surveillance. A 2007 survey of all 124 Association of American Medical Colleges allopathic schools found that of 94 schools responding, 110 student-run clinics were operating from at least 49 medical schools, many involving preclinical and other student health professionals, averaging 16 volunteers per week dealing with acute and chronic illness. The clinics are largely funded by private grants and deal primarily with visible minority populations (Simpson and Long 2007). Since the turn of the century, the number of clinics has been increasing, and there is now an organization for collaboration and exchange of information (SSRFC n.d.).

Student-run free clinics are common internationally. In Germany, over 30 student-administered organizations operate for asylum seekers (see Medibueros, http://medibueros.m-bient.com/). These are based on the "No One Is Illegal" movement, with an underlying premise that all people living in a country have the right to medical care (See Kein Mensch Ist Illegal, http://www.kmii-koeln.de/; and No One Is Illegal, http://www.nooneisillegal.org/). An obligation of all German government employees to report "illegal" migrants, until recently, appeared to include health professionals. This exemption is still unclear to many providers and patients, leading to fear of accessing health services. Students triage, advise, and arrange for referral for free or low-cost professional services from collaborating physicians and hospitals but do not administer services. Non-medical services are often perceived as more important for those whose status in a country is uncertain. At least one refugee law clinic staffed by law students guided by practising lawyers offers free legal advice (See Refugee Law Clinic—Cologne, http://lawcliniccologne.com/english/).

Core learning reported by student-run clinics includes health equity and student leadership. In Canada, the emphasis is on interprofessionalism (Holmqvist et al. 2012).

continued

Students are involved in all aspects of administration: planning programs, triaging patients, budgeting, fundraising, engaging the faculty, and liaising with the community. Compared to the US model, more focus has been placed on team building in Canada through collaborative practice and mentorship by more experienced students and practitioners of different disciplines (Holmqvist et al. 2012). While students engage in health care related activities, the degree of autonomy and supervision by licensed health care professionals helps ensure quality of care and accountability (Holmqvist et al. 2012). In interviews with key stakeholders, Campbell and colleagues (2013) noted that community members perceived students as less distant from themselves and as potential role models. Campbell documented other studies that demonstrated high levels of satisfaction. Benefits derived by students included clinical knowledge, health resource planning, interprofessionalism, social awareness, comfort dealing with marginalized populations, and choice of primary care careers.

However, concerns remain among administrators and communities. Most medical schools outside Western Canada have not developed such clinics, being skeptical about liabilities, risks of inappropriate student behaviour, and inadequate supervision. Furthermore, the service gap is filled in Canada, where universal health insurance includes many groups who are not covered in the US, and where numbers of undocumented migrants are far smaller than in Germany.

Logistical barriers may include university policy or malpractice and liability insurance, or they may be clinic-related. There is also concern over continuity from year to year since the retention of staff and funding for the clinics is challenging.

Some schools have observed merits for their students, as the clinics promote understanding of the needs of those marginalized, but are they merely moving the burden of teaching onto the community? Do clients really have, or know of, alternatives? Communities must be engaged; relationships are key. Furthermore, the clinics should not perpetuate themselves and prevent development of appropriate solutions within the health care systems.

Great care should be taken to avoid creation, or give the perception, of second-rate services. Attitudes that are less respectful, as perceived by clients, can affect clients' experiences. Students, especially preclinical students, need to be oriented around issues and factors such as boundaries, confidentiality, consent, and culture. How should the system deal with students who fail to recognize their own limitations or are insufficiently supervised and act beyond their level of competence, claiming that they had "no choice"?

Beyond the goal of exposure for students, further pedagogical goals are frequently neglected. Where these goals are formalized, they are rarely formally assessed. Opportunities for debriefing, to allow processing of difficult experiences, enhancing professionalism, and supporting student mental health has not been detailed in the literature. Whether such experiences should be mandatory in formal curriculum is generally not debated. Exposure can often lead to transformational experiences, but when the experience is less sought after—that is, when it is made a mandatory part of a curriculum—participants may resent such experiences, perceiving them as ideologically driven, and their preceptors as sanctimonious.

An alternative approach that has been developed through the International Federation of Medical Students' Associations (IFMSA) in Quebec is "INcommunity" in Montreal, a four-week immersion program for preclinical students designed to develop a comprehensive understanding of vulnerable communities (offenders, Indigenous people, inner-city residents, and migrants) by shadowing social workers, stakeholders, and NGOs working with those populations (IFMSA n.d.).

Student-run clinics have the potential to cater to communities of under-served populations and to serve the educational needs of students. The development and fostering of relationships and community partnerships is critical in providing meaningful service and achieving pedagogical goals. Critically asking what the added value is in a particular context, ensuring safety and medicolegal responsibility, and placing trainees in situations with adequate supervision and support must not be neglected. Commitment, purposeful planning, evaluation, and re-evaluation of the impact on each participant and stakeholder are also essential for success. Learning opportunities with the potential for improving care by future professionals need to be balanced with the needs of the community. At the core of the formation of such clinics must be an embodiment of respect.

wide range of creative activities, providing important social outcomes for individuals and communities. Valuable outcomes include learners becoming more socially responsible, participating in community life, and having the ability to reflect on their values and attitudes, freely facilitating transformative learning.

Arya (N. A.) instituted a service-learning project among Master of Public Health (MPH) distance learners at the University of Waterloo in 2007—one chosen by the students themselves but separate from their professional public health career. The students could choose for themselves what was a local marginalized setting (refugee, Indigenous, immigrant, homeless, etc.). Some settings were international (e.g., South Africa [TB, HIV], Peru [remote, Indigenous community]) where students were living and working. A public health's student role might be service provision rather than the administrative or policy role of their day-to-day work. While their public health knowledge might be useful, here they would be "on the other side"—in a clinical or community setting where they could interact more directly with clients. While students initially expressed reluctance as it took them outside their comfort zone, this project became among the most highly rated aspects of the course.

Butin (2010) outlines different perspectives on service learning as both transformative and regressive. Service learning is transformative because it disrupts the banking approach to education (Freire 1972); it provides a visible difference to communities, where students are engaged in learning; and it enables participants to question the dominant norms and hegemonic practices of who controls, defines, and limits access to knowledge and power. On the other hand, service learning can be viewed as a repressive model that does not provide real changes in the communities in which it is practised: "Service-learning becomes yet another means for those in the 'culture of power' to maintain inequitable power relations under the guise of benevolent volunteerism" (Butin 2010, 11–12). It has the potential to enable individual transformation through a process of action and reflection, but it is unlikely to change political inequities at a societal level.

ROLE MODELLING

Learning to become a health professional—maintaining professional skills and competencies—involves transformative learning. This can be achieved through role modelling, mentoring, and professional supervision. A role model is a practitioner or academic able to set a positive example about practice, whether this is behavioural, attitudinal, cognitive, or affective. Providing effective modelling goes beyond how to do the job and skill development; more importantly, it encompasses how professionals think about practice, how they care for and about others, how they enact values and critical reflection. The process involves spiral teaching, whereby a learner is assisted with the support of a mentor or facilitator to make sense of their experience, discover new insights, and deepen understanding of how and why things are the way they are, which lead to key lessons and ultimately new and different actions.

Many students and newly graduated practitioners often find it difficult to work with people who are different to them or where there is little or no common ground. This is evident in feedback from participants in the Mount Sinai study (Lam n.d.). A seasoned practitioner with deep understanding of social accountability and the impact of racism, and who is comfortable in caring for people irrespective of their circumstances, provides a rich socialization experience for practitioners.

Beth Perry (2009) provides an example of how role modelling operates in nursing. In her phenomenological study of exemplary practitioners, she found that it was the little things, and making connections, that made a difference both in practice and to novice practitioners. She provides an illustration of changing bandages while maintaining dignity: it was "the subtle ways she showed respect for her patient. It was the little things, the gentleness of her hands, the confidence of her voice, the extra drape placed discreetly over exposed parts of his body during the dressing change that made her care outstanding" (Perry 2009, 39).

Each health profession prefers its particular professional nomenclature for development of professional identity through supervisory practices. This nomenclature may include role modelling, mentoring, proctoring, or supervising. Without dissecting the differences between these different terms, the common ideas include the importance of psychosocial support for the learner or practitioner, modelling affective and cognitive processes, using this process to think about values, attitudes, and ethics, and ultimately facilitating professional development.

Irrespective of professional nomenclature, all clinical educators help students to problem solve complex practice problems, engage in active teaching and provision of feedback, and develop new ways of thinking to stretch the practitioner's capabilities. Modelling, mentoring, and supervising are regarded as one-on-one processes, usually contained by impermeable professional boundaries preventing opportunities for interprofessional education. One-on-one approaches to mentoring and supervision can be expensive, subject to financial workplace constraints, and are often used managerially as a form of surveillance in the workplace.

Moving beyond individualized clinical learning, focusing on development of professional identity can also be achieved in a community of practice with other professionals. Communities of practice are valuable resources in learning about marginalized populations. Embedding students in a community of practice where other professionals, the community, service users, and carers provide a diversity of role models and exposure to variation in practice is perhaps a richer pedagogical approach.

Communities of practice, first described by Lave and Wenger (1991), enable people to work together in a spirit of partnership and transformation. Core characteristics include connection with people, shared processes for discussion of ideas, stimulating and situated learning environments, and generation of ideas and knowledge. The richness of socialization comes from multiple exposures to a variety of experienced exemplary practitioners rather than unidimensional exposure to the socialization strategies of one person. All professionals have a role to play in how they work with students, patients, colleagues, and the community. Modelling equitable and respectful practice, enacting social justice, and enabling reflection of discrimination, racism, and marginalization can provide a profound learning experience for all professionals.

CONCLUSION

Social accountability that enables equitable health care and education of professionals working in the health area to achieve these goals with marginalized populations is clearly identified in international reports. These goals mean consideration of the best approaches to teach practice and the diversity of knowledge underpinning this practice. Awareness of the impact of our values and tacit perspectives on service users and carers are critical to graduate outcomes.

CRITICAL THINKING QUESTIONS

1. How do principles of equity and social justice impact on health care of vulnerable populations? Can you give examples that advantage some populations and disadvantage others?
2. How would you model good practice to others in working with marginalized populations? Can you provide examples of both good and poor modelling of your professional practice? What is the difference between these two approaches?

3. Identify a marginalized group of people that you are familiar with from your practice. These groups could be refugees, Indigenous peoples, homeless people, transgender and intersex people, or displaced populations. What questions might you ask about the delivery of health care and their journey to receiving health care? If you are teaching, which pedagogical strategies might you employ, and what are potential benefits/drawbacks/enablers/barriers as you seek to sensitize and transform those around you?
4. Health professionals are clear about the core values in the delivery of health care. Are the values of under-served populations the same as those of health providers? What are the similarities and differences, and why is this so?
5. What does empathy mean to you? Reflect on a situation when another person displayed empathy towards you and how that made you feel. What did they say or do that makes you think it was empathy? How might you use this in your own practice/work?
6. Are you aware of overt or tacit discrimination in learning or in your health care practice? How is this manifested, and what strategies are available to discuss these issues?

REFERENCES

Association of Faculties of Medicine in Canada (AFMC), College of Family Physicians of Canada (CFPC), Le Collège des médecins du Québec (CMQ), and the Royal College of Physicians and Surgeons of Canada (RCPSC). 2012. *The Future of Medical Education in Canada: A Collective Vision for Postgraduate Medical Education in Canada.* https://www.afmc.ca/future-of-medical-education-in-canada/postgraduate-project/pdf/FMEC_PG_Final-Report_EN.pdf.

Baba, L. 2013. *Cultural Safety in First Nations, Inuit and Métis Public Health: Environmental Scan of Cultural Competency and Safety in Education, Training and Health Services.* Prince George, BC: National Collaborating Centre for Aboriginal Health. http://cahr.uvic.ca/nearbc/media/docs/cahr5194682829965-cipher_report_en_web.pdf.

Bekemeier, B., and P. Butterfield. 2005. "Unreconciled Inconsistencies: A Critical Review of the Concept of Social Justice in 3 National Nursing Documents." *Advances in Nursing Science* 28 (2): 152–62.

Benbassat, Jochanan, and Reuben Baumal. 2004. "What Is Empathy, and How Can It Be Promoted During Clinical Clerkships?" *Academic Medicine* 79 (9): 832–9.

Boelen, Charles, Shafik Dharamsi, and Trevor Gibbs. 2012. "The Social Accountability of Medical Schools and Its Indicators." *Education for Health* 25 (3): 180–94. https://doi.org/10.4103/1357-6283.109785.

Butin, Dan. 2010. *Service Learning in Theory and Practice.* New York: Palgrave Macmillan.

Campbell, David J. T., Katherine Gibson, Braden G. O'Neill, and Wilfreda E. Thurston. 2013. "The Role of a Student-Run Clinic in Providing Primary Care for Calgary's Homeless

Populations: A Qualitative Study." *BMC Health Services Research* 13: 277. https://doi.org/10.1186/1472-6963-13-277.

Cranton, Patricia. 2010. "A Transformative Perspective on the Scholarship of Teaching and Learning." *Higher Education Research & Development* 30 (1): 75–86. https://doi.org/10.1080/07294360.2011.536974.

Driessen, Erik, Jan van Tartwijk, Cees van der Vleuten, and Val Wass. 2007. "Portfolios in Medical Education: Why Do They Meet with Mixed Success? A Systematic Review." *Medical Education* 41 (12): 1224–33. https://doi.org/10.1111/j.1365-2923.2007.02944.x.

Freire, Paulo. 1972. *Pedagogy of the Oppressed.* Middlesex, UK: Penguin.

Frenk, Julio, Lincoln Chen, Zulfiqar Bhutta, Jordan Cohen, Nigel Crisp, Timothy Evans, Harvey Fineberg, et al. 2010. "Health Professionals for a New Century: Transforming Education to Strengthen Health Systems in an Interdependent World." *Lancet* 376 (9756): 1923–58. https://doi.org/10.1016/S0140-6736(10)61854-5.

Global Consensus for Social Accountability of Medical Schools. 2010. *Global Consensus for Social Accountability of Medical Schools.* December. http://healthsocialaccountability.sites.olt.ubc.ca/files/2011/06/11-06-07-GCSA-English-pdf-style.pdf.

Godkin, Michael, and Judith Savageau. 2001. "The Effect of a Global Multiculturalism Track on Cultural Competence of Preclinical Medical Students." *Family Medicine* 33 (3): 178–86.

Hafferty, F. W. 1998. "Beyond Curriculum Reform: Confronting Medicine's Hidden Curriculum." *Academic Medicine* 73 (4): 403–7.

Harding, Sandra. 2009. "Standpoint Theories: Productively Controversial." *Hypatia* 24 (4): 192–200. https://doi.org/10.1111/j.1527-2001.2009.01067.x.

Hojat, Mohammadreza, Michael J. Vergare, Kaye Maxwell, George Brainard, Steven K. Herrine, Gerald A. Isenberg, Jon Veloski, and Joseph S. Gonnella. 2009. "The Devil Is in the Third Year: A Longitudinal Study of Erosion of Empathy in Medical School." *Academic Medicine* 84 (9): 1182–91. https://doi.org/10.1097/ACM.0b013e3181b17e55.

Holmqvist, M., Carole Courtney, Ryan Meili, and Alixe Dick. 2012. "Student-Run Clinics: Opportunities for Interprofessional Education and Increasing Social Accountability." *Journal of Research in Interprofessional Practice and Education* 2 (3). http://jripe.org/jripe/index.php/journal/article/viewFile/80/61.

International Federation of Medical Students' Associations (IFMSA). n.d. "About INcommunity." Accessed April 5, 2018. http://ifmsa.qc.ca/en/committees/human-rights-peace-scorp/activities/incommunity/.

Kirkham, Sheryl, and Annette Browne. 2006. "Toward a Critical Theoretical Interpretation of Social Justice Discourses in Nursing." *Advances in Nursing Science* 29 (4): 324–39.

Kolb, David. 1984. *Experiential Learning: Experience as the Source of Learning and Development.* Englewood Cliffs, NJ: Prentice Hall.

Lam, Ruby. n.d. *Made in Sinai Health Equity Competencies: Delivering Health Care to Diverse Communities—Community Consultation Summary Findings.* Toronto: Mount Sinai Hospital Joseph and Wolf Lebovic Health Complex. https://www.mountsinai.on.ca/about_us/human-rights/CommunityConsultationMSH.pdf.

Lappano, Jon-Eric. 2011. 8th Annual Guide to Sustainable Education in Canada. *Corporate Knights Magazine*, September 27.

Lave, Jean, and Etienne Wenger. 1991. *Situated Learning: Legitimate Peripheral Participation.* New York: Cambridge University Press.

McIntosh, Peggy. 1988. "White Privilege: Unpacking the Invisible Knapsack." In "White Privilege and Male Privilege: A Personal Account of Coming to See Correspondences through Work in Women's Studies." Working Paper 189. http://www.collegeart.org/pdf/diversity/white-privilege-and-male-privilege.pdf.

Mercer, Stewart, and William Reynolds. 2002. "Empathy and Quality of Care." *British Journal of General Practice* 52 (suppl): S9–12.

Mezirow, Jack. 1991. *Transformative Dimensions of Adult Learning.* San Francisco: Jossey-Bass.

Mill, Judy, Barbara Astle, Linda Ogilvie, and Denise Gastaldo. 2010. "Linking Global Citizenship, Undergraduate Nursing Education, and Professional Nursing: Curricular Innovation in the 21st Century." *Advances in Nursing Science* 33 (3): E1–11. https://doi.org/10.1097/ANS.0b013e3181eb416f.

Newton, Bruce, Laurie Barber, James Clardy, Elton Cleveland, and Patricia O'Sullivan. 2008. "Is There Hardening of the Heart During Medical School?" *Academic Medicine* 83 (3): 244–9.

Papps, Elean, and Irihapeti Ramsden. 1996. "Cultural Safety in Nursing: The New Zealand Experience." *International Journal for Quality in Health Care* 8 (5): 491–7. https://doi.org/10.1093/intqhc/8.5.491.

Perry, Beth. 2009. "Role Modeling Excellence in Clinical Nursing Practice." *Nurse Education in Practice* 9 (1): 36–44. https://doi.org/10.1016/j.nepr.2008.05.001.

Pinto, Andrew, and Ross Upshur. 2009. "Global Health Ethics for Students." *Developing World Bioethics* 9 (1): 1–10. https://doi.org/10.1111/j.1471-8847.2007.00209.x.

Simpson, Scott A., and Judith A. Long. 2007. "Medical Student-Run Health Clinics: Important Contributors to Patient Care and Medical Education." *Journal of General Internal Medicine* 22 (3): 352–6. https://doi.org/10.1007/s11606-006-0073-4.

Society of Student Run Free Clinics (SSRFC). n.d. "Creation of SSRFC." Accessed March 31, 2016. http://studentrunfreeclinics.org/about/.

Starfield, Barbara. 2011. "The Hidden Inequity in Health Care." *International Journal for Equity in Health* 10 (15). https://doi.org/10.1186/1475-9276-10-15.

Strasser, Sheryl, Megan O. Smith, Danielle Pendrick Denney, Matt C. Jackson, and Pam Buckmaster. 2013. "A Poverty Simulation to Inform Public Health Practice." *American Journal of Health Education* 44 (5): 259–64. https://doi.org/10.1080/19325037.2013.811366.

Student Wellness Initiative towards Community Health (SWITCH). n.d. "About SWITCH." Accessed April 5, 2018. http://switchclinic.com/about/.

Trevithick, Pamela. 2012. *Social Work Skills and Knowledge: A Practice Handbook.* Maidenhead, UK: Open University Press.

CHAPTER 25

Thinking Upstream:
A Vision for a Healthy Society

Ryan Meili and Thomas Piggott

LEARNING OBJECTIVES

After reading this chapter, you should be able to:

1. Understand the perspective of shifting thinking on health issues upstream.
2. Describe the "Trinity Trap" in health promotion and the differences between focusing on individual risk factors and the root causes for health conditions.
3. Understand the Health in All Policies approach to health policy planning.
4. Describe ways that health providers can work towards developing healthier societies for under-served populations.

BACKGROUND

Imagine for a moment that you're standing at the edge of a river. You see a kid floating by, and that kid is struggling, drowning. Brave soul that you are, you tear off your shoes, dive into the water, and haul that kid to shore. You feel exhilarated. You saved a life. But then, before you're even dry, another kid comes floating by, and you dive in again. Then along comes kid number three, and four, and five. You're calling everyone you know to help you haul kids out of the river. Eventually, hopefully, one of you is wise enough to ask, "Who keeps chucking these kids in the river?" and heads upstream to try and find out.

This classic public health story is an analogy for how we approach health in general. We spend most of our time dealing with the symptoms of illness rather than the root causes. When discussing health in public policy, we tend to focus on health care services: doctors and hospitals, pharmaceuticals and technology.

A significant body of research has established the concept of the social determinants of health (SDH), the factors influenced by political and economic policies that play a significant role in health outcomes (Raphael 2008; Mikkonen and Raphael 2010). There have been numerous lists of SDH, such as those by Raphael in Chapter 2 in this volume, the Public Health Agency of Canada (see box: Public Health Agency of Canada List of Determinants of Health), and the World Health Organization (see box: Nine Themes from the World Health Organization Commission on the Social Determinants of Health).

Public Health Agency of Canada List of Determinants of Health

1. Income and social status
2. Social support networks
3. Education and literacy
4. Employment/working conditions
5. Social environments
6. Physical environments
7. Personal health practices and coping skills
8. Healthy child development
9. Biology and genetic endowment
10. Health services
11. Gender
12. Culture

Source: Public Health Agency of Canada (2011).

Nine Themes from the World Health Organization Commission on the Social Determinants of Health

1. Employment conditions
2. Social exclusion
3. Priority public health conditions
4. Women and gender equity
5. Early child development
6. Globalization
7. Health systems
8. Measurement and evidence
9. Urbanization

Source: WHO (n.d.).

There are certainly valid academic reasons for exploring and debating among the various lists as to which is the most accurate or helpful in influencing policy decisions, but, when reviewing the various lists of SDH, the overall point is clear. When we look at what influences whether we will be ill or well, whether our lives will be long or short, health services play a minor role. For health care providers that dedicate all their energy towards health services, this work can be difficult. Health care providers don't want to hear that most of the factors that impact health are outside the realm of their clinic or hospital. Certainly, reviewing a high-level list of SDH doesn't make the process of recognizing the factors that really impact health any easier. To better understand this impact, let us consider a single individual's story. Stories are the unit of our everyday encounters in health care, and here we will reflect on the factors outside the realm of health care—the upstream factors that can drive health.

To many of us in health care, Crystal's story (see below) is all too common. Given what she has experienced, given all of the upstream factors that have acted against her, anything we do in the clinic will not really make a substantial impact on Crystal's health. To respond to her health issues, we need to shift our thinking upstream. We need to be thinking about how to get her enough money to live, how to make sure she's got a good place to stay, how to connect her to supports to help her deal with the addictions that resulted from the trauma in her life.

Crystal's Story

I (R. M.) work at the West Side Community Clinic in inner-city Saskatoon, Saskatchewan. I live in the same neighbourhood as I work, and often, on my walk to work, I run into someone who we will call Crystal.

Every time I see Crystal, it makes my day. She's got a big wave and a big smile, and she always has something funny to say. It makes my day, and it breaks my heart, because I'm not seeing her in the clinic. I'm seeing her on the street corner, which is a bad thing, because she's quite sick. She has HIV and her CD4 count—which tells us how well she can fight infection—is really low: around 10. It should be up around 1,000.

As a result of this diminished immune system, she gets frequent bouts of pneumonia and other infections. When she does, she comes in to the clinic and gets treatment for those acute illnesses, but she hasn't been able to take the antiretroviral medications that we know would make a difference in restoring her immune system. The reason is that she's not really sick with HIV. She's sick with poverty. She's sick with a truncated education from becoming a mother when she was still a child, sick with never having had stable housing, sick with the abuse she suffered as a child, and the abuse and marginalization—she's First Nations—of her people over generations and generations.

SALUTOGENESIS AND PROMOTING THE HEALTH OF UNDER-SERVED POPULATIONS

An early health promotion theorist who thought about the "river of health" and the implications of our "downstream" thinking was an Israeli sociologist, Aaron Antonovsky. Antonovsky (1996) wrote about the blossoming of an interest in the prevention of disease, but felt that the focus on preventing disease, pathogenesis, was a downstream approach. He argued that even "health promoters" are focused on preventing disease. This is true to this day. A quick Google search for health promotion will bring up images of diabetes and heart disease prevention programs.

Antonovsky argued that, given the prevalence of diseases, people are more often "diseased" than healthy, and that moving upstream requires moving away from a sole focus on pathogenesis to a salutogenesis orientation (*salutos* is Latin for health). The salutogenic orientation, as is shown in figure 25.1, involves shifting our downstream focus on the disease we see in front of us to an upstream one focused on the factors that lead to health and disease. Microbes, injuries, and genetic mutations are pathogenic, but what factors are salutogenic?

The factors "chucking" the kids into the river upstream, the drivers that have the biggest influence on health outcomes, are not in fact medical. When considered in the light of our understanding of the social determinants of health, it's clear that the causes of Crystal's ill health are political. Therefore, any solutions to improve her health—any salutogenic interventions—must be political as well. But in order to make better political decisions, we need the space for these good decisions to happen.

Unfortunately, political conversations about health still tend to fall into familiar traps. When we talk about health, we return again and again, as if by reflex, to the health care system. This is an understandable impulse, as these tend to be the sorts of activities that fall under the mandates of ministries or departments of health—the areas of government that we imagine are most responsible for keeping us healthy. It's also important to note that health services are still a factor in achieving equitable health, especially in countries with universal health insurance systems. The estimates vary, but health care is described as accounting for less than 25 percent of health outcomes, compared to 50 percent or greater for the social determinants of health (Keon and Pépin 2008). This is not insignificant, but it means that if our goals are optimal population health and helping under-served and marginalized people like Crystal, even the best health care system can only take us so far.

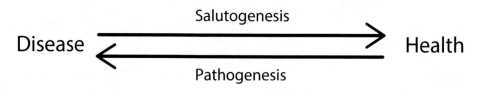

Figure 25.1: The Continuum of Health

THE TRINITY TRAP

When speaking of prevention, even professionals in the field tend to have a difficult time moving beyond what is often referred to as the "holy trinity" (Nettleton 1997) of health promotion: smoking, diet, and exercise. Just as when we think about health, we can be trapped into thinking about health care, when thinking about prevention and health promotion, we can get trapped into thinking only about the most obvious elements of behavioural choices without considering the larger context in which those choices are made.

As a result of this shift in understanding, nods to prevention and health promotion have become a regular element of public discourse on health. This is not to say that these are not important factors in health outcomes. Stopping smoking is one of the most effective means available to an individual to expand his or her lifespan and improve well-being. Despite the fact that most patients are dealing with factors high up on the list of social determinants, whenever possible, we counsel on smoking cessation and frequently discuss diet and exercise at length.

In reality, the problem is not that we talk about these individual choices. The problem is that as clinicians, that's where we stop, and in doing so, we fail to address the factors that will have the greatest impact. Why is that, then, when we know that the social determinants of health are what matter most? Why do we get stuck in the trinity trap?

Some of this may be a matter of health promotion being a victim of its own success. Victories in informing public opinion have had great influence in improving diet and exercise and decreasing smoking, at least in certain segments of the population. Health behaviours tend to improve with rising incomes, as social factors determine not only health but also behaviour. In fact, there's been some argument that in this way, health promotion has actually increased health inequality, as the messages are most effective at reaching those with the least need of help (Rice 2011). People who are already wealthy have higher levels of education or other advantages, have more resources at their disposal, and are more able to increase their level of exercise, buy healthier foods, or take advantage of clinical smoking cessation supports, for example. They may also benefit from social pressures that reinforce healthy choices, a luxury not always available to vulnerable populations whose financial and social circumstances create systemic barriers to healthy choices. This is well characterized by the tongue-in-cheek list of top ten social determinants tips for better health (see the following box).

Of course, the limitations of a health promotion approach do not constitute an argument to stop promoting wise individual choices, but it does demonstrate the way that this approach, taken alone, can actually impede health improvements or worsen health inequities for marginalized populations. These successful campaigns may play a role in crowding the field, acting as a go-to set of prevention points that block us from thinking in greater depth about what really keeps people healthy.

Health is most easily imagined through stories, whether our own or those of patients dealing with specific illnesses. The solutions are, accordingly, most easily imagined at

> ### The Social Determinants—10 Tips for Better Health
>
> 1. Don't be poor. If you are, stop. If you can't, try not to be poor for long.
> 2. Don't have poor parents.
> 3. Own a car.
> 4. Don't work in a stressful, low-paid manual job.
> 5. Don't live in damp, low-quality housing.
> 6. Be able to afford to go on a foreign holiday and sunbathe.
> 7. Practise not losing your job and don't become unemployed.
> 8. Take up all benefits you are entitled to, if you are unemployed, retired or sick or disabled.
> 9. Don't live next to a busy major road or near a polluting factory.
> 10. Learn how to fill in the complex housing benefit/asylum application forms before you become homeless and destitute.
>
> *Source:* Gordon (1999).

the same level. Someone has poorly controlled diabetes? It's far easier to consider what they choose to eat each day than it is to address the prevalence of food insecurity in their region and the macroeconomic policies that influence what choices are available. It's so much simpler and quicker to think of personal agency rather than societal agency. As a result, even public policy measures tend to focus on influencing individual choices through awareness campaigns and incentives.

HEALTH IN ALL POLICIES

The *Closing the Gap in a Generation* report from the World Health Organization's Commission on the Social Determinants of Health (2008), led by social determinants of health pioneer Sir Michael Marmot, has outlined a global agenda for health equity. Three "Principles of Action" give us an understanding of the steps required to achieve health equity, as well as the scope of the challenge:

1. Improve the conditions of daily life—the circumstances in which people are born, grow, live, work, and age.
2. Tackle the inequitable distribution of power, money, and resources—the structural drivers of those conditions of daily life—globally, nationally, and locally.
3. Measure the problem, evaluate action, expand the knowledge base, develop a workforce that is trained in the social determinants of health, and raise public awareness about the social determinants of health.

The list of determinants of health themselves—economics, education, environment, and so on—are by definition linked to policy and politics. At every level of government, there are departments tasked with addressing these issues. This work is also clearly not the role of the Ministry of Health, but really encompasses the whole of government, leading some countries, provinces, and municipalities to apply a new lens that takes into account the health impact of decisions in every area, be it education or economic development, environmental regulations or income supports.

This "Health in All Policies" model has been gradually gaining traction around the world since the latter part of the twentieth century. One of the earliest examples was the North Karelia project in Finland in the 1970s. In order to improve heart health in one of the least healthy parts of the country, policy-makers worked with food producers to reduce the salt and fat in their products, improve workplace menus, and toughen anti-smoking laws. As a result, cardiac disease was reduced in 18- to 65-year-olds by 73 percent over 25 years (Puska 2002).

In 2002, Quebec became the first Canadian province to implement Health in All Policies, and health impact assessments have become routine and influential elements of government decisions (Kickbusch and Buckett 2010). English Canada has been slower to follow suit, but there are signs of progress, with municipalities performing more health impact assessments, and the government of Newfoundland and Labrador announcing an intention to establish a Health in All Policies approach (Government of Newfoundland and Labrador 2015). The World Health Organization (WHO 2015) has recently released a step-by-step guide for governments at various levels to make the shift to Health in All Policies, giving some hope that this model will be more easily accessible and universally applied. If done properly, with a sufficient focus on health equity, a Health in All Policies approach can have significant impacts on the health of vulnerable populations.

CHANGING THE LANDSCAPE

As our understanding of the social determinants of health illustrates, politics is the field of human endeavour with the greatest impact on health outcomes. If we think back to the core purpose of our public decision-making bodies, and the legitimacy on which their authority rests, their role, above all, should be to improve our health and well-being. Political decisions can and should improve our health, and they should be evaluated based on the degree to which they are successful in doing so.

Human health—physical, mental, and social—is the primary metric of the health of our society. It serves as a proxy for a host of meaningful variables. Using the SDH to guide our policies, and health indicators to judge their effectiveness, gives us a much-needed yardstick and an excellent alternative to relying on simple economic measures. It takes us from a situation where the goals of our society are limited to a range of narrow economic indicators that don't reflect the quality of our lives or whether all people within the society have the same opportunities to achieve optimal health and well-being.

Yet, in today's discourse, a narrow and economistic outlook seems to trump any attempts to address those social determinants. Our ability to realize what government is truly for, to improve the lives of people, is hampered by the terms of discussion. Whatever brilliant ideas may come forward to improve lives and health, whatever arguments may be advanced, they are quickly dismissed if they counter the current frame. That frame is informed to a great extent by the "TINA" frame: you may not like the system the way it's working now, but *There Is No Alternative*, so get on with your individual lives and let the market decide.

To get beyond TINA and evade the trinity trap, to create the space for political decisions to be driven by the goal of a healthy society, we need to shift the "Overton's window" of what is politically possible (Lehman 2003). Our current frames don't allow for this; they are about economics as the primary goal, about gross domestic product as the measurement of success, and about austerity rather than abundance.

Starting with the WHO's definition of health as being not just the absence of illness but full physical, social, and mental well-being, we have an inspiring model for a society, for what we would really want our country to be trying to achieve. That frame is there for us—it's something that already matters to us. When one starts to shift the measurement of success in our society, the space of options that are possible changes and the space of damaging decisions that can be made shrinks.

Changing the political landscape isn't something that happens overnight. Such a change takes many years, many voices, many stories. A new movement of advocates and academics, organizations and ordinary citizens, is trying to use the story of upstream thinking to change the political landscape by changing the frame of success, and the terms of the argument, to health. Upstream (http://www.thinkupstream.net) is a movement to build a healthy society through evidence-based, people-centred ideas. This national non-profit organization is intent on changing the current conversation, and it uses the parable of the river and our understanding of the social determinants to try to do so. Upstream aims to make the mainstream look upstream, helping citizens to demand a healthy society and to understand the best ways to get there. This sort of reframing effort is necessary if we're to open up enough space to discuss policies that would make real differences in income inequality, access to quality education, and affordable housing, and help maintain sufficient environmental integrity to safeguard human life. Without such a reframing, we get stuck downstream, focusing on sickness care and personal agency, and the social change needed to improve the lives of marginalized populations remains stubbornly out of reach.

Every time a young person winds up in jail, every time people have to take medicines to make up for the fact that they couldn't afford good food, we're suffering from the results of downstream thinking. Thinking upstream means making smarter decisions based on long-term outcomes. What better goal is there than creating the conditions for all people to enjoy true health—complete physical, mental, and social well-being? And what better measure of its success is there than the health of those people?

FRAMING FORWARD

Putting health outcomes as the lead measure of successful governance opens up space for ideas that now seem impossible. This starts with providing health care in an equitable fashion, providing the highest quality care for under-served populations. But it doesn't end there. Taking into account the principles of action from the *Closing the Gap in a Generation* report, it also means examining the distribution of wealth and power in our society.

An upstream approach also allows us to stop seeing investment in people as a cost. When we consider the economic and social benefits of a healthy, educated population, we see that by doing nothing to address the factors that make people sick, we ensure that more and more kids will fall into the river and that many of them will drown.

This means that ideas like living wages or basic income guarantees, Pharmacare or a national housing strategy, go from the margins of public policy to core mission. Rather than nice things we can have if they don't interfere with the economy, social investment starts to lead our political and policy choices.

Thinking and writing about upstream determinants of health brings a personal tension for me, because it means time spent away from patient care. There are kids in the river right now, and it's really frustrating because we want to be contributing to a healthier political environment, but we also want to be there to help people when they are sick.

Despite that tension, the reason to step away from the bedside to look upstream is a more serious frustration: the frustration of seeing young people such as Crystal coming back to the clinic over and over again with the same illnesses. This frustration is increasingly common among physicians and other health care providers, who realize that while we can give patients medications or advice and refer them to a specialist or a counsellor, we ultimately send them back into the situation that made them sick in the first place. There is a growing movement to recognize that health care providers can play a significant role in advocacy to address the social determinants of health (College of Family Physicians of Canada 2015). This advocacy can take place at the level of the individual patient (micro), the local community level (meso), or a systemic or political level (macro). Given the trusted voice that health professionals enjoy in society, their efforts can be a powerful means of turning attention to the health needs of the populations they serve.

This is incredibly important, because to improve the lives of the people we work with, we need social change. We need food security, adequate housing, and robust income supports. But in order to see that social change, we need a new frame. As American linguist George Lakoff (2004) has said, reframing is itself social change. It's the upstream thinking required for upstream action that leads to better downstream results. Because politics is at the root of many of our problems, it can be at the root of our solutions as well.

Inequities in health outcomes are the avoidable result of political decisions and social policy. Making decisions through a health lens gives us a way of improving the lives of under-served populations and increasing health equity that no health care solution alone could achieve. Returning to the story of Crystal, we see just how mobilizing supports through political action and public policy can make a huge difference in the lives of individuals and communities. Her life has changed considerably for a number of reasons, not least because of the introduction of a Housing First program that now has her living in a stable home. She is also connected with outreach workers who are helping her get to social service and medical appointments. She has started antiretroviral medications, and she is receiving more support for addictions. She's doing so much better now that I (R. M.) actually see her more often in the clinic than I do on my walk to work. And that gives me hope. If we change the frame, we start to invest upstream and address the things that keep people healthy rather than just responding to illness as it occurs. In doing so, we can help those who have fallen to the margins and build a truly healthy society.

CRITICAL THINKING QUESTIONS

1. Describe a health promotion program you have encountered for under-served populations. What orientation does it take: upstream or downstream? Why?
2. What population-level salutogenic factors for improving the health of under-served populations can you think of?
3. You have been tasked with improving health and resiliency with an inner-city, low-income population in your community. What upstream factors could you consider targeting? How might you measure the success of your intervention?

ADDITIONAL RESOURCES

Upstream: http://www.thinkupstream.net/
   Upstream is an independent, non-partisan organization incorporated as a non-profit organization. It is a movement to create a healthy society through evidence-based, people-centred ideas. Upstream seeks to reframe public discourse around addressing the social determinants of health in order to build a healthier society. It does this by sharing stories, actions, and evidence.

Meili, R. 2017. *A Healthy Society: How a Focus on Health Can Revive the Canadian Democracy.* Vancouver: UBC Press.
   This book, now in its second edition, is an important text that draws on evidence and stories to show the critical importance of health to democracy in Canada.

REFERENCES

Antonovsky, A. 1996. "The Salutogenic Model as a Theory to Guide Health Promotion." *Health Promotion International* 11 (1): 11–18. https://doi.org/10.1093/heapro/11.1.11.

College of Family Physicians of Canada. 2015. *Best Advice Guide: Social Determinants of Health.* Mississauga, ON: College of Family Physicians of Canada.

Commission on the Social Determinants of Health. 2008. *Closing the Gap in a Generation: Health Equity through Action on the Social Determinants of Health.* Final Report of the Commission on the Social Determinants of Health. Geneva: World Health Organization.

Gordon, D. 1999. "The Spirit of 1848 Listserv." *Spirit of 1848*, April. http://www.spiritof1848.org/listserv.htm.

Government of Newfoundland and Labrador. 2015. "Premier's Summit on Health Care Lays Foundation for Primary Health Reform." News Release, January 19. http://www.releases.gov.nl.ca/releases/2015/health/0119n06.aspx.

Keon, W. J., and L. Pépin. 2008. *Population Health Policy: Issues and Options.* Ottawa: Senate of Canada.

Kickbusch, I., and K. Buckett. 2010. *Implementing Health in All Policies: Adelaide 2010.* Geneva: World Health Organization.

Lakoff, G. 2004. *Don't Think of an Elephant.* White River Junction, VT: Chelsea Green.

Lehman, J. 2003. "A Brief Explanation of the Overton Window." Mackinac Center for Public Policy. Accessed July 13, 2015. http://www.mackinac.org/12887#Explanation.

Mikkonen, J., and D. Raphael. 2010. *Social Determinants of Health: The Canadian Facts.* Toronto: York University School of Health Policy and Management.

Nettleton, S. 1997. "Surveillance, Health Promotion and the Formation of a Risk Identity." In *Debates and Dilemmas in Promoting Health*, edited by M. Sidell, L. Jones, J. Katz, and A. Peberdy, 314–24. London: Open University Press.

Puska, P. 2002. "Successful Prevention of Non-communicable Diseases: 25 Year Experiences with North Karelia Project in Finland." *Public Health Medicine* 4 (1): 5–7.

Public Health Agency of Canada. 2011. "What Determines Health?" Last modified October 21. http://www.phac-aspc.gc.ca/ph-sp/determinants/index-eng.php.

Raphael, D. 2008. *Social Determinants of Health.* 2nd ed. Toronto: Canadian Scholars' Press.

Rice W. 2011. *Health Promotion through an Equity Lens.* Toronto: Wellesley Institute.

World Health Organization (WHO). n.d. "Evidence on Social Determinants of Health." Accessed April 24, 2018. http://www.who.int/social_determinants/themes/en/.

World Health Organization (WHO). 2015. *Health in All Policies: Training Manual.* Geneva: WHO.

CHAPTER 26

Reforming Health Systems to Promote Equity and Improve the Health of Under-Served Populations

Anne Andermann

LEARNING OBJECTIVES

After reading this chapter, you should be able to:

1. Understand the role of structural factors and systems in creating marginalization.
2. Appreciate the complexity involved and jurisdictional ambiguities in addressing challenges relating to disadvantaged and under-served populations.
3. Identify pathways for creating structural changes to promote more inclusive, equitable, and healthier societies.

BACKGROUND

Improving the health of marginalized populations requires action on the social determinants of health, which is not something that can be achieved through the efforts of the health sector alone (Commission on the Social Determinants of Health 2008). Indeed, the health sector is but a single component in a much larger web of health determinants including education, employment, and housing (Mahamoud et al. 2013). However, either the health sector can be part of the solution by promoting health equity within the health system and beyond, or it can contribute to the regressive structural factors that maintain and widen health gaps from generation to generation.

This chapter will outline some of the ways in which health systems may contribute to health inequities—even if inadvertently—as well as ways in which health systems can become more pro-equity in the future.

THE GOALS OF THE HEALTH SYSTEM

According to the *World Health Report 2000*, "health systems have a responsibility not just to improve people's health but to protect them against the financial cost of illness—and to treat them with dignity" (Musgrove et al. 2000, 8). Multiple objectives are therefore involved, including improving the overall health of the population while at the same time reducing gaps in health outcomes between individuals and groups, preventing catastrophic health expenditure and poverty due to out-of-pocket spending during illness, and treating patients in a way that considers the whole person and promotes their agency and involvement in decisions that affect their current and future well-being.

Improving Overall Population Health

Life expectancy in Canada increased by 24.6 years between the years 1921 and 2011 (Decady and Greenberg 2014). Much of this improvement in health outcomes results from reductions in infant and child mortality, particularly in the first half of the twentieth century, as well as further reductions in mortality in more recent decades due to fewer premature heart disease deaths among younger adults. Moreover, while mortality is now occurring in later age groups (predominantly among persons 75 to 89 years of age), functional health and quality of life continue for longer, with more severe disability occurring after 77 years of age on average. Thus, in Canada, as in many other countries around the world, there have been significant improvements in overall population health in recent generations.

Reducing Health Inequities between Groups

While Canadians are much healthier on the whole than they were a century ago, not all groups fare as well. For instance, homeless persons in Canada have a life expectancy that is almost 40 years less than the population average (Hwang et al. 2009; Condon and McDermid 2014). Babies born to Inuit mothers today have infant mortality rates not much lower than the Canadian rates in the 1920s, which is two to three times higher than current rates in the general population (18.7 infant deaths per 1,000 live births among Inuit babies as compared to 4.9 infant deaths per 1,000 live births among non-Aboriginal babies) (Gilbert, Auger, and Tjepkema 2015). These are simply a few examples, but the list of marginalized groups with worse health outcomes as compared to the general population is vast, including immigrants and refugees, young single mothers, persons who are institutionalized or incarcerated, persons with mental health problems and addictions, persons with disabilities, children living in poverty, and isolated seniors, all of whom not only have greater health needs but tend to "fall through the cracks" of traditional health systems.

Preventing Catastrophic Health Expenditure

Despite health care services in Canada being largely publicly funded via the ten provincial and three territorial health systems that make up our Canadian health system, this is mostly true for services delivered in hospitals or through doctors' offices (Maioni 2014). However, with changing medical practice over the years, as well as the demographic transition resulting in greater chronic disease care required later in life, there is more and more that is often left uncovered by public health insurance, and users therefore must bear the additional costs themselves unless they can afford and access private health insurance. This is true even in Canada, and is particularly challenging for marginalized patients who have difficulties accessing mainstream care and thus take a "double hit"—reduced access to care at a greater cost. For instance, "most vulnerable elderly do not have a coordinated care system they can rely on; instead, they are dependent on office visits, hospital and emergency room care, a family caregiver (for those who have access), or an assisted living situation (for those who can afford it)" (Maioni 2014, 38).

Treating All Patients with Dignity and Respect

The health system is part of the larger society in which it is embedded, and as a result, certain prejudices and structural forms of racism and violence can also be present—overtly or not—within these systems. Despite health professionals learning about person-centred care during their training, there are nonetheless examples, in Canada and beyond, of patients not receiving the attention and care that they deserve; and when they do receive care, it is not always provided in a respectful and dignified way. A recent and disturbing example of this are the findings of a report entitled *First Peoples, Second Class Treatment: The Role of Racism in the Health and Well-Being of Indigenous Peoples in Canada* (Allan and Smylie 2015). In this report, the authors explain that "stereotypes of Aboriginal people impact the care they receive ... being denied treatment or access to hospital care based on assumptions that they were drunk or that they were 'troublemakers' ... [and] how the anticipation or experience of being blamed for one's own health problems prevented some from even trying to access hospital care at all" (27). There is even increasing concern about the way in which power differentials within the doctor-patient relationship can lead to criminal abuses including sexual misconduct (Collège des médecins du Québec 2018). Important needs exist, then, to create safe spaces within health care settings, clarify boundaries, and provide trauma-informed care that considers the whole person, since health workers have more power to promote social accountability than they may realize, starting at the patient level (Goel et al. 2016).

HEALTH SYSTEMS—PART OF THE PROBLEM?

Even though by definition, "health systems consist of all the people and actions whose primary purpose is to improve health" (Musgrove et al. 2000, 1), there are times when these actions are intentionally or inadvertently counterproductive.

The Inverse-Care Law

It has long been recognized that those with the greatest health needs are often less likely to be able to access quality health care, particularly when market forces are at play (Tudor Hart 1971). The inverse-care law can also be found when local conditions are so dire that it is difficult to attract health workers to provide services in areas where people are most in need—for instance, in conflict and post-conflict areas, or in areas with extreme poverty and few resources (Moosa et al. 2013). This also applies to northern, rural, and remote areas of Canada, where health workers are often transient, and recruitment and retention are difficult. Even in heavily populated inner-city settings, there are relatively sparse outreach services to meet the needs of those out in the community who, for various health or social reasons, are less able to navigate often complex and siloed hospital-centric health and social systems.

The Health Care Imperative

Health systems are often focused on acute health care issues, dealing with day-to-day problems and "putting out fires" through diagnosing health conditions and providing patients with treatment and rehabilitation. However, there is generally less time and fewer resources dedicated to preventing disease in the first place and promoting health more broadly using the strategies laid out in the *Ottawa Charter for Health Promotion* (WHO 1986). Often, the focus on prevention only enters the public discourse after some breakdown has occurred and people are looking to understand what went wrong—for instance, after the Walkerton crisis or the SARS outbreak. Only then do people appreciate that neglected and anemic public health systems need to be better funded and strengthened (Naylor et al. 2004), rather than dismantled in the name of greater efficiency and cost-savings, as is the current trend (Guyon et al. 2017). Indeed, more emphasis on prevention can lead to a greater return on investment for each health dollar spent, and prevention provides better value for money; yet all too often, this aspect gets overlooked in favour of acute care services that are often more expensive in the long run than it would be to get the root of the problem and prevent disease and human suffering in the first place (Young and Olsen 2010).

HEALTH SYSTEM REFORM TO INCREASE HEALTH EQUITY

In order to make progress in reducing disparities in health outcomes, health equity needs to be clearly articulated and at the core of every health system, every health worker mandate, and every health action.

Primary Health Care as the Cornerstone of the Health System

A key mechanism through which health systems can contribute to improving health equity, social justice, and the end of exclusion is to move towards universal health coverage and social health protection by making health care services available to all, and to transform conventional health care into primary health care by putting patients at the centre of care and bringing care closer to the people (WHO 2008). At the global level, there is still a long way to go, as 100 million people fall into extreme poverty each year due to health expenses, and 800 million spend more than 10 percent of their annual income on out-of-pocket health expenses (WHO and World Bank 2017).

Indeed, beyond preventing poverty, having a "patient medical home" can also make a major impact on improving health outcomes, especially for marginalized patients (Sugarman et al. 2014). The patient medical home assures that every individual has timely access to a family physician or other primary health care professionals, including nurses, midwives, or community health workers, depending on the context, all working within a patient-centred primary health care team, with coordination and continuity of care, close to where patients live (College of Family Physicians of Canada 2009).

Reorienting Health Systems

In addition to addressing the under-service of marginalized populations in terms of diagnosis and treatment, there is a need for greater "upstream" focus on disease and injury prevention, health promotion, and addressing the social determinants of health (see Meili and Piggott, Chapter 25 in this volume). It is important to ensure that the entire continuum of these strategies is being used to improve health (Andermann 2013).

Even when a new program or service intended to improve health is developed, such as a cancer screening program or a sexual health education curriculum in schools, the consideration of equity is critical, so that those who have the greatest education and ability to navigate the system don't end up as the sole beneficiaries. Even a well-intentioned program can lead to increased inequities if those who are more marginalized are less able to benefit; ongoing vigilance and monitoring are required to ensure that certain population subgroups are not being left behind (Morère et al. 2018).

For instance, a school-based program may not reach students who have already dropped out of school and are even more vulnerable. Thus, it is necessary to always think ahead of ways to increase access for those most in need (e.g., through outreach), as well as ways of evaluating whether marginalized groups are accessing care and benefitting from it.

Supporting a Pro-equity Lens within the Health Workforce

Front-line health workers can make a difference in reducing health inequities, particularly when they attempt to address the root causes of morbidity and mortality, in addition to treating illness (Gilbert, Auger, and Tjepkema 2015). First, health workers can play a key role in improving outcomes for marginalized patients in the way that they organize their clinical practice to make it more accessible (e.g., close proximity to where marginalized patients live, welcoming look and feel, extended open hours after regular working hours and on weekends, no hidden fees, etc.).

> ### Case Study: The CLEAR Toolkit
>
> Established in 2010, an international collaboration of researchers and policy-makers joined together with the goal of creating an evidence-based clinical decision aid to help front-line health workers contribute to raising awareness and tackle the social determinants of health, particularly in low- and middle-income countries. The CLEAR toolkit (available at http://www.mcgill.ca/clear) was developed based on 1) a realist review of the literature on what health workers can do to address the social determinants of health; 2) primary research with vulnerable patients, their health care workers, and community members to determine what patients would find helpful and what health workers have found effective in practice; 3) feedback from key informants and international experts in social determinants and primary health care; and 4) pilot studies in a wide variety of health care settings, ranging from remote Aboriginal communities and inner-city neighbourhoods with a high prevalence of immigrants and refugees in high-income countries, to urban slums and rural areas in low- and middle-income countries. The resulting toolkit is therefore a practical and clinical practice–oriented way of enabling primary health care workers to provide much needed support to disadvantaged patients, as well as to galvanize community mobilization, intersectoral partnerships, and policy change at multiple levels. In particular, the toolkit guides front-line health workers in a) treating the immediate health problem, b) asking about underlying social problems, c) referring to local social support resources, and d) advocating for more supportive environments for health. The toolkit has been translated into over a dozen languages including Arabic, Russian, Chinese, Urdu, French, Spanish, and Portuguese.

In addition, health workers can also ask about and support patients in dealing with complex health and social issues through taking a social history and referring to social support services (Andermann 2011). Health care workers can be made more aware of the issues that marginalized patients face, and of their own background and preconceived notions, to provide more culturally safe care (Macaulay 2009).

There are also numerous opportunities for increased advocacy by health care professionals who come into regular contact with the health effects and human suffering caused by these inequities while working on the front lines (British Medical Association 2011). The role of health care providers engaging in advocacy around issues related to the health of under-served populations will be discussed further in the following chapter.

Promoting Community Development through Intersectoral Action

Improving the health of populations requires intersectoral action and sustainable community development (WHO 2012). Indeed, there are long-standing models of how front-line health workers can help to galvanize intersectoral action and impact social determinants at a grassroots level.

The concept of community-oriented primary care (COPC; discussed at length in Chapter 15 by Guenter, Oudshoorn, and Mancini in this volume) was developed by two family doctors, Sidney and Emily Kark, while they were working in a poor rural community in South Africa in the 1940s. Rather than treating each health problem that presented at their doorstep, the Karks wondered what more could be done to prevent these problems, which were so common in the community. COPC is thus "a continuous process by which primary care is provided to a defined community on the basis of its assessed health needs through the planned integration of public health practice with the delivery of primary care services" (Mullan and Epstein 2002, 1750); it is an important approach that should receive greater emphasis in undergraduate and postgraduate medical training programs to enable future health workers to incorporate COPC in their day-to-day clinical practice.

Partnering with Local Government and Community Groups

While health workers can be important catalysts in the process of community development, many other local partners, including municipal government and community groups, are needed to make this happen. However, the notion of intersectoral action and collaboration towards reducing health inequities may be a rather novel concept in certain spheres. While recreational programming and affordable housing are considered within the remit of local governments in taking action on the social determinants of health, insufficient federal and provincial funding is often perceived to be the biggest constraint on municipal action, raising concerns about "inter-governmental downloading of responsibilities, and behaviour-based assumptions of disease etiology" (Collins and Hayes 2013, e304). Yet, supportive guidance and coaching can help civil servants, managers, and municipal councillors in adopting a "Health in All Policies" approach with the aim of improving health and social outcomes for the community (Steenbakkers et al. 2012).

THE CANADIAN HEALTH POLICY CONTEXT AS IT RELATES TO UNDER-SERVED POPULATIONS

When considering the Canadian health policy context as it pertains to under-served populations, one must necessarily identify the jurisdictional responsibilities in this regard. For instance, in relation to the issue of homeless persons with mental health conditions, who is responsible for creating the social safety net and ensuring adequate and appropriate access to care? There is no simple answer to such complex questions. Addressing these issues often involves "shared responsibility" across multiple government departments and levels of jurisdiction, and as a result, things tend to "fall between the cracks." Health care services clearly fall within provincial and territorial jurisdiction in Canada, and on the whole, the federal government is not involved in social housing (except on reserves and in certain military bases), which is left to provincial and municipal authorities (Munn-Rivard 2014).

This challenge of jurisdictional ambiguity is also a major issue pertaining to Indigenous health. Even within the federal government, there are multiple departments supporting various aspects—for instance, until recently, Indigenous and Northern Affairs Canada dealt with infrastructure for housing and water, Health Canada's First Nations and Inuit Health Branch with health care services on reserve, and the Public Health Agency of Canada with urban Indigenous populations; and then there is the provincial health care system and public health authorities who also provide services and care to varying degrees across the country (National Collaborating Centre for Aboriginal Health 2011). To overcome this complexity and address the challenges of "shared responsibility," mechanisms are needed whereby Indigenous partners and all levels of government come together to see the big picture, define shared goals, and identify who does what to make things work "on the ground" from a person-centred perspective. This requires consultation and a strong voice from those who are most affected by the decisions being made, thus allowing greater self-determination in co-creating the systems that are more responsive to the needs of specific groups, which can in and of itself lead to improved health outcomes (Chandler et al. 2003).

INFLUENCING POLICY TO CREATE SUPPORTIVE ENVIRONMENTS FOR HEALTH

According to theories on influencing policy (Nutbeam, Harris, and Wise 2010), health workers need to better understand who makes policy (e.g., government officials, school boards, etc.), who else is influencing policy (e.g., stakeholders, media, the public), what can be influenced (e.g., the content of policy and the speed at which it is adopted), and how to influence policy change to improve community health (e.g., understanding the context, recognizing who is most influential, determining what different stakeholders stand to win or lose, identifying where they may be willing to compromise). Increasing one's power in influencing policy requires understanding the process, monitoring interests, acting strategically, and building alliances. According to the prominent policy theorist Kingdon (2011), the first step is to ensure that the issue is identified as an important problem and makes it onto the policy agenda. Next, one can influence the various policy options that may be available to address the issue. Finally, one must understand the political forces determining the adoption of policy. Experience has shown that "policy entrepreneurs or champions" (i.e., leaders from professional, political, or interest groups who effectively advocate policy) have played key roles in policy reforms (Brownson, Chriqui, and Stamatakis 2009). While there is some debate about the extent to which health workers should be involved in political activism as opposed to advocating for patient needs in a clinical context (Dobson, Voyer, and Regehr 2012), health workers who are often highly respected members of communities and who have access to privileged information about the health needs of the population are well-placed to encourage local action and to advocate, along with other key stakeholders, for more supportive environments for health.

CONCLUSION

Structural factors, whether intentional or inadvertent, create the emergence and perpetuation of disadvantaged and marginalized populations. Therefore, the key is not only increasing access to care for these under-served groups but also reducing the marginalization itself by creating more transparent, inclusive, and equitable structures. These structures are developed and modified over time, in planned and unplanned ways, and can often be bureaucratic and slow to change, but people can intervene to turn these structures into engines for equity. Within the health system, there are many ways that front-line health workers can become catalysts for such wider change, starting at the patient level, the practice level, and the community level (Andermann 2016). Over a century ago, Virchow remarked that "physicians [and other allied health workers] surely are the natural advocates of the poor and the social problem largely falls within their scope" (quoted in Rather 1985, 4). Understanding how to create structural change, then, is an important lever for creating a more inclusive, equitable, and ultimately healthier society.

CRITICAL THINKING QUESTIONS

1. How can a health worker at the front lines begin to tackle complex and widespread social challenges such as homelessness, poverty, and racism?
2. Who are the key decision-makers involved, and who would be natural partners within your local community that you could join up with to try to create wider social change?
3. Why are inequities perpetuated, and what can be done to undo long-standing social exclusion and discrimination rooted in historical events that no longer reflect today's reality?

REFERENCES

Allan, B., and J. Smylie. 2015. *First Peoples, Second Class Treatment: The Role of Racism in the Health and Well-Being of Indigenous Peoples in Canada*. Toronto: Wellesley Institute. http://www.wellesleyinstitute.com/wp-content/uploads/2015/02/Report-First-Peoples-Second-Class-Treatment-Final.pdf.

Andermann, A. 2011. "Addressing the Social Causes of Poor Health Is Integral to Practising Good Medicine." *CMAJ* 183 (18): 2196. https://doi.org/10.1503/cmaj.111096.

Andermann, A. 2013. *Evidence for Health: From Patient Choice to Global Policy*. Cambridge: Cambridge University Press.

Andermann, A., on behalf of the CLEAR Collaboration. 2016. "Taking Action on the Social Determinants of Health in Clinical Practice." *CMAJ* 188 (17–18): E474–83. https://doi.org/10.1503/cmaj.160177.

British Medical Association. 2011. *Social Determinants of Health: What Doctors Can Do.* London: British Medical Association. https://www.bma.org.uk/-/media/files/pdfs/working%20 for%20change/improving%20health/socialdeterminantshealth.pdf.

Brownson, R. C., J. F. Chriqui, and K. A. Stamatakis. 2009. "Understanding Evidence-Based Public Health Policy." *American Journal of Public Health* 99 (9): 1576–83. https://doi.org/10.2105/AJPH.2008.156224.

Chandler, M., C. Lalonde, B. Sokol, and D. Hallett. 2003. "Personal Persistence, Identity Development, and Suicide: A Study of Native and Non-Native North American Adolescents." *Monographs of the Society for Research in Child Development* 68 (2): 1–130. https://doi.org/10.1111/j.1540-5834.2003.00246.x.

College of Family Physicians of Canada. 2009. *Patient-Centred Primary Care in Canada: Bring It on Home.* Ottawa: College of Family Physicians of Canada. http://www.cfpc.ca/uploadedFiles/Resources/Resource_Items/Bring20it20on20Home20FINAL 20ENGLISH.pdf.

Collège des médecins du Québec. 2018. *Sexual Misconduct.* Montreal: Collège des médecins du Québec. http://www.cmq.org/publications-pdf/p-3-2018-02-28-en-inconduite-sexuelle.pdf.

Collins, P. A., and M. V. Hayes. 2013. "Examining the Capacities of Municipal Governments to Reduce Health Inequities: A Survey of Municipal Actors' Perceptions in Metro Vancouver." *Canadian Journal of Public Health* 104 (4): e304–10. https://doi.org/10.17269/cjph.104.3873.

Commission on the Social Determinants of Health. 2008. *Closing the Gap in a Generation: Health Equity through Action on the Social Determinants of Health.* Geneva: World Health Organization. http://www.who.int/social_determinants/thecommission/finalreport/en/.

Condon, S., and J. McDermid. 2014. *Dying on the Streets: Homeless Deaths in British Columbia.* Vancouver: Street Corner Media Foundation. http://homelesshub.ca/resource/dying-streets-homeless-deaths-british-columbia.

Decady, Y., and L. Greenberg. 2014. *Ninety Years of Change in Life Expectancy.* Ottawa: Statistics Canada. http://www.statcan.gc.ca/pub/82-624-x/2014001/article/1 4009-eng.pdf.

Dobson, S., S. Voyer, and G. Regehr. 2012. "Perspective: Agency and Activism: Rethinking Health Advocacy in the Medical Profession." *Academic Medicine* 87 (9): 1161–4. https://doi.org/10.1097/ACM.0b013e3182621c25.

Gilbert, N., N. Auger, and M. Tjepkema. 2015. "Stillbirths and Infant Mortality in Aboriginal Communities in Quebec." *Statistics Canada Health Reports* 26 (2): 3–8. http://www.statcan.gc.ca/pub/82-003-x/2015002/article/14139-eng.pdf.

Goel, R., S. Buchman, R. Meili, and R. Woollard. 2016. "Social Accountability at the Micro Level: One Patient at a Time." *Canadian Family Physician* 62 (4): 287–90.

Guyon, A., T. Hancock, M. Kirk, M. MacDonald, C. Neudorf, P. Sutcliffe, J. Talbot, and G. Watson-Creed. 2017. "The Weakening of Public Health: A Threat to Population Health and Health Care System Sustainability." *Canadian Journal of Public Health* 108 (1): e1–6. https://doi.org/10.17269/cjph.108.6143.

Hwang, S. W., R. Wilkins, M. Tjepkema, P. J. O'Campo, and J. R. Dunn. 2009. "Mortality among Residents of Shelters, Rooming Houses, and Hotels in Canada: 11 Year Follow-Up Study." *BMJ* 339: 1068–70. https://doi.org/10.1136/bmj.b4036.

Kingdon, J. 2011. *Agendas, Alternatives, and Public Policies*. London: Longman.

Macaulay, A. 2009. "Improving Aboriginal Health: How Can Health Care Professionals Contribute?" *Canadian Family Physician* 55: 334–6. http://www.cfp.ca/content/55/4/334.

Mahamoud, A., J. Snyder, S. Barnes, L. M. Williams, and A. Xie. 2013. *Making the Connections: Our City, Our Society, Our Health*. Toronto: Wellesley Institute. http://www.wellesleyinstitute.com/wp-content/uploads/2013/09/MakingTheConnections-Booklet-Wellesley.pdf.

Maioni, A. 2014. "Chapter 2: A Portrait of Health Care in Canada." In *Health Care in Canada*, edited by A. Maioni, 31–46. Oxford: Oxford University Press.

Moosa, S., S. Wojczewski, K. Hoffmann, A. Poppe, O. Nkomazana, W. Peersman, M. Willcox, M. Maier, A. Derese, and D. Mant. 2013. "Why There Is an Inverse Primary-Care Law in Africa." *Lancet Global Health*, 1 (6): e332–3. https://doi.org/10.1016/S2214-109X(13)70119-0.

Morère J. F., F. Eisinger, C. Touboul, C. Lhomel, S. Couraud, and J. Viguier. 2018. "Decline in Cancer Screening in Vulnerable Populations? Results of the EDIFICE Surveys." *Current Oncology Reports* 20 (suppl 1): 17. https://doi.org/10.1007/s11912-017-0649-7.

Mullan F., and L. Epstein. 2002. "Community-Oriented Primary Care: New Relevance in a Changing World." *American Journal of Public Health* 92 (11): 1748–55. http://ajph.aphapublications.org/doi/pdf/10.2105/AJPH.92.11.1748.

Munn-Rivard, L. 2014. *Current Issues in Mental Health in Canada: Homelessness and Access to Housing*. Ottawa: Library of Parliament. Publication no. 2014-11-E. http://www.lop.parl.gc.ca/Content/LOP/ResearchPublications/2014-11-e.pdf.

Musgrove, P., A. Creese, A. Preker, C. Baeza, A. Anell, T. Prentice, A. Cassels, D. Lipson, D. A. Tenkorang, and M. Wheeler. 2000. *Health Systems: Improving Performance—World Health Report 2000*. Geneva: World Health Organization. http://www.who.int/whr/2000/en/whr00_en.pdf?ua=1.

National Collaborating Centre for Aboriginal Health. 2011. *Looking for Aboriginal Health in Legislation and Policies, 1970–2008: The Policy Synthesis Project*. Victoria, BC: National Collaborating Centre for Aboriginal Health. https://www.ccnsa-nccah.ca/495/Looking_for_Aboriginal_health_in_legislation_and_policies,_1970-2008__The_policy_synthesis_project.nccah?id=28.

Naylor, D., S. Basrur, M. Bergeron, R. Brunham, D. Butler-Jones, G. Dafoe, M. Ferguson-Pare, et al. 2004. *Learning from SARS: Renewal of Public Health in Canada—Report of the National Advisory Committee on SARS and Public Health*. Ottawa: Health Canada. https://www.canada.ca/en/public-health/services/reports-publications/learning-sars-renewal-public-health-canada.html.

Nutbeam, D., E. Harris, and M. Wise. 2010. *Theory in a Nutshell: A Practical Guide to Health Promotion Theories*. North Ryde, Australia: McGraw-Hill Education.

Rather, L. J., ed. 1985. *Rudolph Virchow: Collected Essays on Public Health and Epidemiology.* Canton, MA: Science History Publications.

Steenbakkers, M., M. Jansen, H. Maarse, and N. de Vries. 2012. "Challenging Health in All Policies, an Action Research Study in Dutch Municipalities." *Health Policy* 105 (2–3): 288–95. https://doi.org/10.1016/j.healthpol.2012.01.010.

Sugarman, J., K. Phillips, E. Wagner, K. Coleman, and M. Abrams. 2014. "The Safety Net Medical Home Initiative: Transforming Care for Vulnerable Populations." *Medical Care* 52 (11 suppl I4): S1–10. https://doi.org/10.1097/MLR.0000000000000207.

Tudor Hart, J. 1971. "The Inverse Care Law." *Lancet* 297 (7696): 405–12. https://doi.org/10.1016/S0140-6736(71)92410-X.

World Health Organization (WHO). 1986. *Ottawa Charter for Health Promotion.* Geneva: WHO. http://www.phac-aspc.gc.ca/ph-sp/docs/charter-chartre/pdf/charter.pdf.

World Health Organization (WHO). 2008. *The World Health Report 2008: Primary Health Care—Now More than Ever.* Geneva: WHO. http://www.who.int/whr/2008/08_overview_en.pdf.

World Health Organization (WHO). 2012. *Health in the Post-2015 UN Development Agenda.* Geneva: UNAIDS, UNICEF, UNFPA, and WHO. http://www.who.int/topics/millennium_development_goals/post2015/post2015_UNdevelopment_agenda_think_20120918.pdf?ua=1.

World Health Organization (WHO) and World Bank. 2017. *Tracking Universal Health Coverage: 2017 Global Monitoring Report.* Geneva: WHO and World Bank. http://www.who.int/healthinfo/universal_health_coverage/report/2017/en/.

Young, P., and L. A. Olsen. 2010. *The Healthcare Imperative: Lowering Costs and Improving Outcomes: Workshop Series Summary.* Washington, DC: Institutes of Medicine. http://www.nap.edu/download.php?record_id=12750.

CHAPTER 27

From the Clinics to the Streets: The Fight against Refugee Health Cuts in Canada

Philip Berger, Meb Rashid, Alexander Caudarella, Andrea Evans, and Christopher Holcroft

---

LEARNING OBJECTIVES

After reading this chapter, you should be able to:

1. Have a better understanding of the multitude of strategies that may be pursued to support public policy advocacy (legal, political, media, etc.).
2. Distinguish between different audiences for an advocacy message and prioritize the vehicles for reaching each audience.
3. Recognize the critical role of facts, evidence, and data in supporting an advocacy campaign and building credibility.

On April 5, 2012, the federal Conservative government of Canada quietly authorized an Order-in-Council (OIC) that drastically reduced or eliminated health coverage under the 55-year-old Interim Federal Health Program (IFHP) for refugees and refugee claimants (Government of Canada 2012).

The OIC, which was never debated in Parliament, was to take effect June 30, 2012, and would take away dental, vision, and medication coverage from all refugees. It accorded different degrees of coverage, which depended on the refugee's country of origin and legal status in the refugee determination process. For example, refugee claimants from so-called "safe countries" or "designated countries of origin" (DCOs), who were lawfully within Canada's borders and awaiting their refugee determination hearings, would only receive coverage if their health status was determined to be a threat to public health or safety. That meant that a refugee patient who was homicidal would receive treatment, but not one who was suicidal. The government's own fact sheet on the changes used myocardial infarctions (or heart attacks) to illustrate an example of who was eligible for coverage: the coverage for refugees from DCOs was "none" (Barnes 2013).

On April 26, 2012, an email describing the changes was widely distributed to physicians and other workers who worked with refugees. That email led to conversations among several physicians, sparking a virtual cross-Canada physician insurrection in opposition to the cuts, later to be joined by many other health care professionals.

The fight to reverse the cuts initially broke nearly every rule of, or framework for, advocacy. The effort had no leading organization to coordinate, no overall strategic objective, no well-considered approach, and no specific target for a campaign. The only goal arising out of the first phone call on April 26 was to draw media and public attention to the cuts by a dramatic and immediate action.

A call went out to physician colleagues to join in an occupation of a government office with the hope of having 12 doctors in white coats participate. An ad hoc steering committee was formed, and on May 11, 2012, 90 doctors in white coats with their stethoscopes occupied the constituency office of the highest-ranking Toronto Conservative Cabinet Minister, Joe Oliver (Doc4refugeehc 2012). Quickly, organized protests took place simultaneously in another half-dozen Canadian cities. The action was not without controversy, ranging from accusations of the purported elitism of a doctors-only protest to dismay at supposed unprofessional behaviour of doctors taking over a cabinet minister's office. But the fight was on, with doctors using their stature and voices loudly to resist a policy that was discriminatory and making their patients sick.

The May 11 event led to the first of four annual National Days of Action (DOA) held at the beginning of Refugee Week in June and in 2015 included 20 cities across Canada. The ad hoc group of doctors who organized the first DOA on June 18, 2012, called themselves Canadian Doctors for Refugee Care (CDRC). During the summer of 2012, physicians and medical trainees engaged in disrupting a series of Conservative cabinet ministers' public announcements, interjecting with protests against the cuts, garnering them significant media attention (*CBC News* 2012). The CDRC formed a national steering committee and later incorporated, including the formation of a board of directors for the purposes of being a litigant for a future Canadian Charter of Rights and Freedoms constitutional challenge.

The Quebec Government announced in June 2012 that it would cover gaps in coverage left by the IFHP cuts. On June 29, the day before the cuts were to be implemented, the federal government quietly capitulated to criticism and removed government-assisted refugees from those that were to be affected by the cuts (Government of Canada 2012). Despite previously being informed of the pending decrease in services, government-assisted refugees were no longer included in the list of those with reduced insurance. Privately sponsored refugees and refugee claimants continued to be affected.

The actions over the spring and summer of 2012 and beyond led to hundreds of media articles, including editorial support, in both the *Globe and Mail* (2012, 2014) and the *Toronto Star* (2012, 2014), for the CDRC position. The CDRC had accomplished its first hastily crafted goal of inserting the refugee health cuts into the national political discourse. CDRC was helped enormously by public objections raised to the cuts from over 20 national health organizations, including the Canadian Medical Association and the

Canadian Nurses Association (CDRC 2015). The support of national medical associations enhanced the campaign's credibility and led to crucial and unprecedented support from all provincial premiers representing all sides of the political spectrum.

In June 2012, the CDRC implemented a monitoring system called Refugee Health Outcome Monitoring and Evaluation System (HOMES) (n.d.) to catalogue the consequences of the cuts. In the fall of 2012, CDRC privately submitted a proposal to the federal government, which would have met the government's stated objections to the IFHP while preserving coverage for refugee claimants. The government did not acknowledge the proposal and similarly did not respond to three letters of concern over the cuts sent from the leaders of eight national health associations in 2012, refusing to meet with any health care provider group.

In 2013, CDRC released a public statement signed by prominent artists and community activists calling for an end to the cuts, which generated additional awareness and support. The Ontario Government announced the Ontario Temporary Health Program, effective January 1, 2014, for refugee claimants left uncovered by the IFHP (Ontario Ministry of Health and Long-Term Care 2016). On January 20, 2014, the *Canadian Medical Association Journal*, relying on reports from Refugee HOMES, published a leading editorial calling for the restoration of health coverage for refugees (Stanbrook 2014).

In an attempt to build the argument that the IFHP cuts directly affected a population that was unlikely to be abusing the system, a study was undertaken at the Hospital for Sick Children (SickKids) in Toronto. "The Cost and Impact of the Interim Federal Health Program Cuts on Child Refugees in Canada" (Evans et al. 2014) was published in *PLOS One*, an open access journal, in May 2014, and was later the backbone of newspaper opinion pieces and used for evidence in the Charter challenge. It showed a decrease in the number of child refugee claimants presenting to the emergency room six months after the cuts compared to six months before the changes, that there was nearly a doubling of admissions of refugee children after the cuts, and that the three most responsible diagnoses for the admission of refugee children became urgent and life-threatening conditions.

Published research results, as the ones above, generally reach a selective audience, which does not necessarily contribute to a motivation for change based on the data available. The interpretation of results in a research paper is weighed only on the evidence existing within it, whereas there is often a benefit to interpreting the results in a wider public and civil context. The reaction to the paper highlighted the unique impact of directed research, with hardcore data lending credibility to the advocacy message, persuading media, expanding interpretation of results, urging a course of action, and making academia relevant to a wider public.

A decision on the Charter challenge was rendered on July 4, 2014, by the Honourable Madam Justice Mactavish of the Federal Court of Canada: "The 2012 modifications to the Interim Federal Health Program potentially jeopardize the health, the safety and indeed the very lives, of these innocent and vulnerable children in a manner that shocks the conscience and outrages our standards of decency. They violate Section 12 of the Charter"

(*Canadian Doctors for Refugee Care v Canada* 2014). Justice Mactavish found that the "Canadian government has intentionally set out to make the lives of these disadvantaged individuals even more difficult than they already are in an effort to force those who have sought the protection of this country to leave Canada more quickly, and to deter others from coming here." She found that the OIC and cuts violated both sections 12 and 15 of the Charter and ruled the OIC unconstitutional. The CDRC's position had been vindicated by this scathing judgement arising from the third highest federal court of the land.

Within hours of the court decision, the federal government announced that it would appeal the decision. In October 2014, the government unsuccessfully sought to have the decision stayed at the Federal Court of Appeal, resulting in partially restored coverage for refugee claimants. In early November 2014, the government abolished the 1957 OIC, which created the IFHP and, in the view of many, did so to avoid being compelled to fully restore the 1957 OIC—no IFHP, no program to restore.

On March 29, 2015, the *Toronto Star* reported that the central Government Operations Centre, which coordinates the federal government's response to national emergencies and natural disasters, received a report on the government's monitoring of CDRC's third National Day of Action (Boutilier 2015). The Conservative government viewed the CDRC as a threat to national safety and security just for speaking out on the consequences of the cuts.

Following a final CDRC advocacy push during the federal election campaign in the fall of 2015—in which the cuts to refugee health featured prominently in a Leaders' Debate—the Liberal Party was elected to a majority government, with a promise to fully restore the IFHP (Mas 2015). On December 16, 2015, the Liberal government announced it would drop the appeal of the Federal Court's decision to reverse the cuts. The government also promised to resettle 10,000 Syrian refugees prior to the end of the year, and to provide full medical coverage to them (Levitz 2015). Finally, on February 18, 2016, the federal government announced that it would fully restore the IFHP, effective April 1, 2016 (*CBC News* 2015).

Despite the previous Conservative government's efforts to undermine coverage for refugee health care, by every measure of advocacy work, the refugee health campaign has been a success. The public discourse shifted as media coverage proliferated and editorial support grew. Opposition parties, emboldened by our aggressive advocacy, endorsed the campaign's call to reverse the cuts. We contributed to the legal case that eventually saw the Federal Court of Canada declare the cuts to refugee health care "cruel and unusual" and force the government to introduce, at least temporarily, health coverage for most refugees.

Many of the obstacles that existed at the start of the campaign remained throughout: defence of a vulnerable population in a hostile public discourse; very limited resources, including no CDRC full-time staff; and an obstinate federal government unwilling to even meet with advocates and experts to discuss this issue.

Throughout the campaign, we would regularly receive emails from students, health workers, social activists, and concerned individuals across the country who wanted to express and offer their support. The response of the medical community to the cuts to refugee health insurance is a stellar example of the impact that health care workers can have on public policy, particularly when they work together. CDRC demonstrated that a campaign operating with a disciplined focus of a national political operation could grow organically into something more closely resembling a social movement. Physicians have an obligation to respond to such policies that so obviously violate the right to health care of vulnerable populations. It is our responsibility to speak out, particularly when affected communities may not be able to do so.

The campaign also maintained a robust social media presence, and with each Facebook post and Tweet, we reached more Canadians and reshaped the language around the issue. Frequently, government members, the minister, and his staff presented fodder online that the campaign used to highlight the issue and the inconsistency of the government's position with anything resembling informed or fair policy.

Ultimately, the campaign against the cuts succeeded by creating opportunities to promote the cause while reacting quickly to events as they arose in order to strategically promote its messaging. Initiatives such as the annual DOA; regular commentary pieces in a variety of newspapers, magazines, online forums, and the *Canadian Medical Association Journal*; frequent news releases highlighting cases of health coverage denied; and provocative announcements such as challenging the citizenship and immigration minister to a public debate all helped draw attention to, and support for, the cause.

CRITICAL THINKING QUESTIONS

1. What is the role of health professionals in advocating for systemic change?
2. Do people make history, or does history make people? In other words, are advocacy efforts successful because of individuals or because the conditions are right?
3. How might the dialogue of fair and just access to health services for refugees be maintained so that future governments/political parties are less likely to target this community?
4. Which campaign tactics did you find most surprising? Were those the same tactics you found most or least effective? How important is the development of broad coalitions, and what are some of the challenges in such developments?
5. Reflect on the communications approaches you would pursue if faced with a situation where legislators refused to meet to discuss your/your group's position.

REFERENCES

Barnes, Steve. 2013. "The Real Cost of Cutting the Interim Federal Health Program: Policy Paper." October. Toronto: Wellesley Institute. http://www.wellesleyinstitute.com/wp-content/uploads/2013/10/Actual-Health-Impacts-of-IFHP.pdf.

Boutilier, Alexander. 2015. "List of Protests Tracked by Government Includes Vigil, 'Peace Demonstration.'" *Toronto Star*, March 29. http://www.thestar.com/news/

canada/2015/03/29/list-of-protests-tracked-by-government-includes-vigil-peace-demonstration.html.

Canadian Doctors for Refugee Care (CDRC). 2015. "Canadian Doctors for Refugee Care." Accessed August 23, 2017. http://www.doctorsforrefugeecare.ca/.

Canadian Doctors for Refugee Care v Canada (Attorney General) 2014 FC 651 (CanLII). http://canlii.ca/t/g81sg.

CBC News. 2012. "Refugee Health Cuts Protest Cuts Off Oliver Announcement." Video recording. June 22. 5:19. http://www.cbc.ca/news/politics/refugee-health-cuts-protest-cuts-off-oliver-announcement-1.1269431.

CBC News. 2015. "Syrian Refugee Plan Goes to Liberal Cabinet Thursday." November 10. http://www.cbc.ca/news/politics/syria-refugees-canada-susan-ormiston-1.3311786.

Doc4refugeehc. 2012. "90 Canadian Physicians Protest Dangerous Cuts to Refugee Health Care at MP Joe Oliver's Office" YouTube, May 12. 5:33. https://www.youtube.com/watch?v=RiNDtUaNudk.

Evans, A., A. Caudarella, S. Ratnapalan, and K. Chan. 2014. "The Cost and Impact of the Interim Federal Health Program Cuts on Child Refugees in Canada." *PLOS One* 9 (8): e106198. https://doi.org/10.1371/journal.pone.0096902.

Globe and Mail. 2012. "Amid Kenny's Worthy Reforms, a Misstep on Refugee's Health." August 23. http://www.theglobeandmail.com/globe-debate/editorials/amid-kennys-worthy-reforms-a-misstep-on-refugees-health/article4496184/.

Globe and Mail. 2014. "Cruel to Take Health Care Away from Refugee Claimants." July 6. http://www.theglobeandmail.com/globe-debate/editorials/cruel-to-take-health-care-away-from-refugee-claimants/article19473711/.

Government of Canada. 2012. "Order Amending the Order Respecting the Interim Federal Health Program, 2012." *Canada Gazette* 146 (15). http://canadagazette.gc.ca/rp-pr/p2/2012/2012-07-18/html/si-tr49-eng.html.

Levitz, Stephanie. 2015. "Liberals Drop Lawsuit over Refugee Health-Care Cuts, Speed Up Settlement." *Globe and Mail*, December 16. http://www.theglobeandmail.com/news/politics/liberals-formally-drop-lawsuit-over-refugee-health-care-cuts/article27780258/.

Mas, Susanna. 2015. "Spin Cycle: Are Only 'Bogus' Refugees Affected by Federal Health Cuts?" *CBC News*, September 22. http://www.cbc.ca/news/politics/canada-election-2015-spin-cycle-refugees-health-benefits-1.3234080.

Ontario Ministry of Health and Long-Term Care. 2016. "Ontario Temporary Health Program for Refugee Claimants." Last modified March 23. http://www.health.gov.on.ca/en/pro/programs/othp/.

Refugee HOMES. n.d. "Refugee HOMES Data Entry Form." Accessed March 27, 2018. https://www.surveymonkey.com/r/66KPGVS?sm=c4J2w%2fXbmQcsutKTgoSEow%3d%3d and http://www.doctorsforrefugeecare.ca/further-reading-survey.html.

Stanbrook, Matthew. 2014. "Editorial: Canada Owes Refugees Adequate Health Coverage." *CMAJ* 186 (2): 91. https://doi.org/10.1503/cmaj.131861.

Toronto Star. 2012. "Chopping Health Coverage for Refugees Is a False Saving." June 23. http://www.thestar.com/opinion/editorialopinion/2012/06/23/chopping_health_coverage_for_refugees_is_a_false_saving.html.

Toronto Star. 2014. "Harper Government Should End Its Attack on Refugees Health: Editorial." November 5. http://www.thestar.com/opinion/editorials/2014/11/05/harper_government_should_end_its_attack_on_refugees_health_editorial.html.

CHAPTER 28

The Ws of Successful Advocacy for the Under-Served: Lessons from Days of Action for Refugee Health

Neil Arya

LEARNING OBJECTIVES

After reading this chapter, you should be able to:

1. Define *advocacy*.
2. Enunciate benefits and risks of different advocacy strategies for varied populations and contexts and with different actors.

Advocacy involves an entity with greater power speaking out for one with lesser power, with social justice and equity as central principles. The great German anatomist and social reformer Rudolf Virchow termed physicians "natural attorneys of the poor" (Virchow [1848] 2006). In 1996, advocacy was recognized as one of seven essential physician roles by the Royal College of Physicians and Surgeons of Canada, and in 2001, the Association of Faculties of Medicine of Canada adopted a vision of social accountability (Health Canada 2001; Royal College of Physicians and Surgeons of Canada 2014). Physicians can be advocates to help promote the health of individuals, communities, or populations; however, collaborations are critical, and it is hoped that this book has conveyed the importance of other health care personnel, academics, researchers, and students, each with positions of influence to advocate for our populations.

Indeed, Virchow, when sent to investigate a typhus outbreak in Upper Silesia, determined that while the immediate causes of mortality appeared to be famine and malnutrition, as well as the typhus disease, the true cause was a lack of democracy and governance, education, employment, and housing. Civil servants, he said, could not help the "poor, ignorant and apathetic population" without dealing with social conditions (Virchow [1848] 2006).

Advocacy for change can be direct, or it can happen at a policy level, but at any level, it may trigger violent opposition. Dr. Salvador Allende, one of the major founders of Latin American Social Medicine, on being elected president of Chile, attempted to act for social justice, something that threatened various interests, including US corporate interests, resulting in his overthrow and death and Augusto Pinochet's assumption of power. Dorothy Day, founder of the Catholic Worker movement, worked in solidarity in inner cities causing her and many of her followers (priests, nuns, and lay Catholics) to be put under surveillance. So too was Helen Keller, blind and deaf, who became a renowned speaker for people with disabilities, but also for justice for women, minorities, and the labour movement (Dreier 2012).

Recent public advocacy efforts, from the global Occupy movement to Idle No More (INM), have focused, broadly speaking, on determinants of health. Sometimes such movements as Occupy appear to have no explicit results in the form of direct change, except that they spark conversation—for example, about income inequality. However, discussion of the "one percent" may have launched Bernie Sanders in the United States, the Indignados to the electoral success of Podemos in Spain, and the debt crisis to Syriza's election in Greece. More recently, we have seen the stage given to Piketty in France and Jeremy Corbyn and Momentum in Britain; meanwhile in Ontario, the raising of the minimum wage, the launch of Pharmacare, and the inception of living wage projects represent actual policy change. INM is mirrored by Indigenous movements throughout the Americas, including the Indigenous governance leadership of Bolivian president Evo Morales.

In the preceding chapter, the creation of Canadian Doctors for Refugee Care (CDRC) and the Days of Action on Refugee Health was chronicled. This was one of the most successfully coordinated modern-day movements by health professionals in Canada. Such massive support from mainstream health professional organizations was unique, attaining serious attention and ultimately contributing to a partial reversal of the funding cuts by the federal government. Understanding this success may guide health advocacy for other at-risk populations. This chapter will analyze the Ws of this campaign: **who**, **what**, **when**, **where**, and **why**, as well as how. The *where* is rather simple—in Canada—and so the *why* is a good place to begin.

WHY?

Why? What drove the physicians involved in the care of refugees to shout out, "We're not going to take it any more"? Their basic motivation was empathy for their patients who would be harmed, but also outrage at the scale and arbitrary nature of such cuts, the lack of consultation, and the vilifying of their patients.

Why did they achieve success? What were some of the reasons (what seemed fortuitous, unpredictable)? Sometimes, it is merely an accident of history, a momentary decision, an idea whose time has come. Rosa Parks, though an activist, having grown tired both of racism and standing, refused to yield her seat as the bus filled up. Sometimes it is strategy and a lifetime of work. Mahatma Gandhi, transformed by racist experiences in South Africa decades prior, worked against colonialism in India. More germane to this volume than driving factors for individuals is why the message caught on. The message from the Days of Action was not easy to convey. Initially, the government was able to portray refugee health cuts as an issue of fairness for other Canadians who don't receive supplemental benefits, as well as in relation to cost-saving or lowering taxes. That the economic argument was a canard that would be difficult to appreciate since it was the provinces that would eventually bear the burden of downloading, but the immediate savings, however minor, were tangible. It was challenging to explain to Canadians, who did not have drug, optometry, or dental benefits, that giving refugees such "rights" was " just" as well as cost-effective social policy. Going beyond this, making the argument that equal access to health care does not balance roadblocks placed by limitations to their social determinants of health is an even harder sell. The barriers faced by refugees or other disadvantaged populations, and their underlying personal deficits, require them to have more resources, a "hand up," at least at the beginning, to do well (Arya, McMurray, and Rashid 2012). Further, providing health care (medications, prostheses, etc.) may be a matter of fairness, not privilege, particularly for those whom Canada had invited from camps where they may have had such benefits. Similar arguments may relate to Indigenous and homeless populations. But such arguments do not make simple, succinct sound bites for the media or elevator speeches to governmental bureaucrats.

The government thus logically perceived cutting back as a political winner, where it could portray itself as fiscally responsible, with an added bonus that those subject to the crackdown had no vote. How could this movement capture the imagination of health professionals and sufficient support from the general public to at least partly change government policy? To understand this, we might look at three remaining W's—the *who*, *what*, and *when*, as well as the *how*.

WHO?

The chill of retaliation or retribution placed on individuals and agencies working within the sector did not allow them to speak. But the ones leading this movement were the grey suits or white lab coats—the heads of family medicine at major teaching hospitals, and physicians with status, authority, wealth, education—and connections could not be cowed. Nor could they be labelled as foreign-funded extremists, as has occurred with environmentalists concerned about the tar sands or advocates for peace and human rights. Beyond this, they were able to mobilize the grassroots, the "baby docs" attractive to media, and other professionals to come out on those warm June days. The presence of Chris, a dedicated consultant to keep the movement united and on message, was essential.

WHAT?

Students and younger members creatively used social media to inform; they also created videos and art (FiftyNine Cents Campaign 2012; Miller 2013). In another era, the

Raging Grannies were able to confront Prime Minister Mulroney directly; INM used social media starting from an effective hashtag, #IdleNoMore (Kossick 2012; Kreindler 2012; students4refugeehth 2012).

People prefer charity to service, and service to asking hard questions. People often mistrust those engaged in direct action. The reaction to the Latin America liberation theology movement resulted in arrests, disappearances, torture, assassinations, and war. Brazilian archbishop Dom Helder Camara said, "When I give treatment to the poor, they call me a saint. When I ask why the poor are untreated, they call me a communist" (quoted in Rocha 2000, 53).

The tactic of direct action, occupying ministers' offices or interrupting their ribbon-cutting ceremonies, as was used by CDRC, had the potential to turn off people who would see this as disrespectful and political. But physicians, who were selflessly sacrificing office hours, were able to turn this around so that it was the government that was seen as disrespectful (Docs4refugeehc 2012).

Gandhi's Hindu roots and Martin Luther King's Christian pacifism led them to use non-violence as a tactic. These only became effective with administrative overreach, when the British arrested those with Gandhi's salt march for illegally harvesting salt from the sea, and or when police in the US South violently broke up peaceful demonstrations, making themselves look cruel, but even more ridiculous.

WHEN?

In history, the *when* has always been critical. Circumstances sometimes even make the individual. The landmines campaign took off with the death of Princess Diana. Days of Action against refugee health cuts erupted in the late spring of 2012, a year and a half after the election of a majority government. The honeymoon phase had passed, and people were beginning to tire of the ideology of the arrogant incumbent government. This probably contributed to many health organizations' willingness to take a stand.

HOW?

How can a movement be sustained? A campaign based on compassion alone would have limited success; the base needed to be mobilized and broadened. The CDRC movement was able to build momentum after the initial success of the federal government quietly reversing itself on June 30, 2012, by giving lie, on its website on government-assisted refugees, to their argument that the decision to remove coverage of care for refugees had been thought out (Government of Canada 2012).

The next phase was evidence-building, tracking refugees who had been denied care and sharing their stories, and trying to develop cost estimates on burdened hospitals. This evidence convinced provincial governments to make up for the slack, but it may also have resonated in the minds of the general public, with what was seen at the Death of Evidence rallies (Death of Evidence n.d.; Pedwell 2012), where the federal government was observed to choose ideology over scientific evidence, muzzling civil servants on issues from gun control, to climate change, to the long-form census, to nuclear isotopes. The credibility of physicians in disseminating such data easily outshone that of the government. The campaign attempted to be responsible and inclusive, eschewing shaming; soon, editorial boards and reporters appeared universally supportive, and even the conservative *Calgary Herald* in Prime Minister Harper's home base came out against the cuts, though letters to the editor were less sympathetic. In time, even the comments sections of newspapers, with stories of the vulnerability of children and pregnant women, became more balanced.

ARE LESSONS FOR ACTION FOR INNER-CITY OR INDIGENOUS POPULATIONS PROVIDED? WHAT ARE THE CHALLENGES?

In Chapter 14 (Goel and Bloch in this volume), the authors describe "hunger clinics," where physicians filled out forms to get recipients of Ontario Works and Ontario Disability Support programs the full 250-dollar-a-month diet top-up to their monthly cheque, which caused numbers to burgeon from 5,300 recipients in 2002 to 31,000 in 2007 (Mandel 2009; Ontario Coalition Against Poverty 2005). The province responded, specifying 41 conditions to qualify for this top-up, including chronic constipation or allergies to eggs, milk, soy, and/or wheat, to qualify putting a burden on physicians, some of whom determined that all patients should qualify. One such physician, Roland Wong, was reprimanded by the College of Physicians and Surgeons of Ontario for failing to properly assess patients or keep proper records. "'The temptation to exaggerate in order to maximize financial benefit for a patient is entirely understandable,' the committee wrote. 'Advocacy for a patient, however, should not trump one's professional integrity'" (Gerster 2013). The Canadian Medical Protective Association (CMPA 2014) also issues some cautions on advocacy, especially for physicians working in institutions, as it might lead to conflict. Direct action against cuts to welfare, disability benefits, and public housing, as well as resistance from the Ontario Coalition Against Poverty, mentioned by Goel and Bloch in Chapter 14, may have turned off potential supporters. In Dr. Wong's case, he actually billed substantial amounts for his services, further throwing this "selfless advocacy" into question. However, this advocacy was seen as necessary to get poverty recognized as a disease requiring intervention, triggering the gathering of evidence and the development of the Poverty Tool (Bloch 2013).

Violations of Indigenous rights with reports from commissions, Supreme Court decisions granting rights to resources, reports of displacements due to lack of water or housing, and the seemingly daily assault and murder of young, urban Indigenous women rarely registered on the radar. However, Chief Theresa Spence's Parliament Hill protest and hunger strike galvanized the Idle No More movement (Wingrove 2013). Despite some successes publicizing exploration, invasion, and colonization, as well as the violation of treaty-right lands and resources, once again on the back page are wealth exploitation of natural resources on Indigenous lands, and limitations to finance, education, housing, and water, perhaps requiring another catalyst. Are we any more advanced in recognizing Indigenous rights than half a century ago, during the aftermath of the ill-considered 1969 White Paper recommending abolishing the Indian Act (see Freeman, Chapter 3 in this volume), or the 1974 Berger Commission declaring that Aboriginal rights had to be respected when considering the Mackenzie Valley Pipeline? Even advocating for control of one's data or the telling of one's stories has had limited success, let alone participating in each facet of research (see Healey, Chapter 20, and Salsberg et al., Chapter 23 in this volume). How can we advance First Nations Principles of OCAP (ownership, control, access, and possession), so that First Nations control data collection processes in their communities, and own, protect, and control how their information is used (Schnarch 2004)?

For each of these populations, lessons may be learned from the Days of Action in order to advance stalled agendas. But to achieve success, timing must be right, or another catalyst may be required; advocates need to look at their particular strengths in terms of who, what, where, and why, and find the right timing—sometimes, though, change comes when least expected, and villains become heroes. From slavery and the landmines to smoking cessation and seatbelts, societal attitudes and policies can transform rapidly. The following quote is attributed to Arthur Schoepenhauer (and in modified form to Gandhi and George Bernard Shaw): "All truth passes through three stages. First, it is ridiculed. Second, it is violently opposed. Third, it is accepted as being self-evident" (Wikiquote 2018). Radicals from Helen Keller and Martin Luther King become mainstreamed (Dreier 2012); the Occupy movement and Che Guevara become commodified.

Advocacy is a medical responsibility (Arya 2013) that requires persistence and people working at different levels, before the wall comes tumbling down, to motivate society to pass through its stages of change to action. We hope that these stories move you forward as you consider your own journey to advocacy.

CRITICAL THINKING QUESTIONS

1. What are the specific capacities that sectors of society other than medicine possess to advocate for the under-served? What capacities do you have personally?
2. Many advocacy campaigns, particularly when they involve the defence of a vulnerable population, are low resourced. What organizational strategies would you recommend to maximize opportunities for success in such a situation? And what are the challenges in dealing with a population less able to advocate for itself?
3. What can be learned from advocacy movements for the health of other populations (e.g., Idle No More, Indigenous land claims, water rights, guaranteed income, open health care)? Compare the campaigns mentioned here, or elements of them, with other advocacy initiatives you may have been involved with.

REFERENCES

Arya, Neil. 2013. "Advocacy as Medical Responsibility." *CMAJ* 185 (15): 1368. https://doi.org/10.1503/cmaj.130649.

Arya, Neil, Josephine McMurray, and Meb Rashid. 2012. "Enter at Your Own Risk: Government Changes to Comprehensive Care for Newly Arrived Canadian Refugees." *CMAJ* 184 (17): 1875–6. https://doi.org/10.1503/cmaj.120938.

Bloch, Gary. 2013. "Poverty: A Clinical Tool for Primary Care in Ontario." Toronto: Ontario College of Family Physicians. http://ocfp.on.ca/docs/default-source/poverty-tool/poverty-a-clinical-tool-2013-(with-references).pdf?sfvrsn=0.

Canadian Medical Protective Association (CMPA). 2014. "The Physician Voice: When Advocacy Leads to Change." *CMPA Perspective* 6 (2): 10–13. https://www.cmpa-acpm.ca/en/advice-publications/browse-articles/2014/the-physician-voice-when-advocacy-leads-to-change.

Death of Evidence. n.d. "The Death of Evidence: No Science, No Evidence, No Truth, No Democracy." Accessed March 27, 2018. http://www.deathofevidence.ca/what.

Docs4refugeehc. 2012. "90 Canadian Physicians Protest Dangerous Cuts to Refugee Health Care at MP Joe Oliver's Office." Youtube, May 12. 5:33. https://www.youtube.com/watch?v=RiNDtUaNudk.

Dreier, Peter. 2012. "The Radical Dissent of Helen Keller." *YES! Magazine*, 12 July. http://www.yesmagazine.org/people-power/the-radical-dissent-of-helen-keller?utm_source=YTW&utm_medium=Email&utm_campaign=20150410.

FiftyNine Cents Campaign. 2012. "59 Cents Campaign." Youtube, June 24. 2:14. https://www.youtube.com/watch?v=TQiSe00HOec.

Gerster, Jane. 2013. "'Dr. Robin Hood' Has No Regrets about Helping Welfare Patients Get Extra Money." *TheStar.com*, 30 July. http://www.thestar.com/news/gta/2013/07/30/dr_robin_hood_has_no_regrets_about_helping_welfare_patients_get_extra_money.html.

Government of Canada. 2012. "Order Amending the Order Respecting the Interim Federal Health Program, 2012." *Canada Gazette* 146 (15). http://canadagazette.gc.ca/rp-pr/p2/2012/2012-07-18/html/si-tr49-eng.html.

Health Canada. 2001. *Social Accountability: A Vision for Canadian Medical Schools*. Ottawa: Health Canada. https://www.afmc.ca/pdf/pdf_sa_vision_canadian_medical_schools_en.pdf.

Kossick, Don. 2012. "Voices on Parliament Hill for Refugee Health Rights 2." Youtube, October 29. 4:26. https://www.youtube.com/watch?v=S2aJEI0Ck80.

Kreindler, Adi Sara. 2012. "Thank You Jason Kenney—by Just Theatre." Youtube, July 17. 2:29. https://www.youtube.com/watch?v=FC9EUhuiWfA.

Mandel, Michele. 2009. "Welfare's Dirty Little Secret: Special-Diet Subsidy Has Gone from $2M in 2002 To $55M This Year, Sources Say." *Toronto Sun*, 18 October. http://www.torontosun.com/news/columnists/michele_mandel/2009/10/18/11438551-sun.html.

Miller, John. 2013. "University of Saskatchewan Refugee Health Advocacy Video." Youtube, April 6. 3:00. https://www.youtube.com/watch?v=MIVJLS6hQ24.

Ontario Coalition Against Poverty. 2005. "News Articles about the Mass Hunger Clinic." http://www.ocap.ca/node/385.

Pedwell, Terry. 2012. "Scientists Take Aim at Harper Cuts with 'Death of Evidence' Protest on Parliament Hill." *Global and Mail*, July 10. http://www.theglobeandmail.com/news/politics/scientists-take-aim-at-harper-cuts-with-death-of-evidence-protest-on-parliament-hill/article4403233/.

Rocha, Zildo. 2000. *Helder, O Dom: uma vida que marcou os rumos da Igreja no Brasil* [*Helder, the Gift: A Life that Marked the Course of the Church in Brazil*]. Petrópolis, Brazil: Editora Vozes.

Royal College of Physicians and Surgeons of Canada. 2014. "We Actively Influence Health System Public Policy." http://www.rcps.ws/what-we-do/policy-advocacy.

Schnarch, Brian. 2004. "Ownership, Control, Access, and Possession (OCAP) or Self-Determination Applied to Research: A Critical Analysis of Contemporary First Nations Research and Some Options for First Nations Communities." *Journal of Aboriginal Health* 1 (1): 80–95. https://doi.org/10.18357/ijih11200412290.

students4refugeehth. 2012. "Thank You MP Kelly." Youtube, November 11. 2:31. https://www.youtube.com/watch?v=tLh28yf3QvE.

Virchow, Rudolf Carl. (1848) 2006. "Report on the Typhus Epidemic in Upper Silesia." In *Archiv für pathologische Anatomie und Physiologie und für klinische Medicin*, Vol. 2, 143–332. Berlin, Germany: George Reimer. Reprint, *American Journal of Public Health* 96 (12): 2102–5.

Wikiquote. 2018. s.v. "Arthur Schopenhauer." Last modified March 15. https://en.wikiquote.org/wiki/Arthur_Schopenhauer.

Wingrove, Josh. 2013. "Chief Spence: Idle No More must keep momentum." *Globe and Mail*, February 8. http://www.theglobeandmail.com/news/national/chief-spence-idle-no-more-must-keep-momentum/article8421487/.

Conclusion

Thomas Piggott and Neil Arya

There are many reasons why you might have chosen to read this text. You may have read it as part of a course—a component of your mission to become a competent health care, public health, or policy professional. You could have picked up this book because you had limited exposure to the social determinants of health and were interested in exploring the field further. Or, possibly, you work with one or more of the under-served populations that have been discussed in the book and decided to delve deeper into understanding the needs of your clients. For many of you, this book may represent an important stepping stone at the beginning of your career. For others, it might be a reflective pause in a journey that has long since started. Whatever the reason you've come to this book, as it reaches its conclusion, we hope that for you, this might just be a new beginning.

We hope that you have derived meaning from the stories and profited as much from the academic content as we, as editors, have. During our journey of producing this text, we have been honoured to learn from, and be inspired by, our book's contributors. We have benefitted from their diverse experiences and academic expertise, but, equally importantly, we have been transformed through respectful dialogue—not just with them but also with the populations we each try to serve.

The book has focused on a number of special populations in Canada, all of whom face a high degree of marginalization and poorer health outcomes than the Canadian average. A principle we hope to have conveyed is that the three under-served populations in Canada that we have focused on—Indigenous, refugee, and inner-city—are tremendously heterogeneous. There are over 60 languages spoken by First Nations groups in Canada alone. Refugees have come to Canada from an incredibly diverse mix of countries and contexts. In inner-city settings, poverty and marginalization may have diverse roots, including mental health and addiction, but also others. It is often said that everyone is only a couple of steps, bad choices, or instances of bad fortune away from being in poverty or homeless themselves; yet we continue to "other" people in these circumstances. Such othering may fuel punitive social policy, which in turn entrenches marginalization. We also acknowledge in this book that certain demographics within the populations we discuss may be more under-served than others, particularly those with the multiple burdens that a lens of intersectionality may highlight.

You may feel that we have forgotten or insufficiently dealt with other groups that are socially, economically, or politically marginalized, or whom our health care system may under-serve. It would have been impossible to present an encompassing perspective of all populations. Further, we hope the focus on the populations in this book will allow for application of the concepts discussed to other populations and other contexts.

Common across all populations discussed in this book are health inequities resulting from diverse factors leading to social, political, and economic discrepancies. We have introduced a number of barriers to health and health care for the marginalized and under-served populations discussed in the book. These factors are both contributors to and resultant from ill-health. The cyclical nature of the social determinants of health, as well as consideration of the intergenerational transmission of their impacts, complicates solutions and any attempts at helping people to merely "change their circumstances." Their circumstances and conditions are not immutable; people should not be defined by their current state of experience. A theme that resonated across all chapters is that efforts to assist with health improvements must be advanced in solidarity and collaboration with these populations themselves.

For Indigenous populations, this must begin with an understanding and recognition of the history of colonization and sustained trauma. For refugees and migrants, this requires consideration of their origins, migration experiences, and culture. Their experiences prior to arriving in Canada and the persisting challenges after arrival may continue to shape them and their children in lasting ways—physically, mentally, emotionally, and spiritually. With respect to inner-city under-served populations, as the stories and research presented has demonstrated, individuals experience states of homelessness and poverty from far-ranging roots.

Throughout the book, we have striven to be solutions-focused, without neglecting important discussions of the history and background that is needed to appreciate context. The varied solutions promoted here centre around actions at the individual health care encounter level, at the level of the health care system, and at the wider population level.

Although the opportunities presented are many, five solutions echo throughout the chapters. First, income and secure housing may be important first steps to empowering individuals. Second, education and fostering positive relationships early can interrupt intergenerational impacts and improve childhood development. Third, fostering resiliency can help individuals to help themselves. Fourth, community-driven approaches to engaging individuals in health care and health research can be positive for health. Finally, health care and health care practitioners can have a major influence on health through advocacy efforts.

These considerations should be embraced by health care providers in the provision of health care for special populations. In the same fashion that clinical guidelines and evidence-based medicine are now embraced by health care providers broadly, evidence must be broadly embraced for the health care of special populations by policy-makers and administrators.

However, we argue that employing evidence-based practice does not always go far enough. We should reflect on the values and biases of what we deem to be evidence, and what that may overlook. The health care system must undergo deep self-examination on the harms that we can cause and propagate. There are instances where the best-intentioned health care providers and institutions convey the same racist assumptions and judgements—the lack of respect prevalent in the dominant culture—which furthers marginalization. Cultural safety approaches and innovative service models can counter this. But even our embrace of reformed health care is not sufficient—some of the populations explored rarely have a voice, even among discussions specifically focused on the health care of special populations in Canada. Health care service and research must be community-driven and participatory, and it must embrace other models of thinking, including other conceptions and models of health. We must shift the lens from "disease care" to "health care," and in so doing, acknowledge and foster resilience among special populations. Finally, as health care providers, our duties should not end at "the bedside." As described in Chapters 27 and 28, in relation to the advocacy by health care providers in response to refugee health cuts, where injustices are witnessed, we should advocate in solidarity with the affected groups. Beyond activism "on the streets," we must also continue our work to improve health by shifting our orientation towards public health policy solutions that address health upstream, as described by Meili and Piggott in Chapter 25.

Public health, at its essence, is about population-level improvements in health involving policy-making, programming, research, education, or advocacy. But as with health providers, those leading public health initiatives for under-served populations may take comfort in stability and homeostasis. For the various health inequities we've discussed throughout the course of this book, the stage of recognition they reside in may vary. For action on the social determinants of health common to all populations discussed—such as access to health care, with medications and services as a right, guaranteed basic income, or living wage and cultural safety—their acceptance as truths is inconsistent outside of certain circles in the health and socially oriented communities.

The German philosopher Arthur Schoepenhauer wrote that "all truth passes through three stages. First, it is ridiculed. Second, it is violently opposed. Third, it is accepted as being self-evident" (quoted in Shallit 2005, 5). Those who upset the applecart of inertia are rarely viewed positively. When it comes to major change, most of us, like the proverbial frog in the slowly boiling pot, remain in a pre-contemplation phase most of the time. Sometimes we need to jump out of the pot into cooler surroundings in order to adopt solutions—living wage, guaranteed income, and Pharmacare are a few—where governments may have to work without large-scale randomized controls but a few small-scale projects before taking the plunge.

Progress on some of the determinants of health, such as strategies to reverse the opioids crisis, remains seemingly distant visions. For these, radical change may be needed, but the solutions may not be clear, or they may be multi-factorial. While waiting is difficult and frustrating, particularly as people are dying before our eyes, radical haste may end up being counterproductive. At other times, a more radical rights-based approach, such as in the campaign for access to essential HIV medicines, which helped lead to a substantial reduction in price, may be required. Maybe that is required to achieve clean water for all First Nations living on reserves. Or maybe each approach has its place, and a balance between the two will be best.

We are confident that this book has provided you, as practitioners or policy-makers, with tools to practise culturally safe and comprehensive care for under-served populations in Canada. If you are an educator, we trust that you better understand the learning needs of, and pedagogical strategies for, these populations. If a researcher, our intention was to provide you with guidance in reflecting on ethics, research questions, and approaches. Finally, regardless of your field, we are optimistic that you can use the lessons from successful campaigns, and individual stories of transformation presented, to be effective advocates and changemakers.

Through the exploration of the presented groups, you should be able to apply a critical lens to the issues of other marginalized and under-served populations. Through our collective work as health care providers, collaborating within our field and across disciplinary boundaries, we can lead and inspire action to improve the health of those who are underserved. As this book comes to a close, do not look upon it as a finish line, but rather use the book as the starting block for further dialogue, debate, and action.

REFERENCE

Shallit, J. 2005. "Science, Pseudoscience, and the Three Stages of Truth." Department of Computer Science, University of Waterloo. https://cs.uwaterloo.ca/~shallit/Papers/stages.pdf.

Glossary

Source chapter listed in brackets.

Ableism: Discrimination against people who are differently abled, or the presumption of a particular norm of abilities. (Chapter 10)

Addiction: Behaviour out of an individual's control; often but not always used to refer to lack of control over substance use. (Chapter 12)

Adverse childhood experiences: Potentially traumatic events that can have negative, lasting effects on health and well-being. (Chapter 11)

Attachment Theory: Also known as the Theory of Attachment; developed by John Bowlby, who proposed the importance of the parent-child bond for developmental outcomes. Based on the nature of early relationships with primary caregivers, the theory states that children develop internal working models that guide thoughts, feelings, and behaviours. (Chapter 11)

Census Agglomeration (CA): A geographic designation used by Statistics Canada to identify smaller cities. A CA is an urban area with a core population of at least 10,000. (Chapter 5)

Census Metropolitan Area (CMA): A geographic designation used by Statistics Canada to identify large cities. A CMA is an urban area with a total population of at least 100,000, of which 50,000 or more live in the core area. (Chapter 5)

Cisheterosexism: The social privilege afforded by mainstream society to those who are heterosexual and those whose gender identity and expression are congruent with their biological sex and society's norm of a gender binary. (Chapter 13)

Colonialism: In the Canadian context, colonialism refers both to the historic act of the take-over of Indigenous lands by white settlers and to current processes of implicit and explicit discrimination enacted against Indigenous people. (Chapter 10)

Corporate power and influence: Refers to the dominance of corporate views in shaping public policy. It represents an imbalance between the influence of citizens, labour, and governments, and results in skewed government and societal priorities. Addressing the social determinants of health is low on the public policy agenda in large part due to this dominance. (Chapter 2)

Cultural/behavioural explanations of health: These explanations are about how health-related behaviours are associated with poverty and come to influence health. (Chapter 2)

Cultural humility: Relates to a reflective process of understanding one's own individual and systemic biases (both implicit and explicit) and managing power imbalances. It involves humbly acknowledging our role as learners in seeking to understand the complexity of another's experience. (Chapters 4, 6, 17)

Cultural safety: This has its roots in nursing education in New Zealand in response to Maori nursing students. It seeks to disrupt damaging power imbalances and emphasizes the importance of building respectful, bicultural exchange, in which knowledge is shared. It focuses on respecting the cultural identities of others and providing care that safely meets their needs and priorities within the values and norms individuals define for themselves. Like cultural humility, it also involves critical reflection on the part of the health care provider on one's own power, privilege, and perspectives. Cultural safety strives to create an environment free of racism where people feel safe receiving care. The safe place and practice is defined by the Indigenous patient. The health care provider starts by understanding the historical roots of racism, how they are nourished, where racism takes place, and when to recognize its detrimental effects on the Indigenous patient. Challenging its existence, no matter how benign or lethal its consequences appear for victims or perpetrators, takes courage and honest self-reflection. (Chapters 4, 6, 17, 24)

Delinquent behaviours: Anti-social behaviours (e.g., aggression) that may or may not be illegal acts. These behaviours may cause harassment, alarm, or distress to one or more persons. (Chapter 11)

Dose effects: Refers to differences in the nature or magnitude of the effect based on the frequency or duration of the event or experience. (Chapter 11)

Friendship centre: One of a national network of urban organizations that provide a range of social and health services to Indigenous peoples in Canadian cities. (Chapter 5)

Government-assisted refugees (GARs): Individuals approved as refugees overseas and who are sponsored for the first year of resettlement by the government of Canada or Quebec. (Chapter 17)

Harm reduction: Policies or programs focused on reducing harms associated with drug use, without an emphasis on discontinuing drug use. (Chapter 12)

Hidden curriculum: A set of influences that implicitly transmits specific values and attitudes to support oppressive power structures. It functions at the levels of organizational structure and culture that affect learning, teaching, and clinical practice and may well conflict with the institution's stated educational mission. (Chapters 4, 24)

Housing First: This is both a philosophy and a model of service delivery. The model is based on best evidence that has found that best health and housing outcomes are achieved when people are moved rapidly from homeless to housed, with no pre-conditions (such as treatment or sobriety) required. Principles of Housing First include participant choice, harm reduction, housing with supports, no pre-conditions to housing, and community integration. (Chapter 10)

Housing selection worker: A part of the Housing First model, the housing selection worker works with landlords to identify potential units, ensure payment of rent, and address landlord concerns as they arise. (Chapter 10)

Housing stability worker: A part of the Housing First model, the housing stability worker works with program participants to maintain housing, enhance life skills, and connect to community supports. (Chapter 10)

Indian Act: The Canadian federal statute that identifies who is and who is not legally an "Indian" and sets out the fiduciary responsibilities of the federal government to "Registered Indians." (Chapter 5)

Integrated knowledge translation: This form of knowledge translation engages stakeholders or potential research knowledge users in the entire research process. By doing so, researchers and research users work together to make all important research decisions, including the following: determining the research questions; deciding on the methodology, data collection, and tools development; interpreting the findings; and disseminating research results. This approach improves knowledge uptake by producing findings that are more likely to be relevant to the end-users. (Chapter 23)

Intergenerational trauma: Legacy trauma from adverse historical events passed on from one generation to the next. The legacy of the residential school system in Canada (1884–1996) continues to affect the health of its victims and their families, communities, and children today. The system, which lasted for the better part of Canada's nationhood, was designed exclusively to assimilate school-age Indigenous children into Canadian society by destroying their cultural ties. Physical, emotional, and sexual abuse; deprivation; humiliation; and social isolation were often employed to break the Indigenous person. Many children died in school custody. The trauma suffered by these victims has led to tremendous suffering that is passed on to families and communities.

Post-traumatic stress response is common in Indigenous people who went through the residential school system. Subsequent generations also suffer from post-traumatic stress syndrome from intergenerational trauma. (Chapter 4)

Internal working models: Internal representations that guide an individual's thoughts, emotional regulation, and behaviours. Bowlby proposed that the valency of children's internal working models was developed based on the nature of early parent-child relationships and remain stable across the lifespan. He proposed that children develop two internal working models: one for the self and one for others. (Chapter 11)

Intersectionality: A social justice approach that considers power, privilege, and marginalization through the critical junctures of people's multiple co-occurring social locations, such as their race, class, and sexual orientation. (Chapter 13)

Knowledge Translation: A dynamic and iterative process that includes synthesis, dissemination, exchange, and ethically sound application of knowledge. This process takes place within a complex system of interactions between researchers and knowledge users. (See reference Graham and Tetroe 2007; Chapter 23)

Low-Income Cut-Off: A measure of poverty that considers the proportion of family income spent on basic necessities. (Chapter 10)

Managed Alcohol Program: These programs are designed to support those with chronic experiences of alcoholism who are not currently treatment-ready. These residential programs provide residents with a small and regular quantity of alcohol to reduce harms to the resident from drinking non-beverage alcohol, as well as harms of severe drinking to the broader community, such as theft, in the maintenance of addiction. (Chapter 10)

Market Basket Measure: A measure of poverty that considers the total costs within a particular community of a variety of necessities. (Chapter 10)

Materialist (analyses): Analyses about how poverty leads to differential exposures to health-damaging or health-enhancing elements in living and working conditions; both positive and negative aspects of the world. (Chapter 2)

Mortality rate: Mortality rate is the number of deaths in a particular size of population over a period of time (such as 23/10,000); the mortality rate *difference* is for a particular population compared to the average (such as a rate difference of 43, where the particular population has a rate of 66/10,000 and the general population has a rate of 23/10,000). (Chapter 10)

Mortality rate ratio: A ratio of the death rate for a particular cause for a particular subpopulation compared to that of the general population. (Chapter 10)

Narcotic: The term for a non-medical drug used for illegal purposes; not the preferred term for opioids by many health providers and people who use drugs in part due to the overlap of the crisis with sanctioned prescription opioids. (Chapter 12)

Opioids: A group of pain relieving drugs that induce euphoria contributing to addiction. Includes, among others, codeine, fentanyl, heroin, hydromorphone, morphine, and oxycodone. (Chapter 12)

Parental incarceration: Having a mother and/or father (i.e., biological or step-parent) who has been accused of a criminal offence and as a result has been held in correctional facility for a period of time. (Chapter 11)

Participatory research: An approach to research, rather than a methodology; the co-construction of knowledge through equitable partnerships between researchers and those affected by the issues under study or who must apply the results. The approach fosters self-determination through engaging individuals and communities to contribute their knowledge and expertise in shaping scientific inquiry leading to action or change. We follow Cargo and Mercer, and Green and colleagues in using *participatory research* as an umbrella term to include all partnered research, including community-based participatory research, action research, participatory action research, participatory evaluation, and community and patient engagement. (See references Cargo and Mercer 2008; Green et al. 1995; Chapter 23)

People who use drugs: Individuals who use non-medical drugs as a result of personal choice or addiction. It is the preferred terminology as it places the emphasis on people, not their medical condition. (Chapter 12)

Poverty: When individuals or families lack or are denied the economic, social, or cultural resources to participate in their community. This includes both absolute poverty, or the inability to meet basic needs, and relative poverty, meaning social disadvantage and exclusion. (Chapter 10)

Privately sponsored refugees (PSRs): Individuals approved as refugees overseas and who are sponsored for the first year of resettlement by groups of private sponsors. (Chapter 17)

Privilege: As coined by Peggy McIntosh, this is an invisible package of unearned assets, an invisible weightless knapsack of special provisions, maps, passports, codebooks, visas, clothes, tools, and blank cheques that one can count on cashing in each day, but about which one was "meant" to remain oblivious. (Chapter 24)

Psychosocial pathways: The explanations related to either (a) the experience of belonging to a particular social class, or (b) the experiences of stress associated with living in poverty, and how these come to be related to health. (Chapter 2)

Public policy: "A course of action or inaction chosen by public authorities to address a given problem or interrelated set of problems." It is anchored in a set of values regarding appropriate public goals and beliefs about the best way of achieving those goals. Public policy assumes that an issue is not private but rather a societal affair. (See reference Pal 2006, 2; Chapter 2)

Queer: Catchall term used by some to defy gender or sexual restrictions. (Chapter 13)

Quintile: When a population or sample is divided into five equal groups. This is often used to allow for a statistical comparison. (Chapter 10)

Racialized people: All people who are non-Caucasian or non-white in skin colour. This terminology replaces that of "visible minority," recognizing that non-white is the majority population in some communities. (Chapter 10)

Refugee: A person forced to flee their home country and who cannot return home due to fear of persecution. (Chapter 17)

Refugee claimant: A person who has fled from their home country due to fear of persecution and is seeking protection in another country but has not yet had their claim assessed (also known as *asylum seeker* in some contexts). (Chapter 17)

Resiliency: The natural, human capacity to navigate life well; positive adaptation in the face of severe adversities. (Chapter 8)

Sexual Orientation: One's preference for sexual and romantic partners. (Chapter 13)

Social determinants of health: The economic and social conditions that shape the health of individuals, communities, and jurisdictions as a whole. Canadian researchers have outlined several of these: Aboriginal status, disability status, early life, education, employment and working conditions, food security, health services, housing, income and income distribution, race, social exclusion, social safety net, and unemployment and employment insecurity. (See reference Mikkonen and Raphael 2010; Chapter 2)

Stages of Change model: Also known as the transtheoretical model, a health promotion theory, advanced by Prochaska and DiClemente in 1983, stating that behavioural change (e.g., relating to substance use) may occur temporally in stages. The stages include pre-contemplation, contemplation, preparation, action, and maintenance. (Chapter 12)

Timing effects: Refers to differences in the nature or magnitude of the effect based on the timing of the event or experience. Timing effects can also be referred to as a sensitive period. (Chapter 11)

Transgender: Someone whose gender identity differs from their physical sex characteristics, as expected by society. (Chapter 13)

Tri-Council Policy Statement for Ethical Conduct on Research Involving Humans: The core principles of this document include (1) respect for the person, (2) concern for welfare, and (3) justice. (Chapter 21)

Under-served population: A population whose health inequities are not met due to insufficient health care resources dedicated to their need. (All chapters)

Welfare state: The typology of welfare state describes clusters of wealthy developed nations grouped according to their approach to social provision. These are "liberal," "conservative," "Latin," and "social democratic." Esping-Andersen's typology and revisions of it offer a "reconceptualization and re-theorization of the basis of what can be considered important about the welfare state." The major difference between the regimes is whether the state (social democratic), the market (liberal), or the family (conservative and Latin) is expected to provide for the welfare needs of its citizens. (See reference Esping-Andersen 1990, 2; Chapter 2)

Contributor Biographies

EDITORS

Akshaya Neil Arya is a family physician in Kitchener, Ontario. He is President of the Canadian Physicians for Research and Education in Peace (CPREP) (http://www.cprep.ca), and Chair of the PEGASUS Global Health Conference (www.pegasusconference.ca). He remains Assistant Clinical Professor in Family Medicine at McMaster University (part-time) and Adjunct Professor in Environment and Resource Studies at the University of Waterloo, and recently became an Adjunct Professor and Scholar in Residence in Health Sciences and a Fellow at the International Migration Research Centre at Wilfrid Laurier University.

Dr. Arya is a former Vice-President of International Physicians for the Prevention of Nuclear War (IPPNW), which won the 1985 Nobel Peace Prize, and President of Physicians for Global Survival (PGS). He has written and lectured around the world about Peace through Health. He was Founding Director of the Global Health Office at Western University and chair of the Ontario College for Family Physicians Environmental Health Committee. He recently edited two books on international health experiences, as well as conducted research on the impact of overseas electives on host communities and students.

Dr. Arya continues as founder/director of the Kitchener/Waterloo Refugee Health Clinic in collaboration with the Waterloo Region Reception House, where he provides case-specific care to newcomers and those in need of specialized care. He was lead physician developing the Psychiatric Outreach Project, providing mental health for those homeless or at risk in St. John's Kitchen in Kitchener, tasks which led to him receiving the 2009 College of Family Physicians of Canada Geeta Gupta Award for Equity and Diversity. In 2011, Dr. Arya received a DLitt (Honorary) from Wilfrid Laurier University and the Mid-Career Award in International Health from the American Public Health Association. In 2013, he was given an Ontario College of Family Physicians (OCFP) Award of Excellence.

Thomas Piggott is currently pursuing specialty training in Public Health and Preventive Medicine at McMaster University. He completed his MD at McMaster University, his Masters in Public Health Economics at the London School of Hygiene and Tropical Medicine, and a BScH at the University of Guelph. He is interested in public health issues as they concern under-served populations in Canada and abroad. His research has focused on Indigenous health issues, climate change and health, the politics of public health, and conflict and health. Internationally, he has been involved in research on Indigenous health issues relating to alcohol abuse policy in Botswana and has worked clinically in Uganda. In Canada, he has worked clinically with the inner-city homeless and new Canadian refugee populations.

In public health, Dr. Piggott has worked with the Population Health Assessment and Scenarios Team of the Public Health Agency of Canada, being involved in scenario planning to inform policy and in assessing neglected diseases in under-served populations. He led a research project looking at the political context of adaptations to climate change in a number of Indigenous populations. An additional research project has looked at the impact that the political climate has on conflict and health outcomes.

Dr. Piggott has presented research on engagement in medical education and has been involved in numerous academic committees and community organizations. He is involved on the planning committee of the PEGASUS conference and the Canadian Conference on Global Health. He sits on the Board of Directors of Canadian Physicians for Research and Education in Peace, and on the council of the Public Health Physicians of Canada, and he provides policy input to the Royal College of Physicians and Surgeons of Canada's Health and Public Policy Committee. He is also a Governing Councillor of the World Federation of Public Health Associations.

CONTRIBUTORS

Shpresa Aliu-Berisha was born in Prishtina, Kosovo, where she graduated from medical school in 1998 at the University of Prishtina. Arriving in Canada as a war refugee in the spring of 1999, she became actively involved in helping others in the Kosovar community to settle in this adopted land. In 2011, she graduated from McMaster University's Family Medicine Residency Program and is now a practising family physician in Ontario.

Anne Andermann is a family doctor, public health physician, and founding director of the CLEAR Collaboration (http://www.mcgill.ca/clear). She has previously worked at the World Health Organization in Geneva, and has been a visiting lecturer at major universities in the United States, Brazil, Germany and the United Kingdom. Currently, Dr. Andermann is an Associate Professor at McGill University where she does research on caring for hidden homeless, is piloting a community outreach clinic at a local food bank, and teaches medical students and residents about taking action on the social determinants of health. Dr. Andermann is a member of the Social Accountability Working Group of the College of Family Physicians of Canada. Her book *Evidence for Health: From Patient Choice to Global Policy* is available from Cambridge University Press (http://www.cambridge.org/9781107648654).

Kelly Anderson completed a postgraduate degree in International Project Management and spent nearly a decade working in the non-governmental HIV/AIDS sector before seeking more training through medical school. She completed a fellowship in HIV Medicine through the Ontario HIV Treatment Network and is now a family physician at St. Michael's Hospital within the Department of Family and Community Medicine at the University of Toronto. Beyond her general and HIV primary care practices, she is a part-time emergency physician in Georgetown, Ontario.

Neil Andersson is Professor of Family Medicine and Director of Participatory Research at McGill University (PRAM). His work focuses on structural intervention trials that address social determinants. He is concerned about the system implications of participatory research and research techniques that engage stakeholders across cultural and educational divides.

Anna Banerji, the Faculty Lead for Indigenous and Refugee Health, Post-MD Education, Faculty of Medicine, University of Toronto, is a pediatric infectious tropical disease specialist and global health specialist. She has trained in Toronto, Ottawa, and Montreal, and at Harvard University, where she completed her MPH in International Health. She is the Chair of the Indigenous Health Conference and the North American Refugee Health Conference (Canadian site). Dr. Banerji has been studying lower respiratory tract infections in Inuit children for over two decades, and her research has changed national policy for the Inuit children. Dr. Banerji uses a human rights framework for her work, research, and education and is often an advocate for vulnerable populations. In January 2012, she was inducted into the Order of Ontario.

Philip Berger is an Associate Professor in the Department of Family and Community Medicine at the University of Toronto. From 1997 to 2013, he was Chief of the St. Michael's Hospital, Department of Family and Community Medicine. Dr. Berger co-founded the Amnesty International Canadian Medical Network and the Canadian Centre for Victims of Torture. He has been involved in the treatment of people with HIV/AIDS since the epidemic began. In December 2004, Dr. Berger began a seven-and-a-half month assignment as Team Leader of the Ontario Hospital Association's AIDS initiative (OHAfrica Project) at the Tšepong (Place of Hope) Clinic in Leribe, Lesotho. In 2012, he co-founded Canadian Doctors for Refugee Care, helping to lead physicians and others in national protests against government cuts to refugee health care.

Gary Bloch is a family physician with St. Michael's Hospital and an Associate Professor at the University of Toronto. His clinical practice focuses on the health of people who live in poverty and without adequate housing. His advocacy, research, curriculum development, and program creation focuses on health provider–based interventions into social challenges to health. He regularly teaches health providers, trainees, and the general public, and has designed and implemented core medical school curricula on poverty interventions. Dr. Bloch founded and co-chairs the Ontario College of Family Physicians' Committee on Poverty and Health. He has stimulated the development of a series of primary care–based social determinants and health equity–focused interventions at St. Michael's Hospital. He was instrumental in the establishment of Inner City Health Associates, a group of over 80 physicians working with individuals experiencing homelessness in Toronto, as well as the advocacy group Health Providers against Poverty.

Erin Bryce completed her PhD in Anthropology in 2014. Her research interests include biometeorology, social and environmental determinants of health, numerical modelling of large data sets, and frailty in elderly populations.

David Butler-Jones was the Chief Public Health Officer of Canada and Deputy Minister for the Public Health Agency of Canada from its inception in 2004 to 2014. He has worked in many parts of Canada in both public health and clinical medicine as well as working and advising internationally. He is a Professor in the Faculty of Medicine at the University of Manitoba and Clinical Professor in Community Health and Epidemiology at the University of Saskatchewan. He has served as President of the Canadian Public Health Association, Vice President of the American Public Health Association, Chair of the Canadian Roundtable on Health and Climate Change, and Co-Chair of the Canadian Coalition for Public Health in the 21st Century. He has received honorary degrees (LLD) from Carleton University and York University. He is also a recipient of the Canadian Public Health Association Defries Award, the Medal of Service from the Canadian Medical Association, and the President's Award from the Public Health Physicians of Canada. He continues to work, teach, and mentor in practice, policy, and leadership.

Alex Caudarella is a family physician and addiction medicine physician, and lecturer at the University of Toronto. He has various experiences working abroad, including in Haiti, Ecuador, and South Africa. He is the co-founder, along with Andrea Evans, of an NGO in Ecuador providing primary health care in the rural Andean mountains to Indigenous populations. In addition to his clinical work at St. Michael's Hospital, he works in Nunavut.

Martin Cooke is Associate Professor in the Department of Sociology and Legal Studies and the School of Public Health and Health Systems at the University of Waterloo, and an Affiliated Scientist with the Propel Centre for Population Health Impact. His major research interests are social demography and health over the life course. Dr. Cooke has done research for and with First Nations and other Indigenous organizations, as well as for several federal government departments. He is currently the principal investigator of the Canadian Student Tobacco, Alcohol and Drugs Survey (CSTADS), implemented on behalf of Health Canada.

Lesley Cooper has extensive professional and academic experience as a social worker, community worker, researcher, and educator in Australia, New Zealand, and Canada. These positions have taken her to work with rural and remote communities in Queensland, the Northern Territory, and Western Australia. She has worked closely with Aboriginal communities in Australia in the areas of housing, sustainable tenancy, family violence, and diabetes education. She worked at Wilfrid Laurier University as Dean of the Faculty of Social Work and Vice-President of the Brantford Campus, and is now the Foundation Professor of Social Work at the University of Wollongong. In her academic work, she has a strong interest in research with marginal populations. In her teaching, she has provided leadership in work-integrated learning, winning a National Teaching Award in the Social Sciences and Education.

Treena Wasonti:io Delormier is Kanien'kehá:ka (Mohawk) from Kahnawake. She has been involved with the Kahnawake Schools Diabetes Prevention Project (KSDPP) since 1994. Dr. Wasonti:io is an Associate Professor in the School of Human Nutrition and Associate Director of the Centre for Indigenous Peoples Nutrition and Environment at McGill University.

Thomas Dignan, OOnt, is the Chair of the Royal College Indigenous Health Advisory Committee. Dr. Dignan of Thunder Bay, Ontario, a Mohawk from Six Nations of the Grand River Territory, is a tireless advocate for eradicating disparities in health outcomes and inequities in the quality of health care facing Indigenous people. Dr. Dignan is a past Council Member of the Royal College, and he was appointed to the Board of the First Nations University of Canada, based in Saskatchewan. Dr. Dignan originally trained in nursing and was the inaugural President of the Native Nurses Association of Canada. He subsequently attended medical school at McMaster University and was, to that point, the oldest graduate of the program. As a practising physician specializing in community medicine in Health Canada's First Nations and Inuit Health Branch, Dr. Dignan has dedicated his life to improving the health of Indigenous Peoples in Canada—particularly drawing attention to "institutional racism."

Angela Di Nello is a research coordinator at McMaster University and has over 15 years of experience in research administration and coordination. She has her Master of Arts in Political Science, Bachelor of Arts in Psychology and Criminal Justice and Public Policy, and Bachelor of Education.

James R. Dunn is a Professor in the Department of Health, Aging and Society at McMaster University, and is Director of the McMaster Institute for Healthier Environments. He is also the principal investigator for the studies referred to in Chapter 21.

Andrea Evans is a consultant pediatrician and assistant professor at the University of Toronto. She has various experiences in working abroad, including in Haiti with the NGO Partners in Health, Ecuador, and multiple countries in sub-Saharan Africa. In addition to her clinical work at SickKids, she frequently works in Nunavut and the Northwest Territories, providing acute pediatric care. Her research interests are in health services access and health outcomes in vulnerable populations such as refugee children. She is an executive committee member of the Canadian Paediatric Society's section on Global Child and Youth Health.

Bonnie M. Freeman is Algonquin/Mohawk from the Six Nations of the Grand River Territory in Ontario, Canada. Bonnie is currently an Assistant Professor in the School of Social Work at McMaster University. She brings many years of practice experience in student services, as well teaching experience from several universities. Her research and work are rooted in connections to Six Nations, the Hamilton Aboriginal Community, and many other Aboriginal communities throughout Canada and the United States. Bonnie focuses her work and research on cultural interventions in social work practice, community healing approaches, anti-oppressive practices and decolonization, and Indigenous–non-Indigenous relations and alliances. Her PhD dissertation research examined the journey of Six Nations Haudenosaunee youth as they travelled on foot through their ancestral lands promoting the message of peace and unity. The outcome from this research provided an understanding of the transformation through journeying and how it promotes health, well-being, and cultural identity for Indigenous youth by connecting to land, the natural environment, and Haudenosaunee knowledge and practices. Bonnie is also certified in Equine Assisted Growth and Learning and has worked with the Hamilton Métis Women's Circle developing and implementing programs for Indigenous high school students and Indigenous women with horses.

Patricia Gabriel is a full-service family physician in Coquitlam, British Columbia. She has completed additional training in primary care research through the Clinical Scholar Program at the University of British Columbia, a Master's degree in Health Sciences at Simon Fraser University, and a Canadian Institutes for Health Research fellowship through Transdisciplinary Understanding and Training on Research—Primary Health Care (TUTOR-PHC). Her research focus broadly examines access to primary health care for refugees in Canada.

Jacqueline Gahagan, PhD, is a Medical Sociologist and a Full Professor (Health Promotion) at Dalhousie University. Jacqueline holds research associate positions with the European Union Centre of Excellence, the Health Law Institute, the Beatrice Hunter Cancer Research Institute, and the Atlantic Health Promotion Research Centre, among others. Professor Gahagan's program of research focuses on intersectional approaches aimed at addressing gender-based health inequities in health programs, interventions, and policies. Her funded research projects include an examination of the breast and gynecological cancer experiences among LBQ women and trans people; promoting resilience among LGBTQ youth; gender- and equity-based analyses of HIV/HCV prevention policies and programs aimed at youth; end-of-life preparedness among older LGBTQ populations; and access to and uptake of HIV testing innovations such as point-of-care HIV testing among socially marginalized populations.

Ritika Goel is a family physician with the Inner City Health Associates in Toronto and a lecturer at University of Toronto. She completed medical school at McMaster University, family medicine residency at St. Michael's Hospital in Toronto, and a Master's of Public Health from Johns Hopkins School of Public Health. Ritika's clinical work is with people experiencing or at risk of homelessness, as well as migrants with precarious immigration status. She has served as the Lead Physician for the Inner City Family Health Team and the Population Health Lead for the Inner City Health Associates, and is currently Chair of the College of Family Physicians of Canada Social Accountability Working Group. Ritika is also involved in grassroots advocacy work as a board member of Canadian Doctors for Medicare, and organizer with the OHIP for All campaign. She is an active contributor to print, online, and social media.

Hanna Gros is a Toronto-based lawyer and the Immigration and Refugee Advocate at the International Human Rights Program (IHRP) at the University of Toronto's Faculty of Law. Hanna co-authored three IHRP reports on immigration detention. The first report focused on mental health issues: *"We Have No Rights": Arbitrary Imprisonment and Cruel Treatment of Migrants with Mental Health Issues in Canada* (2015); the second two reports focused on children: *"No Life for a Child": A Roadmap to End Immigration Detention of Children and Family Separation* (2016), and *Invisible Citizens: Canadian Children in Immigration Detention* (2017).

Dale Guenter is a Family Physician and Associate Professor at McMaster University. His clinical, teaching, and research interests include HIV care, chronic pain, mental health, addiction, and population determinants of health. He is co-founder and member of the board of directors of Hamilton Shelter Health Network, addressing health and social needs of Hamilton's precariously housed individuals. He is a collaborator with the Ateneo de Zamboanga University School of Medicine in the Philippines. He is the primary care lead for the Health Links initiative of Ontario's Ministry of Health and Long-Term Care.

Gwen K. Healey was born and raised in Iqaluit, Nunavut, and it is in this community that she continues to work and live with her family. Gwen is the Executive and Scientific Director of the Qaujigiartiit Health Research Centre in Iqaluit, NU. She holds a PhD in Public Health from the Dalla Lana School of Public Health at the University of Toronto. Gwen co-founded the Qaujigiartiit Health Research Centre in 2006 to enable health research to be conducted locally by northerners and with communities in a supportive, safe, culturally sensitive, and ethical environment, as well as to promote the inclusion of both Inuit Qaujimajatuqangit and Western sciences in addressing health concerns, creating healthy environments, and improving the health of Nunavummiut. Qaujigiartiit has supported and/or initiated community research projects examining climate change and health, food security, child and youth mental health and wellness, women's health, sexual health, and public health.

Karen Hill is from the Mohawk Turtle Clan living in her home community of Six Nations of the Grand River Territory in Southern Ontario, where she works as the Lead Physician with the Six Nations Family Health Team. Karen's vision is to see traditional Indigenous knowledge and ways of healing return to the centre of health care in her community and other Indigenous communities in Canada. Her work in family medicine is carried out in relationship with the traditional helpers and healing system within the community. Karen has been learning from the traditional knowledge keepers in her community for nearly 20 years and has recently completed an academic paper for the special edition of the National Aboriginal Health Organization's (NAHO) *Journal on Aboriginal People's Health* on Traditional Medicine, in collaboration with Elva Jamieson, traditional healer, and Bernice Downey, PhD candidate and former CEO of the NAHO.

Christopher Holcroft launched Empower Consulting in 2008 to provide professional communications and public advocacy services for non-profit and labour organizations, including many health care groups. As principal of Empower, Christopher draws on his more than 15 years of strategic communications, media relations, and political campaign management experience in the private, public, and non-profit sectors. Christopher is also a frequent media commentator on public policy issues and has written several op-ed articles for major Canadian newspapers. Christopher has a BA in Political Science from the University of Toronto and was nominated for the Rodrigue-Pageau Scholarship in 1993 for academic excellence and community involvement while attending the University of Ottawa. His extensive community involvement includes leadership roles on issues related to civic participation, the environment, health care, and youth.

Richard Hovey, PhD, is an Associate Professor in the Division of Oral Health and Society, Faculty of Dentistry, at McGill University in Montreal, Quebec. He has extensive experience as a qualitative researcher and over 35 years of experience as an educator and course/curriculum developer, and in the assessment of students in a wide range of academic situations. His research explores the complexity of living with chronic illness, trauma, and suffering; interprofessional/interdisciplinary collaborations; and the application of adult learning for enhanced person-centred health care.

Andrea Hunter is an Associate Professor of Pediatrics at McMaster University and a Consultant Pediatrician at McMaster Children's Hospital and St. Joseph's Healthcare, Hamilton. She completed both medical school and pediatric residency training at McMaster University, followed by a Diploma in Tropical Medicine and Hygiene in London, UK. Dr. Hunter maintains a consulting pediatric practice in addition to outreach clinics with newcomer children/youth and the Hamilton Shelter Health network. Dr. Hunter is a recognized educator, and she transitioned in June 2016 to the role of Program Director of the pediatric residency program. Her clinical and research interests include pediatric refugee and immigrant health, social determinants of health, and global child health. She has coordinated community-based pediatric refugee/immigrant health clinics in Hamilton since 2004 and is an editor and task force member of Caring for Kids New to Canada, a Canadian Pediatric Society peer-reviewed guide to health professionals working with immigrant and refugee children and youth. Internationally, she has been involved in ongoing global child health education programs in Uganda and is co-program director of a pediatric residency program in Guyana.

Michaela Hynie is a Cultural Psychologist in the Department of Psychology and the Centre for Refugee Studies at York University. Her research in Canada, Kenya, Rwanda, India, and Nepal explores social inclusion and resilience in situations of social conflict and displacement, and interventions that can strengthen these relationships to improve health and well-being in different cultural, political, and physical environments.

Sharon Koivu has been a practising physician for over 25 years. For 12 years now, she has had a focused practice as a Palliative Care Physician Consultant in London, Ontario. She has previously worked as a Family Physician, Acting Medical Officer of Health, and Chronic Pain Physician. Leadership roles include Site-Chief for the Department of Family Medicine at University Hospital in London currently, and previously, President of Medical Staff at St. Thomas Elgin General Hospital. She has been a lifelong volunteer on boards including the London Association for International Development, Violence against Women Services Elgin County, and the Sexual Assault Centre, London. She has been involved in teaching residents and medical students and with curriculum development in Ethics in End-of-Life at Western University, Schulich School of Medicine and Dentistry. Her career and volunteer path has giving her a strong interest in working with patients who are marginalized, particularly those with intravenous drug addictions.

Nathan Lachowsky is an Assistant Professor and Michael Smith Foundation for Health Research Scholar in the School of Public Health and Social Policy at the University of Victoria in British Columbia. He is an epidemiologist using interdisciplinary community-based participatory research approaches to address health inequities and promote sexual health among gender and sexual minorities. His research has spanned Canada and Aotearoa, New Zealand, having received scholarship and grant support from the Canadian Institutes of Health Research, Rotary International, the Canadian Foundation for AIDS Research, and Canadian Blood Services. He is an avid community volunteer, serving on governance boards and with front-line community-based organizations.

Barry Lavallée is acting director of the University of Manitoba's Centre for Aboriginal Health Education. He is a member of the Saulteaux and Métis communities of Manitoba, and he is a descendent of the Bear Clan. Barry is currently the past president of the Indigenous Physicians Association of Canada. He graduated from the Faculty of Medicine (University of Manitoba) and completed his postgraduate training in Family Medicine with an emphasis on rural/Aboriginal health in 1990. He completed his Master of Clinical Sciences in Family Medicine at the University of Western Ontario in 2004. His research focuses on the experiences of First Nations and Métis patients within the patient-physician therapeutic relationship. He acts as medical lead for the Diabetes Integration Project and teaches about factors influencing First Nations, Métis, and Inuit health to various health faculties at the Health Sciences Campus.

S. Luckett-Gatopoulos is currently pursuing specialty training in Emergency Medicine at McMaster University and training in Narrative Medicine at Columbia University. She previously completed her MD at Queen's University and holds a BSc in Psychology and Music Studies from the University of Toronto, a diploma in American Sign Language and Deaf Studies from George Brown College, and an MSc from the Institute of Medical Science at the University of Toronto. Her academic interests include free open access medical education (FOAMed), curriculum development, and literacy as a determinant of community and individual health. Her work can be found at http://sluckettg.org.

Ann C. Macauley is a Professor of Family Medicine at McGill University, Scientific Director of the Kahnawake Schools Diabetes Prevention Project (a long-standing participatory research health promotion project in partnership with the Kanien'kehá:ka [Mohawk] community of Kahnawake, Quebec), and Inaugural Director of Participatory Research at McGill University. She has also had many years practising as a family physician in Kahnawake. She has received the Order of Canada for contributions to Indigenous health, foreign membership of the National Academy of Medicine (formerly Institute of Medicine), and honorary membership of the Royal College of Physicians of Canada.

Soultana Macridis, PhD, is a Research Associate and Knowledge Translation Specialist at the Alberta Centre for Active Living within the Faculty of Kinesiology, Sport, and Recreation at the University of Alberta in Edmonton. She is also a member of the board of directors of SHAPE Alberta. Soultana completed her doctorate in Kinesiology and Physical Education from McGill University, working with the Kahnawake Schools Diabetes Prevention Project (KSDPP) and participatory research at McGill University. She has expertise in community-based participatory research and health promotion programming and policies in schools and communities to support physical activity, nutrition, and active transportation.

Joe Mancini began the Working Centre with his wife, Stephanie Mancini, in 1982 as a project that would give people the respect and dignity they deserve, provide multiple community supports, and expand the concept of access to tools. Thirty-six years later, more than 1,000 people use 40 different services and projects of the Working Centre every day. During this time, over 73,000 square feet of underutilized heritage buildings have been renovated into thriving community space that provides a web of essential services and supports through food, health, housing, employment, hygiene, and community tools. These projects and more are sustained by over 120 staff members and 500 active volunteers. *Transition to Common Work: Building Community at the Working Centre* (Wilfrid Laurier University Press, 2015) by Joe and Stephanie Mancini describes how this alternative organization rooted itself in downtown Kitchener. Joe and Stephanie were made Members of the Order of Canada in 2016.

Alex M. McComber, DSc (Hon), MEd, is Kanien'kehá:ka (Mohawk) from Kahnawake Territory, Quebec. He works with the Kahnawake Schools Diabetes Prevention Project and is an Assistant Professor with Family Medicine, McGill University. He is a teacher, community researcher, facilitator, and co-investigator on several health promotion research projects.

Janet McLaughlin is an Associate Professor of Health Studies and Research Associate with the International Migration Research Centre, based at Wilfrid Laurier University. For over a decade, she has researched and published in the area of migrant farm worker health, specializing in social determinants of health, sexual and reproductive health, occupational health and safety, workers' compensation, and health care access. Dr. McLaughlin is co-founder of the Migrant Worker Health Project (http://www.migrantworkerhealth.ca), which aims to promote accessible health care for migrant workers in Canada, and she has served as a volunteer and adviser to several community-based migrant health initiatives.

Ryan Meili is the NDP member of the legislative assembly for Saskatoon Meewasin and the leader of the official opposition in Saskatchewan. A family doctor by profession, he practised at the Westside Community Clinic in Saskatoon and worked as an Assistant Professor in the Department of Community Health and Epidemiology at the College of Medicine, University of Saskatchewan, where he served as head of the Division of Social Accountability, director of the Making the Links Certificate in Global Health, and co-lead of the Saskatchewan HIV/AIDS Research Endeavour. Ryan has published numerous articles in academic journals and the popular press and is the author of *A Healthy Society: How a Focus on Health Can Revive Canadian Democracy* (Purich Press, 2012).

Mona Negoita graduated from Western University as a physiotherapist and is currently practising in Kitchener-Waterloo with a passion for post-stroke rehabilitation. She has completed a Master's in Medical Education through the Karolinska Institute in Stockholm with a project regarding the attitudes and behaviours supported by international health placements. She helped found and is volunteering with the charity Abrazos Canada. Mona is travelling to Mexico and Ecuador to support the organization's projects and encourage the international involvement of Canadian allied health students.

Aaron Orkin is a family, emergency, and public health physician and Assistant Professor in the University of Toronto Department of Family and Community Medicine. He is a researcher at the Schwartz/Reisman Emergency Medicine Institute at Mount Sinai Hospital, Clinical Public Health Fellow at the University of Toronto Dalla Lana School of Public Health, and a doctoral candidate in clinical epidemiology at the University of Toronto Institute of Health Policy, Management and Evaluation. He practises emergency medicine at Mount Sinai Hospital and family medicine at Seaton House with Toronto's Inner City Health Associates. Aaron's work is mostly about enhancing health equity and redistributing medical power by equipping members of marginalized populations to deliver life-saving clinical services.

Abe Oudshoorn is an Assistant Professor in the Arthur Labatt Family School of Nursing at Western University, as well as the Department of Psychiatry Schulich School of Medicine and Dentistry, Associate Scientist with Lawson Health Research Institute, and a member of the Centre for Research on Health Equity and Social Inclusion. Having worked as a nurse with people experiencing homelessness, Abe's research focuses on health, homelessness, gender, trauma, housing policy, and poverty. Outside the University, Abe is past Chair of the London Homeless Coalition and a board member with the United Way of London and Middlesex, and he sat on the Mayor's Advisory Panel on Poverty. Abe is the recipient of Western University's 2016 Humanitarian Award.

Ngan Pham recently obtained a Master of Science in Global Health at McMaster University. She has been involved in research on teaching around vulnerability and is interested in refugee health, having had a father and brother who were refugees. Ngan coordinated two multinational studies related to the prevalence of intimate partner violence (IPV) and perceptions of screening for IPV among women attending orthopedic clinics.

Kevin Pottie is an Associate Professor in the Departments of Family Medicine and Epidemiology and Community Medicine at the Faculty of Medicine, University of Ottawa. He is a Principal Scientist at Elisabeth Bruyère Research Institute and at the Centre for Global Health, Institute of Population Health. He is a leader of the Canadian Collaboration for Immigrant and Refugee Health (CCIRH) and a member of the New Canadian Task Force on Preventive Health Care, and he practises as a family physician as part of the Champlain Immigrant Health Network. He is co-founder of the Bruyère Gallery: Culture, Art and Healing. He has worked in the Republic of Georgia as a Medical Coordinator with Médecins Sans Frontières and has taught in several Latin American countries including Bolivia, Dominican Republic, Guatemala, and Venezuela, and has also worked in Thailand, Indonesia, Republic of Congo, and Benin.

Dennis Raphael is Professor of Health Policy and Management at York University, as well as the author of over 250 publications that speak to topics in public policy, poverty, and social determinants of health. Raphael's extensive list of publications includes *Poverty in Canada* (2011) and *Health Promotion and Quality of Life in Canada* (2010). He is the editor of *Tackling Health Inequalities: Lessons from International Experiences* (2012), *Immigration, Public Policy, and Health: Newcomer Experiences in Developed Nations* (2016), and *Social Determinants of Health: Canadian Perspectives* (2016), and co-editor of *Staying Alive: Critical Perspectives on Health, Illness, and Health Care* (2010). He is co-author of *Social Determinants of Health: The Canadian Facts*, a primer for the Canadian public, which has been downloaded over 750,000 times from http://thecanadianfacts.org.

Meb Rashid is the Medical Director of the Crossroads Clinic, a medical clinic that serves newly arrived refugees in Toronto. He is a co-founder of the Canadian Doctors for Refugee Care, an organization founded to advocate for refugees to access health insurance. He was on the steering committee of the CCIRH, a group that developed evidence-based guidelines for the assessment of newly arrived immigrants and refugees. He also co-founded the Christie Refugee Health Clinic, a health clinic located in a refugee shelter. He is on the steering committee of the Canadian Refugee Health Conference. He has brought together clinicians across Canada with an interest in refugee health through a web-based project called the Canadian Refugee Health Network and through a group called the Refugee Health Network of Southern Ontario. He recently was awarded an Award of Excellence from the College of Family Physicians of Ontario. He is on staff at the Women's College Hospital in Toronto and is affiliated with the Department of Family and Community Medicine at the University of Toronto.

Vanessa Redditt is a family physician at the Crossroads Clinic at the Women's College Hospital, where she focuses on the care of newly arrived refugees in Toronto, and a lecturer at the University of Toronto. She holds a BA in International Development Studies from McGill University and an MD from Harvard Medical School. She completed family medicine residency and fellowships in global health and vulnerable populations and in low-risk obstetrics at the University of Toronto. Vanessa is interested in improving the health of marginalized individuals and communities through clinical care, health system strengthening, and tackling social inequities. Vanessa has also worked in health worker training and health systems strengthening initiatives in resource-limited settings, including with Partners in Health/Inshuti Mu Buzima in rural Rwanda.

Jessica Reid co-founded Fostering, Empowering and Advocating Together (FEAT) for Children of Incarcerated Parents in 2012 after being separated from her father for 24 years and witnessing the devastating effects of parental incarceration as an educator. Currently, FEAT is the only organization in Canada providing supportive programming for children of prisoners. Jessica has developed several programs, including Peer Mentorship, Girls Empowerment Retreats, and a Family Visitation program. Jessica has spoken widely as an advocate and educator and organized Feet for FEAT, an annual 400-kilometre walk, to raise awareness of these issues. Jessica has received the prestigious SSHRC Nelson Mandela Award for her work in the community and her research on the impact of parental incarceration on internalizing symptoms and externalizing behaviours. She is currently completing her PhD at the University of Guelph where she continues to explore possible protective factors that may help to mitigate the effects of parental incarceration. Jessica also represents Canada as Director on the Board of the International Coalition of Children with Incarcerated Parents.

Jon Salsberg, PhD, is Senior Lecturer in Primary Healthcare Research—Patient and Public Involvement, at the Graduate Entry Medical School, University of Limerick, Ireland. His experiences in Indigenous community health research shaped his interest in understanding the theory and practice of participatory engagement, particularly in how communities come to take ownership over academic research. He is also interested in how engaging patients and health care providers in the evidence-creation process leads to practice improvement and better health outcomes in primary care.

Michelle Tew is an occupational health nurse with a background in clinical practice, administration, research, and education. For the past 10 years, in her role with the Occupational Health Clinics for Ontario Workers, she has been engaged in program planning, evaluating, research, lobbying, and providing (occupational) health services to address the needs of migrant agricultural workers and other vulnerable worker populations.

Paul Tomascik, MBA, BSc, is a senior analyst in health policy and partner relations with the Office of Health Policy at the Royal College of Physicians and Surgeons of Canada. As a member of the policy team, he has produced a number of discussion papers, workshops, and research reports on Indigenous health in support of the Royal College's commitment to advance culturally safe medical education and practice. He was a major architect in developing the Royal College Indigenous health values and principles statement, which was co-authored by members of the Royal College Indigenous Health Advisory Committee (IHAC). The statement is a foundational document that guides the Royal College's strategic plan for Indigenous health. He works closely with members of IHAC and other organizations to raise awareness of racism and how it affects the health of Indigenous peoples. He regularly informs other areas of policy, including quality improvement and advocacy, and has written a number of federal government committee briefings supporting principles of the Royal College as expert witnesses representing specialty medicine.

Biljana Vasilevska is a writer and researcher living in Hamilton, Ontario. She specializes in qualitative methods and conducting research with vulnerable populations. A former English as a Second Language instructor, she has offered training on teaching survivors of psychological trauma and worked with program staff and funders to make language programs more responsive to students' emotional and psychological needs.

Piotr Wilk is an Assistant Professor in the Department of Epidemiology and Biostatistics and Paediatrics at Western University and a Scientist at the Children's Health Research

Institute in London, Ontario. His research is focused on the health and well-being of children, particularly obesity among Aboriginal children and youth. Previously, Dr. Wilk was a community health researcher and educator at the Middlesex-London Health Unit, where he was responsible for studies of maternal and child health. Dr. Wilk is currently conducting a number of studies on child-, family-, and neighbourhood-level determinants of childhood obesity and is the Academic Co-lead of the *Healthy Weights Connection*, a PHAC-funded intervention to improve service delivery to Métis and First Nations children and families. He is also the Co-director of the Statistics Canada Research Data Centre at Western University.